Systems Immunology
An Introduction to Modeling Methods
for Scientists

Foundations of Biochemistry and Biophysics

This textbook series provides teaching and learning resources at the advanced undergraduate and graduate levels. It covers all areas of intersection between physical and biological sciences, for example, where physical tools are being used by researchers to elucidate understanding and help to solve problems in biology.

Systems Immunology
An Introduction to Modeling Methods
for Scientists

Edited by
Jayajit Das
Ciriyam Jayaprakash

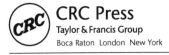

CRC Press
Taylor & Francis Group
Boca Raton London New York

CRC Press is an imprint of the
Taylor & Francis Group, an **informa** business

CRC Press
Taylor & Francis Group
6000 Broken Sound Parkway NW, Suite 300
Boca Raton, FL 33487-2742

First issued in paperback 2021

© 2019 by Taylor & Francis Group, LLC
CRC Press is an imprint of Taylor & Francis Group, an Informa business

No claim to original U.S. Government works

ISBN 13: 978-0-367-78092-0 (pbk)
ISBN 13: 978-1-4987-1740-3 (hbk)

Visit the Taylor & Francis Web site at
http://www.taylorandfrancis.com

and the CRC Press Web site at
http://www.crcpress.com

To my parents and teachers.

Jayajit Das

To Fernand Hayot, scientist, scholar, and friend.

Ciriyam Jayaprakash

Contents

Series preface

Biophysics encompasses the application of the principles, tools, and techniques of the physical sciences to problems in biology, including determination and analysis of structures, energetics, dynamics, and interactions of biological molecules. Biochemistry addresses the mechanisms underlying the complex reactions driving life, from enzyme catalysis and regulation to the structure and function of molecules. Research in these two areas is having a huge impact in pharmaceutical sciences and medicine.

These two highly interconnected fields are the focus of this book series. It covers both the use of traditional tools from physical chemistry such as nuclear magnetic resonance (NMR), x-ray crystallography, and neutron diffraction, as well as novel techniques including scanning probe microscopy, laser tweezers, ultrafast laser spectroscopy, and computational approaches. A major goal of this series is to facilitate interdisciplinary research by training biologists and biochemists in quantitative aspects of modern biomedical research, and teaching core biological principles to students in physical sciences and engineering.

Proposals for new volumes in the series may be directed to Lou M Chosen, Executive Editor (lou.chosen@taylorandfrancis.com).

Foreword

It is becoming increasingly clear that the immune system is critically important for maintaining health and is implicated in mediating various states of disease. The desire to combat infectious diseases since antiquity, the more recent interest in deploying the immune system to combat cancer, the untold amount of suffering caused by autoimmune diseases, and the desire to understand how the remarkable immune system works has led to a great deal of experimental and clinical research aimed toward understanding how immunity is regulated. Some spectacular discoveries have been made over the years. In spite of these major advances, our understanding of how a systemic immune response develops, and how it can be mis-regulated to cause diverse diseases remains incomplete. The ability to collect large amounts of data in a high throughput manner combined with computational inference of patterns in this data, mechanistic modeling to generate appropriate hypotheses to explain these patterns, and experimental/clinical tests of these hypotheses is beginning to change this situation. This convergence of approaches and people from different disciplines may lead us to a future where a person's immune health can be monitored, corrected when it goes awry, and manipulated for therapeutic and prophylactic purposes with precision. This edited book reviews progress in some aspects of ongoing work pertinent to this goal. The first chapter by Salvatore Valitutti and co-workers aims to introduce the basics of how the immune system works to individuals not trained as biologists. There is also an interesting chapter by Steven R. Abel that summarizes the various approaches that are being pursued to construct theoretical and computational models of processes pertinent to the immune system across a range of spatio-temporal scales. Other chapters discuss topics that cover a wide range that includes statistical analyses methods, rule-based modeling of immune cell signaling, characterizing vulnerabilities of mutable viruses to immune attack, importance of spatial heterogeneities in regulating immune responses across scales, the key challenges that remain in understanding immune synapses, etc. Taken together, the body of information contained in this book provides readers with a bird's-eye view of different aspects of exciting work at the convergence of disciplines that will ultimately lead to a future where we understand how immunity is regulated, and how we can harness this knowledge toward practical ends that reduce human suffering. I commend the editors for putting this volume together.

Arup K. Chakraborty
MIT

Preface

I have done this to illustrate that the approach being used is not meaningless speculation but has real possibilities of suggesting experiments that may lead to its modification or rejection.

Frank M. Burnet
Nobel lecture, 1960

The discipline of immunology has undergone transformative changes in the last few decades. Driven by intense research efforts aimed at combating infectious diseases such as HIV infection and by technological advances in experimental approaches our knowledge of the immune system now spans from the scales of single molecules to human communities. To put the above range of scales in a perspective, a similar range in length scale relates the size of a human to the average distance of Saturn from the Sun. The major challenges in immunology are usually multiscale problems where dynamical processes occurring on such a wide range of scales interact with each other to generate responses that affect our health. Take the example of the progression of an epidemic where interactions between viral peptides and immune receptors in the microscale propagate to larger scales infecting individuals and then human communities residing in many geographical regions. The complexity and the multi-scale nature of the immune system have necessitated the use of sophisticated modeling and theoretical techniques to construct mechanistic and data-driven models and then use the models to make predictions and design experiments or hypotheses. Techniques from physical and engineering sciences, in particular physics, have been proven valuable for building such models. Some of these models have led to the development of life saving clinical strategies besides providing basic understanding of the underlying biochemical processes. This interdisciplinary effort has led to a small but steadily growing field loosely designated as computational immunology or systems immunology.

However, it is still difficult for a researcher with a background in physical sciences or immunology to readily start working in this interdisciplinary area. On the one hand, a researcher from physical sciences is often overwhelmed by the vast immunology literature; on the other hand, biologists are intimidated by mathematical jargon and seemingly complicated computational methods. Another common difficulty is that even a well-trained Ph. D. in the physical and mathematical sciences will not know all of the different mathematical techniques required in modeling immunology. Some of these issues are dealt with in review articles published in professional journals; however, these reviews often have a very narrow focus depending on the target audience of the specific journal and fail to provide a holistic picture of the entire field. Thus, there is an acute need for a book that can be used by physical scientists or biologists who are interested in using quantitative methods to develop predictive mechanistic models in immunology.

This book is designed to address some of the above problems and provide a solid foundation for students and researchers in physical and biological sciences who would like to start working in the interdisciplinary field of systems or computational immunology. The nineteen chapters, written by leading experts in the field, cover a wide range of computational and mathematical methods employed in mechanistic and data driven modeling of immune responses at the scales of single cells to organs to individual organisms to populations. In addition, a basic introduction to the immune system is provided to help a newcomer get started. The chapters on fundamentals of statistical data analysis, and, on the approximations and assumptions that are usually made in mechanistic modeling should help students critically assess models presented in the literature where such discussions are often omitted.

Graduate students and advanced undergraduate students in physics, biophysics, chemistry, applied mathematics, chemical engineering, bioengineering, systems biology, ecology, molecular biology, and immunology departments will find this book useful as a textbook for courses pertaining to quantitative methods in immunology or biology. We hope the book will also serve as a useful introduction for modeling approaches to researchers with physical sciences or biology background.

We appreciate the time and effort of the authors who made room in their busy schedules to contribute to this effort. The book would not have been possible without the valuable help from Rhonda Purcell and Gail White, who assisted us with organizing the chapters and coordination between the contributors, the editors, and the publisher.

Jayajit Das

Ciriyam Jayaprakash

MATLAB® is a registered trademark of The MathWorks, Inc. For product information, please contact:

The MathWorks, Inc.
3 Apple Hill Drive
Natick, MA 01760-2098 USA
Tel: 508 647 7000
Fax: 508-647-7001
E-mail: info@mathworks.com
Web: www.mathworks.com

About the editors

Jayajit Das, Ph.D., is an Associate Professor in the Department of Pediatrics at the Wexner Medical Center, The Ohio State University, and Battelle Center for Mathematical Medicine, The Research Institute at Nationwide Children's Hospital, both in Columbus, Ohio. He obtained his Ph.D. in statistical physics from The Institute of Mathematical Sciences and Raman Research Institute, India. He was a postdoctoral research associate at Virginia Tech, University of California, Berkeley, and Massachusetts Institute of Technology prior to joining OSU. He is a member of the American Physical Society, author of many published journal articles, and invited speaker at numerous international conferences. His current research efforts funded by the National Institutes of Health (NIH) and private foundations include modeling responses of single immune cells, bacterial biofilms, and bacterial and viral infections in pediatric diseases.

Ciriyam Jayaprakash, Ph.D., is a Professor in the Department of Physics at The Ohio State University. He earned his doctorate in physics from the University of Illinois at Urbana-Champaign, and was a postdoctoral associate at Cornell University as well as a visiting scientist at the IBM Watson Research Center prior to joining the faculty of OSU. He is the recipient of the prestigious Alfred P. Sloan Foundation Fellowship and the NSF Presidential Young Investigator Award and is an elected Fellow of the American Physical Society. His current research interests include modeling of viral antagonists and immune system response, stochastic effects in subcellular processes, and applications of nonlinear dynamics.

Contributors

Steven M. Abel
Department of Chemical and Biomolecular Engineering
University of Tennessee
Knoxville, Tennessee

Derya Altıntan
Department of Mathematics
Selçuk University
Konya, Turkey

Kelly B. Arnold
Department of Biomedical Engineering
University of Michigan
Ann Arbor, Michigan

Barbara A. Baird
Department of Chemistry and Chemical Biology
Cornell University
Ithaca, New York

Lily A. Chylek
Department of Systems Biology
Harvard Medical School
Boston, Massachusetts

Daniel Coombs
Department of Mathematics and Institute of Applied Mathematics
University of British Columbia
Vancouver BC, Canada

Jayajit Das
Department of Pediatrics
The Ohio State University
and
Battelle Center for Mathematical Medicine
The Research Institute at Nationwide Children's Hospital
Columbus, Ohio

Jascha Diemer
Department of Electrical Engineering and Information Technology and Department of Biology
Technische Universität Darmstadt
Darmstadt, Germany

Elena Dimitrova
Department of Mathematical Sciences
Clemson University
Clemson, South Carolina

Michael L. Dustin
Kennedy Institute of Rheumatology
Nuffield Department of Orthopedics, Rheumatology and Musculoskeletal Sciences
The University of Oxford
Headington, United Kingdom

James R. Faeder
Department of Computational and Systems Biology
University of Pittsburgh School of Medicine
Pittsburgh, Pennsylvania

Andrew L. Ferguson
Department of Materials Science and Engineering and
Department of Chemical and Biomolecular Engineering
University of Illinois at Urbana-Champaign
Urbana, Illinois

Michael Flossdorf
Quantitative Immunology Group
Institute for Medical Microbiology, Immunology and Hygiene
Technical University of Munich
Munich, Germany

Paul François
Department of Physics
McGill University
Montréal QC, Canada

Byron Goldstein
Theoretical Biology and Biophysics Group
Los Alamos National Laboratory
Los Alamos, New Mexico

Gregory R. Hart
Department of Physics
University of Illinois at Urbana-Champaign
Urbana, Illinois

Mathieu Hemery
Department of Physics
McGill University
Montréal QC, Canada

William S. Hlavacek
Theoretical Biology and Biophysics Group, Theoretical Division
Los Alamos National Laboratory
Los Alamos, New Mexico

David A. Holowka
Department of Chemistry and Chemical Biology
Cornell University
Ithaca, New York

Thomas Höfer
Division of Theoretical Systems Biology
German Cancer Research Center (DKFZ)
Heidelberg, Germany

Roxana Khazen
Dynamics of Immune Responses
Institute Pasteur
Paris, France

Heinz Koeppl
Department of Electrical Engineering and Information Technology and Department of Biology
Technische Universität Darmstadt
Darmstadt, Germany

Reinhard Laubenbacher
Center for Quantitative Medicine
UConn Health
Jackson, Laboratory for Genomic Medicine
Farmington, Connecticut

Ramit Mehr
The Mina & Everard Goodman Faculty of Life Sciences
Bar-Ilan University
Ramat-Gan, Israel

Miri Michaeli
The Mina & Everard Goodman Faculty of Life Sciences
Bar-Ilan University
Ramat-Gan, Israel

Kathryn Miller-Jensen
Department of Biomedical Engineering
Yale University
New Haven, Connecticut

Thierry Mora
Laboratoire de physique statistique
Centre national de la recherche scientifique, Sorbonne Université, Université Paris-Diderot, and
École normale supérieure
Paris, France

Christopher R. Myers
Department of Physics and Center for Advanced Computing
Cornell University
Ithaca, New York

Alan S. Perelson
Theoretical Biology and Biophysics
Los Alamos National Laboratory
Los Alamos, New Mexico

Ruy M. Ribeiro
Theoretical Biology and Biophysics
Los Alamos National Laboratory
Los Alamos, New Mexico

John A.P. Sekar
Department of Computational and Systems Biology
University of Pittsburgh School of Medicine
Pittsburgh, Pennsylvania

Amber M. Smith
Department of Pediatrics
University of Tennessee Health Science Center
Memphis, Tennessee

William C. L. Stewart
Department of Pediatrics and
Department of Statistics
The Ohio State University
and
The Research Institute at Nationwide Children's Hospital
Columbus, Ohio

Salvatore Valitutti
Inserm, Université de Toulouse,
Center for Research on Cancer of Toulouse (CRCT)
Toulouse, France

Aleksandra M. Walczak
Laboratoire de physique théorique
Centre national de la recherche scientifique, Sorbonne Université, and École normale supérieure
Paris, France

Introduction to basic concepts in immunology

ROXANA KHAZEN AND SALVATORE VALITUTTI

1.1 SUMMARY

The immune system is a complex network of cells and soluble mediators that evolved to defend its host organism from pathogenic microbes. Since immune responses are endowed with high complexity and plasticity, the understanding of complex immunological networks can strongly benefit from the interdisciplinary work of physicists, applied mathematicians, and experimental immunologist. For successful interdisciplinary collaboration, it is of primary importance that basic concepts are shared in a simplified fashion. In this chapter, we outline some basic concepts to introduce immunology to non-biologists. We provide fundamental knowledge and nomenclature, which is essential to understand the complexity of immunological networks. For a more complete understanding of immunology, the readers can refer to excellent reference texts (Abbas et al., 2015; Murphy et al., 2012; Paul, 2012). We detail T cell antigen recognition and cytotoxic T lymphocyte (CTL) function more than other aspects of immunology. These topics are chosen as examples to illustrate the complexity of the molecular and cellular interactions taking place in the immune system.

1.2 INTRODUCTION

1.2.1 GENERAL VIEW OF THE IMMUNE SYSTEM

The immune response is based on interactive networks of numerous cellular and molecular effectors that evolved to protect a host against infections, to control tumor growth, as well as to maintain the homeostasis of tissues.

1.2.1.1 CELLS

Development of cells of the immune system starts in the bone marrow from a common precursor cell (called pluripotent hematopoietic stem cell) that then differentiates into more specialized cells to form a heterogeneous group of immune cells called leukocytes, or white blood cells (Figure 1.1).

1.2.1.2 CYTOKINES AND CHEMOKINES

Cytokines and *chemokines* are essential components of the immune system. They can be considered "molecular messengers" that cells of the immune system exchange among each other. More than one hundred different cytokines have been identified so far. Cytokines are secreted in the extracellular milieu or are bound on the surface of the cell. They are responsible for complex intercellular communication since each cytokine can be produced by more than one type of cell and acts on different cells of the immune system (remarkably, each cytokine can exert different effects on different cells). Different types of cytokines include: tumor necrosis factor-α (*TNF-α*), interferons (*IFN-α, IFN-β,* and *IFN-γ*), interleukins (*IL-1, IL-2, IL-3,* etc.), and chemokines. All cytokines accomplish their functional role by binding to specific receptors expressed on the surface of a cell. Some cytokines, such as TNF-α and interferons, have the role of alerting the immune system and of promoting immune responses. Others, such as TGF-β and IL-10, are instead inhibitory cytokines and suppress immune responses.

The chemokines are a family of small cytokines involved in *chemotaxis* (directed movement) of cells. Chemokines are therefore chemotactic cytokines. The main role of chemokines is to guide the migration of immune system cells so they may reach the organs or tissues where their function is required.

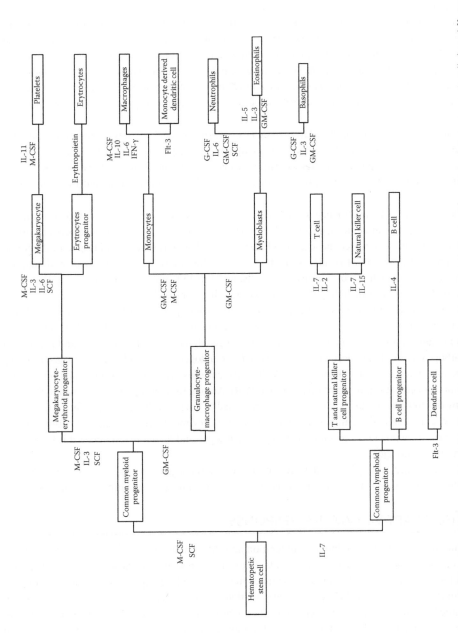

Figure 1.1 Development of cells of the immune system. Development starts from a common pluripotent hematopoietic precursor cell that differentiates into more specialized progenitor cells in the bone marrow to form a heterogeneous group of immune cells called leukocytes, or white blood cells. The main cytokines involved in the differentiation of the different immune cells are indicated in blue. Neutrophils, monocytes, macrophages, and immature dendritic cells (DC) originate from common myeloid precursor cells, whereas B and T lymphocytes and natural killer (NK) cells arise from common lymphoid progenitors.

1.2.2 THE INNATE IMMUNE RESPONSE

Studies over the past three to four decades characterize the immune system as consisting of two main categories: innate immunity and adaptive immunity. Although these two components of the immune response mainly differ in terms of specificity, rapidity, duration, and biological functions, they are complementary and deeply interconnected.

Innate immunity plays an essential role in the immediate defense of the host organism. It allows the discrimination of *self/nonself* by a system that consists of soluble proteins and relatively invariant cellular receptors. By *self*, immunologists mean the molecular patterns that the immune system has learned to recognize as components of the host organism. The immune system does not react against these components. This phenomenon is named *immunological tolerance*. By *nonself*, immunologists mean the molecular structures that do not belong to the host organism and that therefore trigger immune responses when penetrating the organism.

Innate immunity is composed of three layers of defense: (1) the physical barriers composed of epithelial cells and antimicrobial agents; (2) cells such as neutrophils, macrophages, and dendritic cells (*DC*), which uptake pathogens and cell fragments and release antimicrobial agents, and natural killer cells (*NK*), which kill virus-infected cells; and (3) plasma proteins, including cytokines, chemokines, and the *complement system*.

It is important to note that macrophages and DC do not only intervene in early steps of innate immune responses but also present antigenic ligands to T lymphocytes, therefore acting as a bridge between innate and adaptive immune responses (see the legend to Figure 1.2). Other cells that are implicated in the initial protection against pathogens and that play a functional role at the interface between innate and adaptive immune responses are basophils, eosinophils, mast cells, and innate lymphoid cells (*ILC*) as well as some subpopulations of lymphocytes including B-1 B cells, natural killer T cells (*NKT*), and γδT cells.

Cells that are part of the innate immunity category reside in various parts of the body and are in particular located at potential entry sites of pathogens, such as skin and mucous membranes, where they are ready to rapidly respond upon recognition of danger signals. The danger signals are common structural patterns of microbes (pathogen-associated molecular patterns, *PAMP*) or endogenous byproducts of damaged or dying cells (damage-associated molecular patterns, *DAMP*); these patterns are recognized by evolutionary conserved receptors named pattern recognition receptors (*PRR*). Among these receptors, an important family is represented by the Toll-like receptors (*TLRs*) that are expressed by various cells of the immune system.

A peculiar characteristic of the innate immune cells is that they rapidly respond against pathogens, but they do not "learn" from previous encounters with a given pathogen and therefore respond evenly to repeated exposure to an infectious agent.

A typical innate immune response is depicted in Figure 1.2. The legend of Figure 1.2 summarizes, in a schematic fashion, the cascade of cellular and molecular steps constituting innate immune responses.

1.2.3 THE ADAPTIVE IMMUNE RESPONSE

Adaptive immunity is characterized by the proliferation and differentiation of specific cells called *lymphocytes* that recognize antigens. The main feature of adaptive immune responses is the usage of antigen specific receptors expressed by the two main subsets of lymphocytes, the B and T lymphocytes. Pathogens, infected cells, and tumor cells express on their surface antigens that are recognized by B and T lymphocytes. An *antigen* is defined as a molecule that is recognized by the adaptive immune system. More precisely, the receptors expressed by B and T lymphocytes recognize, with high specificity, a small molecular structure named *epitope* within the antigen. A pathogen, such as bacteria, can therefore be seen as a mosaic of antigens (each antigen is made of various epitopes) that triggers different B and T lymphocytes, each one expressing on their surface approximately 30,000-50,000 identical antigenreceptors that are specific for a given epitope.

Adaptive immunity takes longer to get involved when compared to innate immunity and constitutes the second line of the host organism's defense. Although adaptive immunity requires several days or weeks to develop, it can eventually elicit the specific elimination of antigens, infected cells, and cancerous cells. It is

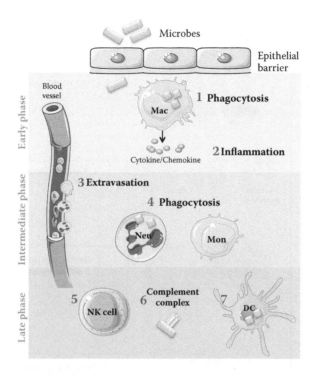

Figure 1.2 Schematic description of an innate immune response and of its relation with the initiation of the adaptive immune response. When epithelial barriers fail to block microorganisms, pathogen entrance and replication activates the innate immune system. (1) The first line of defense is composed of tissue macrophages that engulf microorganisms and destroy them through recognition of pathogen-associated patterns via their receptors. Pathogen clearance is either mediated through the fusion of the phagosome with lysosomes that contain antimicrobial compounds or through the generation of oxygen radicals via a "respiratory burst." (2) Activated macrophages are also capable of secreting cytokines and chemokines, causing inflammation and recruitment of other immune cells. (3) Such inflammatory responses increase the local blood flow, reduce blood flow velocity, and induce up-regulation of adhesion molecules on activated endothelial cells with consequent extravasation of circulating leukocytes into the infected tissues. (4) Neutrophils are the first to arrive to the site of infection followed by monocytes. Monocyte differentiation leads to the generation of additional macrophages ready for in innate response. (5) During viral infection, NK cells play an important role in providing a primary defense by releasing lytic molecules when contacting target cells. (6) The further complement system is activated by microbial products, contributing to the creation of an inflammatory environment. Inflammatory responses also increase the flow of antigens from infected tissues to draining lymph nodes, a mechanism that will help to mount an adaptive immune response. At this stage, innate immunity might succeed in infection removal. Alternatively, infection might be kept under control to prevent dissemination, while adaptive immune response develops to provide a stronger level of defense. (7) Dendritic cells are key effectors in the development of adaptive responses. They capture antigens in tissues, migrate to draining lymph nodes, and present antigens to naive T cells in order to activate adaptive immunity.

called adaptive since this type of immunity is capable of generating memory. Thus, repeated exposure to the same antigen leads to more vigorous and rapid responses and provides long-lasting protection.

The adaptive responses are based on two components: (1) *Humoral immunity*, mediated by B lymphocytes (also named B cells) that produce and secrete molecules called immunoglobulins (*Ig*) or antibodies and (2) *Cellular immunity*, mediated by the T lymphocytes (or T cells). T lymphocytes are divided in two major subsets: T helper (*Th*) cells that coordinate the action of other cells of the immune system and cytotoxic T cells (*CTL*) that destroy infected or cancerous cells.

Before the entry of an antigen in the host organism, there are very few B and T cells that are called naive cells due to their lack of encounter with antigen. Upon antigenic stimulation these cells are activated and proliferate to generate a progeny of activated cells. Therefore, both humoral and cellular adaptive immune responses require several days or weeks to develop. This time is required to allow both B and T lymphocytes to proliferate in order to increase their number and to differentiate into effector cells able to eliminate pathogens

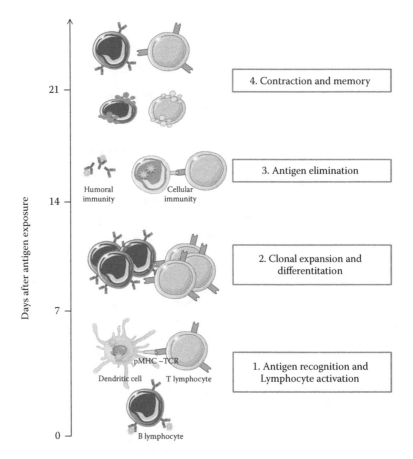

Figure 1.3 Development of an adaptive immune response. The adaptive immune response is made of various phases: antigen recognition, lymphocyte activation, antigen elimination, contraction, and memory. The duration of the different phases can change in the different immune responses. This scheme applies to both humoral and cell-mediated immunity.

(Figure 1.3). The capacity of lymphocytes specific to a given antigen to proliferate after stimulation is named *clonal expansion*. Through this process, the number of antigen-specific B or T cells increases to create a large cohort of cells that are then able to cope with rapidly replicating microbes. Remarkably, in some immune responses the number of T cells specific to a given antigen can increase up to 50,000 fold.

1.2.4 B LYMPHOCYTES

1.2.4.1 B CELL DEVELOPMENT AND FUNCTION

B cell maturation occurs via a series of molecular and cellular events taking place in the bone marrow. This process allows a progenitor of a B cell to proceed along the steps to maturation and results in a mature B cell that expresses a B cell receptor (*BCR*). The BCR is an Ig or antibody expressed on the B cells surface where it is associated with molecules involved in signal transduction. Antibodies are multimeric proteins composed of two heavy chains and two light chains joined to form a "Y" shaped molecule (see scheme in Figure 1.4). Each of the two short arms of the Y is formed by the juxtaposition of one light chain with one heavy chain. They are identical and bind two identical epitopes. The long arm binds other proteins or cellular receptors and confers the biological function to the antibody. There are five main *classes* or *isotypes* of antibodies that differ in their heavy chain and function: *IgM*, *IgD*, *IgG*, *IgA*, and *IgE*. During the various steps of differentiation in the bone marrow, precursor cells mature to the stage of naive B cells that express both IgM and IgD on their surface. The encounter with a specific antigen will lead to the activation of these naive B cells that will then start to

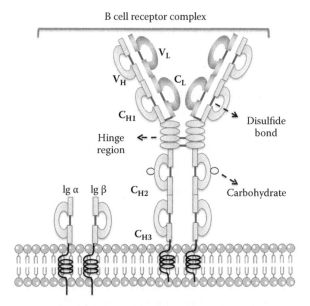

Figure 1.4 Structure of B cell receptor (BCR). Cell bound antibodies are composed of two identical light chains (indicated by subscript L) and two identical heavy chains (indicated by subscript H). Each of these chains is composed of a variable region (V), determining the specificity of the antibody for the antigen, and of a constant region (C), defining the functional properties of the antibody or immunoglobulin. Each BCR is associated with a heterodimer of immunoglobulin superfamily proteins: Igα and Igβ. The terms BCR, antibody, and immunoglobulin can be considered as synonyms, keeping in mind that BCR is the cell bound form of an antibody.

express on their surface antibodies belonging to the other Ig classes (IgG, IgA, and IgE) and will also start to release those antibodies in the extracellular milieu.

Antibodies of different isotypes have different functions. As mentioned above, the different functions are conferred to the antibody by the constant portion of the heavy chain. For example, IgMs play a major role at the beginning of the immune response and are able to activate the *complement system* (a number of small proteins that, when activated, contribute to the amplification of the immune response), while IgGs intervene later in the immune response and are the main virus and toxin neutralizing antibodies in the blood. Another example is the IgA that can be transported through the epithelial cells of gut, airways, and other mucous membranes. They are, therefore, the antibodies present in tears, saliva, mucous, etc.

1.2.4.2 BCR STRUCTURE

Specific antigen recognition by B lymphocytes is mediated by BCRs or membrane bound immunoglobulins. BCRs recognize unprocessed antigens in soluble form or bound to cell surface. BCRs do not possess an intrinsic signaling function. On the surface of a B cell, each BCR is associated with a heterodimer of proteins belonging to the immunoglobulin superfamily: *Igα* and *Igβ*. These proteins bear a cytoplasmic tail containing the ITAM motifs (Immunoreceptor Tyrosine-based Activation Motifs, *YxxL/I-X-$_{6-8}$-YxxL/I*) that are responsible for signal transduction (Figure 1.4).

1.2.4.3 B CELL ACTIVATION

BCR interaction with antigens causes BCR internalization. This allows B cells to process captured antigens within their lysosomal or late endosomal compartments and to express on their surface antigenic peptides bound to *major histocompatibility complex (MHC,* see below) molecules for antigen presentation to a specific type of T lymphocytes: the *helper T (Th)* lymphocytes. This event establishes a cascade of signaling processes that lead to the activation of B cells. Helper T cells induce robust proliferation of the specific naive B cells (*clonal expansion*) and direct their differentiation into antibody-secreting plasma cells or memory B cells. During this differentiation phase, B cells ameliorate their capacity to recognize the antigens. A key antigen binding property of the BCR (that is, the BCR affinity for the antigen) is enhanced via a mutation/selection process named *somatic hypermutation*. Cytokines released by Th cells determine the antibody isotype that better fits the ongoing immune response (*isotype switch*). Once activated, B cells become antibody producing cells and release into the extracellular milieu antibodies that have an affinity for the antigen and an isotype that reflect those exhibited by the BCR mounted on the B cell surface. As a consequence, with the ongoing immune response, B cells release antibodies exhibiting increasing affinities for their antigens. The main purpose of vaccinations is to stimulate B cells repetitively in order to allow them to produce and release antibodies of "better quality."

The biological functions of antibodies are various. A main function of the antibodies is to block (that is, neutralize) the antigen. The neutralizing capacity of an antibody is strictly dependent on its affinity for the antigen. This function is crucial to neutralize toxins released by bacteria (such as tetanus toxin, pertussis toxin, and more) and to neutralize viruses in order to impede their entry in target cells (poliomyelitis virus, measles virus, and others).

1.3 T LYMPHOCYTES

In this and in the following sections, we provide a more detailed description of the biology of T lymphocytes since these cells are the central players in adaptive immune responses. They have a broad range of functions that include the activation and control of several other cells of the immune system. We believe that understanding the complexity of T cell functional interactions with other cells can be useful for mathematicians and physicists and can allow them to become familiar with the complexity of the immune system.

1.3.1 OVERVIEW OF T LYMPHOCYTE ACTIVATION

A T lymphocyte activation requires a sequence of events. The foreign antigen is captured and processed by antigen presenting cells (*APCs*) such as dendritic cells. Antigen fragments are transported to the cell surface in order to be recognized by specific pre-existing T lymphocytes that harbor the complementary receptor for that given antigen (*T cell antigen receptor*, or *TCR*). TCRs are highly specific and each T lymphocyte normally carries only a single form of TCR. Antigen recognition together with signals provided by accessory molecules named the *co-stimulation molecules* (CD80/86 on APC and CD28 on T lymphocytes) will lead to the activation of the selected T lymphocytes that will then undergo vigorous rounds of division (*clonal expansion*). Antigen presentation to T lymphocytes is a complex process that can be considered the key event in the development of an adaptive immune response and is described more in detail below. It is important to know that T lymphocytes are unable to recognize antigens in their original form. Antigens must be processed and degraded in intracellular compartments and then expressed on the cell surface associated to specialized molecules belonging to the MHC. These molecules have the function of binding fragments of antigens (named *antigenic peptides*) and to "present" them to the TCR. In other words, TCR binding to an antigen can only occur when the antigen is processed and a portion of it is bound to an MHC molecule of the host organism. This complex mechanism provides T lymphocytes with a dual specificity: one for the antigenic peptide and one for the MHC molecules (Figure 1.5).

1.3.2 T LYMPHOCYTE SUBSETS

T lymphocytes that express the αβ TCR constitute the majority of T lymphocytes population ανδ αρε called αβ T lymphocytes. As result of gene rearrangements during their development, individual T lymphocytes expresses a unique TCR, responding to a specific antigen-derived peptide.

T lymphocytes are divided into two main subsets: the CD4+ T helper T (Th) lymphocytes and the CD8+ cytotoxic T lymphocytes. Helper T lymphocytes are divided into several functional subsets including *Th1* cells, *Th2* cells, *Th17* cells, *follicular Th (Tfh)* cells, and a heterogeneous group of *regulatory T cells (Treg)*. Thus, the current picture of αβ T cell biology postulates that T lymphocytes are a very diverse family of cell subsets. Table 1.1 summarizes some phenotypic and functional characteristics of these cell subsets.

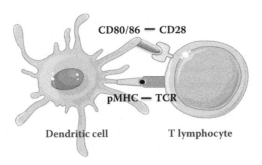

Figure 1.5 A schematic representation of T cell/APC interaction and antigen recognition. The initial encounter of between naive T cells and DCs occurs in secondary organs such as lymph nodes. Activated T lymphocytes will then differentiate into effector cells. During the activation phase, T lymphocytes down-regulate the expression of adhesion molecules and chemokine receptors that retain them in the lymph nodes and in the mean time they acquire receptors that allow their traffic towards the peripheral tissue were their function is requested. T cell response then declines (contraction phase) due to death of antigen specific effector T lymphocytes. At the end of the response a fraction of the antigen specific T cells will remain alive and will constitute a reservoir of memory T cells, ready to be re-activated by a second round of antigenic stimulation (see Figure 1.3).

Table 1.1 Example of various T cell subsets

T cell subset	Specific markers	Cytokine expressed	Some of their function
Th1	CD4	IFN γ	Activates macrophages phagocytosis
	T-bet		Enhance antibody-mediated opsonization
	STAT1		Helps CTL activation
			Inhibits Th2 differentiation
Th2	CD4	IL-4	Activates antibody secretion by B cells
	GATA3	IL-5	Enhances mast cells chemotaxis and function
	STAT6	IL-13	Activates Eosinophils
			Inhibits Th1 differentiation
Treg	CD4	IL-10	Inhibits Th1/Th2 differentiation
	FOXP3	TGF-β	Inhibits effector T cell function
		IL-35	Promotes immune tolerance
			Maintains lymphocytes homeostasis
Tfh	CD4	IL-4	Helps B cells for humoral immunity
	BCL-6	IL-21	
	CXCR-5		
Th22	CD4	IL-22	T cell proliferation
	AhR		Tissue inflammation
			Elimination of extracellular parasites
Th17	CD4	IL-17A	Neutrophil recruitment
	RORγO	IL-17F	Induce antimicrobial peptide production
	STAT3	IL-22	
Th9	CD4	IL-9	Mucosal immunity, autoimmunity, and cancer
	PU.1		
CTL	CD8	IFN γ	Cell mediated cytotoxicity
	T-bet	TNF α	
	EOMES		

1.3.3 T LYMPHOCYTE DEVELOPMENT AND MATURATION

T cell development takes place in the thymus, a lymphoid organ located behind the sternum. T cell development undergoes a strict selection process: only a small fraction of *thymocytes* (thymus resident immature T lymphocytes) that undergo the maturation process survive the different steps of selection and leave the thymus as mature T cells. In the thymic parenchyma, immature thymocytes initially do not express TCR, neither of the TCR co-receptor molecules CD4 or CD8, and they are therefore named double negative (*DN*) thymocytes. Under various cellular contacts and soluble factor-mediated signals, DN thymocytes begin to assemble pre-TCR structures. Successful surface expression of pre-TCRs induces proliferation of thymocytes and triggers further development into double positive (DP) thymocytes, which express both CD4 and CD8 co-receptors. DP thymocytes express αβ TCR and undergo a complex sequence of stimulation/selection steps that are known as *positive* and *negative selection*.

Positive selection leads to the death of thymocytes that express TCRs on their surface that do not bind to self MHC and are therefore useless for immune response. Only cells expressing TCRs with some affinity for self will pass the selection and become single positive (SP) thymocytes that express either the CD4 or the CD8 co-receptor. These SP thymocytes undergo negative selection, which eliminates potentially harmful T cells that express on their surface TCRs that have too high of an affinity for self antigens (complexes formed by self antigenic peptides bound to MHC molecules). For sake of clarity, we described positive and negative selection as sequential steps; however, in reality these steps of selection occur simultaneously. Thus, negative selection can occur both at the DP and SP stage. The combination of positive and negative selection finally allows T cells to be not self-reactive, but expressing at the same time useful TCRs, to leave the thymus as mature T cells. In conclusion, the complex cascade of events involved in the development of T lymphocytes can be summarized in this sentence: "Thymus selects the useful, neglects the useless and destroys the harmful" (von Boehmer et al., 1989).

It should be noted that, as are many other biological processes, the above-described cellular development in the thymus is not totally efficient. Therefore, the thymus does not succeed in eliminating all the potentially self-reactive cells. Other mechanisms, globally named *"peripheral tolerance"* keep the self-reactive cells that escaped thymic selection under control. Among the mechanisms of peripheral tolerance, Treg plays a central role in the control of self-reactivity. This specialized T lymphocyte subset acts to suppress other T cells. Tregs develop in the thymus where they are selected based on their specificity for self-antigens. Once in the periphery they inhibit the responses of other T lymphocytes that might react against self-antigens leading to a potentially harmful immune responses. Tregs are therefore key players in protecting the organism from autoimmune diseases.

It should be noted that the above-described sequence of cell maturation events is an oversimplification of the extremely complex process of T cell development. Readers can find more detailed and updated information about this process in recent review articles (Chyi-Song Hsieh et al., 2012; Klein et al., 2014).

1.3.4 TCR GENE ORGANIZATION

The organization and expression of genes that encode TCR chains are perfectly suited to their particular receptor function. Although important exceptions exist (Valitutti et al., 1995), we can consider for simplicity's sake that each T lymphocyte expresses a unique TCR type on its surface with single antigen specificity, i.e., each T lymphocyte is able to recognize mostly a unique peptide-MHC complex. In order to recognize the immense diversity of peptide antigens, evolution has developed a system that permits the formation of a large number of different TCR. This process randomly generates specificity of TCR for antigenic peptides. It takes place during thymic development and involves a process of gene recombination very similar to that used for rearrangements of the heavy and light chains of the Ig during B cell development.

In its germline configuration, the locus encoding the α chain of the TCR is composed of numerous segments: *V* for *Variable*, *J* for *Joining*, and a *C* for *Constant* domains. In addition, two *D* domains for *Diversity* are present in the locus encoding the β chain of TCR. The C domain encodes the constant, hinge, transmembrane region, and cytoplasmic tail of TCR chains. Once rearranged the VJ and VDJ segments code variable regions of TCR chains (Abbas et al., 2015; Murphy KM, 2012; Paul, 2012).

These gene rearrangements are governed by *Recombination Signal Sequence (RSS)*. These are palindromic sequences, heptameric and nonameric, separated by 12 or 23 pairs of bases, and they serve as anchors to the corresponding machinery of *RAG-1/RAG-2* recombinase (Mombaerts et al., 1992; Shinkai et al., 1993). The β chain genes rearrange first during thymic selection. First, there is the association of one of the D segments with a J segment; then a V segment will be added to the previously created DJ segment producing a VDJ segment. At this point, all segments of genes located in the V-D-J complex intervals are eliminated and the synthesized primary transcript contains the Vβ-Dβ-Jβ-Cβ σεγμεντs. Introns are eliminated and translation of messenger RNA generates TCR β-chain. This protein is then associated with a substitute of α chain of TCR to form the pre-TCR and is expressed on the surface of the DN thymocytes. If rearrangement of TCR β chain is functional, cells proliferate, and subsequently the rearrangement of genes encoding α chain takes place. A V segment will rearrange with a J segment and then, upon transcription and translation, the α chain of TCR is expressed. During these gene recombination processes several mechanisms induce variability at the sites of gene junction, thus generating extremely high variations in the structure of the region of the TCR that will bind the antigen (*complementary determining region*, see below). It has been estimated that via such processes of *somatic recombination* more than 10^{15} TCR can be theoretically generated during thymic development. However a large number of thymocytes that express a given TCR is eliminated during positive and negative thymic selection. Accordingly, it has been estimated that the TCR αβ repertoire of human naive T lymphocytes is of about 2.5×10^7 different TCR in the periphery (Nikolich-Zugich et al., 2004).

1.3.5 TCR STRUCTURE

αβ T lymphocytes recognize antigenic peptides in the context of MHC molecules via their TCRs. The TCR complex is composed of the αβ dimer (which consists of two transmembrane glycosylated polypeptide chains α and β that are linked through a disulfide bond), by the *CD3* γ, δ, and ε chains and by the ζζ homodimer (Garcia et al., 1996; Schumacher, 2002) (Figure 1.6). These glycoproteins belong to the immunoglobulin (Ig) superfamily. α and β chains consist of an amino-terminal extracellular domain containing a variable region (V), a constant region (C), and a short hinge region with a cysteine residue necessary for the formation of

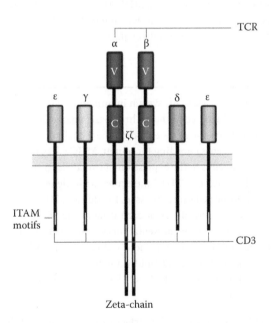

Figure 1.6 αβ T cell receptor structure. α and β chains form a complex with the CD3 signaling molecules that are composed of a γ and ε complex, a δ and ε complex and a ζζ homodimer (written as CD3γε, CD3δε, and ζζ, respectively). CD3 chains contain one ITAM motif in their cytoplasmic region, while each ζ chain that plays a central role in TCR signal transduction contains three ITAM motifs.

disulfide bonds. These two chains contain a short intracytoplasmic tail of 5-12 amino acids and a hydrophobic transmembrane domain composed of positively charged amino acids allowing TCR to stably associate with the CD3 molecules (endowed with a negatively charged transmembrane domain) (Figure 1.6) (Alarcon et al., 1988; Rudolph et al., 2006; Schumacher, 2002).

While C domains are invariant for each chain of TCR, independently of the T lymphocyte on which they are expressed, V domains vary considerably from one individual T cell to another. This variability mainly resides in three regions known as *hyper-variable regions* or *complementary determining regions (CDR)* (Chothia et al., 1988). Crystallographic studies have shown that CDR regions are projected outside of a V domain to bind pMHC complexes. In TCR the variable regions of α and β chains are disposed side by side to form a unique site for antigen recognition. The CDR1 and CDR2 regions mainly bind to MHC molecules, while CDR3 (where most of TCR variability is concentrated) binds preferentially to the antigenic peptide (Jorgensen et al., 1992; Sant'Angelo et al., 1996).

All three proteins of CD3, ε, γ, δ, have an extracellular domain that contains an Ig type domain, followed by a transmembrane region and a cytoplasmic domain of 40-80 amino acids containing an ITAM motif for signal transduction. ζ chains have a very short extracellular portion; thus, they do not contain an Ig domain. On the other hand, ζ chains have an important cytoplasmic region made of 113 amino acids and containing three ITAM motifs (Figure 1.6).

1.3.6 ANTIGEN PRESENTATION TO LYMPHOCYTES

The recognition of antigenic peptides by T lymphocytes requires antigen processing and presentation by APCs. Antigens are presented to T cells on the surface of the APCs in the form of peptides that are bound to the MHC molecules. CD4 or CD8 co-receptors are also involved in recognition of these peptide MHC (*pMHC*) complexes. Whereas CD4[+] T lymphocytes recognize antigenic peptides associated with MHC Class II molecules, CD8[+] T lymphocytes recognize those associated with class I molecules.

Most of the cells are able to present antigens to CD8[+] T lymphocytes in the context of their MHC Class I molecules. Conversely, only cells expressing MHC Class II can present antigens to the CD4[+] T cells: they are called professional APCs. Professional APCs include DC, B lymphocytes, and macrophages. Additional cells that can express, under certain circumstances, MHC-II molecules and serve as unconventional APC for CD4[+] T cells include mast cells (Gaudenzio et al., 2009), endothelial cells (Collins et al., 1984), and basophils (Perrigoue et al., 2009; Sokol et al., 2009; Yoshimoto et al., 2009).

1.3.7 MHC GENES

The MHC or *HLA (Human Leukocyte Antigens)* system in humans is a set of more than 200 genes located on chromosome 6. The molecules of MHC genes have three basic characteristics: *polygenicity, co-dominance,* and *polymorphism*. There are three classic genes encoding the α chain of the MHC Class I in humans: *HLA-A, -B,* and *-C*. There are also three genes encoding for human MHC Class II α and β chains: *DP, DQ,* and *DR* (polygenicity). The co-dominance refers to the expression of two alleles of a certain gene in a single cell. This property allows individual cells to express MHC molecules with higher ranges of specificity for peptides, since two different alleles of the same gene are expressed. In addition, MHC molecule genes are polymorphic genes, referring to the presence of many alleles of each gene in the whole population. This feature, when combined with co-dominance, allows for the presentation of a large pattern of antigenic peptides of a given antigen by the different individuals of the same species. In this way, it allows the whole population to mount a robust response against pathogens that tend to rapidly mutate.

Even though molecules of MHC Class I and Class II have the common property of binding to antigenic peptides, they differ in two key aspects:

1. The MHC Class I molecules are present on the surface of all nucleated cells in the body. The presentation of endogenous peptides by MHC Class I molecules leads to specific activation of CD8[+] T cells. These peptides are products of enzymatic degradation of intracellular molecules by *proteasome* and are constituted of 8-10 amino acids (Bouvier, 2003).

2. The MHC Class II molecules are present only on the surface of professional APCs. The association of the α1 domains with β1 domains of α and β chains forms a groove that can accommodate 12-24 amino acid long peptides to be presented to CD4+ T lymphocytes (Pieters, 2000). These peptides are derived from degradation of extracellular proteins internalized via endocytosis.

Figures 1.7 and 1.8 depict schematically the Class I and Class II MHC molecule structure and how TCR and co-receptors interact with pMHC complexes at the contact site between T lymphocytes and APCs.

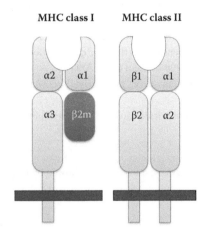

Figure 1.7 Structure of MHC molecules. Left, MHC Class I molecules are composed of a 45 kDa chain with three domains (α1, α2, and α3, similar to those of immunoglobulins) associated to the β2-microglobulin. α1 and α2 domains form a pocket, which is the site where antigenic peptides bind to MHC molecules and where the polymorphism of the molecule is mostly represented. Right, MHC Class II molecules are heterodimeric molecules, composed of two transmembrane glycoproteins: a 30-32kDa α chain that is non-covalently associated to a 27-29 kDa β chain. The peptide-binding pocket is formed by the α1 domain of the α chain and the β1 domain of the β-chain.

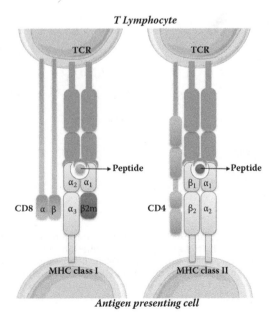

Figure 1.8 Schematic representation of MHC molecule interaction with TCR. The peptides bound to the pocket of MHC interact with CDR (Complementarity Determining Region) regions of the TCR. These interactions are stabilized through association of CD8 or CD4 co-receptor with MHC Class I and MHC Class II molecules respectively.

1.4 T CELL AND APC INTERACTION

T cell and APC cognate interaction is a key step in the initiation of T cell activation and therefore in tuning the adaptive immune response. This interaction is accompanied by the formation of a specialized signaling area called the *immunological synapse (IS)*. In its original definition, the IS was described as a specialized signaling domain formed at the contact site between T cells and APCs, characterized by large-scale molecular segregation of surface receptors and signaling components (Monks et al., 1998). Further research led to an expansion of this term, where the IS consists of a multitude of structures with a common feature of mediating intercellular communication (Trautmann and Valitutti, 2003). IS formation between T lymphocytes and APCs can turn the T cell on or off depending on the type of presented antigen, type of APC, and duration of cell-cell interaction (Benvenuti et al., 2004; Friedl et al., 2005).

A typical sequence of events occurring during productive T cell/APC interaction and IS formation is summarized in Figure 1.9.

T cell/APC interaction can be schematically divided into three phases (Friedl et al., 2005):

1. Initiation of cell-cell contacts
2. Duration and stability of contacts
3. T cell detachment after a few minutes or a few hours, followed by migration resumption.

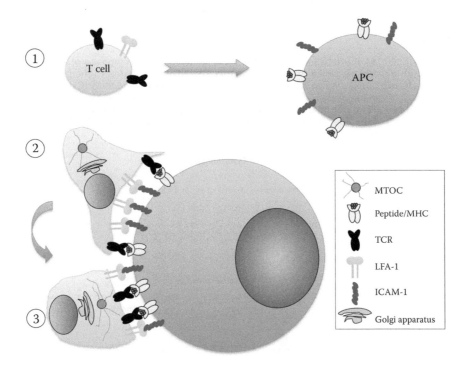

Figure 1.9 Encounter between T cells and APC and initiation of IS formation. (1) T cells form random conjugates with APC that are mediated by the engagement of adhesion molecules such as LFA-1 and ICAM-1. (2) Following productive TCR engagement with peptide/MHC complexes, the adhesion between the two cells increases and they form stable conjugates. (3) T cells change shape, stop migration, polarize secretory machinery towards the APC, and start to rearrange the molecular components of the IS. Reproduced with permission from S. Valitutti et al. (2006) "Immunological Synapse", in *Encyclopedia of Life Science*, Wiley. All rights reserved.

1.4.1 INITIATION OF CELL-CELL CONTACTS

The first step in the interaction between T cells and APCs is their physical contact, which frequently takes place in lymph nodes for naive T cells or in tissues for effector T cells. This step is initially independent of the presence of antigens. T cell motility and DC probing of the intercellular milieu with their highly motile dendrites encourages the random encounter of the cells. T cells scan the APC surface to detect antigens. The average migration speed of T lymphocytes is approximately 10 μm/min with peaks of more than 25 μm/min (Bousso and Robey, 2003; Miller et al., 2003; Miller et al., 2002). APCs, such as DC, are less motile (Lindquist et al., 2004) and their average speed of migration is 6 μm/min (Bousso and Robey, 2003; Miller et al., 2002; Okada et al., 2005). The high migration capacity of T cells *in vivo* allows them to serially scan a large number of APC. M.J Miller et al. estimated that, in the absence of an antigen, approximately 5000 CD4$^+$ T cells can encounter a given DC per hour (Miller et al., 2004) while P. Bousso and E. Robey estimated that about 500 CD8$^+$ T cells can scan a single DC in one hour (Bousso and Robey, 2003). Such rapid and frequent contacts enable recognition of rare antigens by the pool of T cells in a lymph node within a reasonable timeframe. In fact, fewer than 100 DCs in a lymph node are sufficient to initiate a response with very rare naive antigen-specific T cells (Celli et al., 2012). During this first phase, T cells are therefore highly mobile and move from one APC to another. The binding of their TCR with pMHC complexes initiates a process of activation and begins the second phase of specific interaction (Miller et al., 2004; Stoll et al., 2002).

1.4.2 STABILITY AND DURATION OF CONTACTS

T cell responses require the integration of signals derived from receptors engaged at the T cell/APC contact site over prolonged time: two models have been proposed.

The first, defined as "single encounter model," postulates a "stable" T cell/APC interaction and stems from the initial observation of firm adhesion between T cells and APCs. This model describes T cell "stop signal" as a consequence of TCR engagement and a subsequent adhesion molecule-mediated stabilization of cell-cell contact. Such stable interactions are paralleled by the formation of IS which may last for hours (Dustin et al., 1997; Grakoui et al., 1999; Hauss et al., 1995; Monks et al., 1998). Accordingly, full T lymphocyte activation and proliferation has been shown to require stimulation over several hours (Iezzi et al., 1998).

Real time monitoring of T cell movements in 3D collagen during interaction with DCs provided support for a second model, which postulates "sequential" T cell/APC interactions. This model proposed by P. Friedl et al. is based on the observation that several successive transient interactions of about 6-12 minutes are formed between motile T cells and their cognate DCs (Faroudi et al., 2003; Friedl et al., 2005; Gunzer et al., 2000). Even though T cell interactions were rather dynamic, short lived, and sequential, they resulted in T cell activation. The capacity of T cells to be activated by multiple contacts suggests the existence of a short-memory that allows T cells to accumulate signals over time (Friedl et al., 2005).

In vivo experiments showed that the balance between "stable" and "sequential" modes of T lymphocyte activation by cognate APCs can be influenced by the strength and quality of antigenic stimulation and by the type of APC (Hugues et al., 2004; Skokos et al., 2007). It is tempting to speculate that there are two main scenarios of T cell interaction with cognate APCs. First, APCs displaying high affinity pMHC at high density provide a "stop signal" to T cells and lead to the formation of stable IS. Second, a low or intermediate strength of antigenic stimulation leads to dynamic cell-cell interactions due to weak signal transduction and failure to completely arrest T cells (Dustin, 2008; Moreau et al., 2015). Several lines of evidence indicate that additional factors—including the presence or absence of Tregs (Tadokoro et al., 2006) and of chemokines (Asperti-Boursin et al., 2007; Okada and Cyster, 2007; Woolf et al., 2007; Worbs et al., 2007)—can influence the "stable" and "sequential" modes of T cell/APC interaction.

1.4.3 TERMINATION OF CELL INTERACTION

T cell detachment from APC and reacquisition of a migratory phenotype is the terminal phase of cell-cell cognate interaction for antigen recognition. To date, this step has not been studied as much and, therefore, is not fully understood.

1.5 TCR/pMHC INTERACTION

TCRs display a remarkable ability to specifically recognize a wide array of structurally and chemically diverse antigens. The understanding of the molecular basis of TCR interaction with pMHC has been greatly advanced by a number of studies that elucidated key contacts and binding modes of several of these interactions.

1.5.1 AFFINITY OF BINDING

Several studies performed in different T cell models demonstrated that, to achieve full activation, T cells require TCR-mediated sustained signaling (Huppa et al., 2003; Mempel et al., 2004; Valitutti et al., 1995). This concept is difficult to reconcile with several studies performed using isolated TCR and pMHC molecules. These studies based on the measurement of TCR/pMHC binding parameters in solution revealed a low affinity of TCR/pMHC binding (dissociation constant, Kd approximately 1-100 μM) as well as a very short dwell-time of binding (seconds) (Matsui et al., 1991; Weber et al., 1992). This was a paradoxical finding considering the specificity and efficacy of TCR that can recognize one single foreign antigen among a sea of self-pMHC complexes displayed on the APC surface. The high specificity of TCR binding is also shown by the fact that although a given pMHC complex may act as a strong agonist capable of triggering full activation of a T cell through TCR engagement, other related peptides will serve as weak or null agonists and may have no or at best partial effects on T cell activation. Moreover, substitution of a single amino acid in the sequence of the antigenic peptide presented by MHC can render T cells unresponsive to subsequent stimulation with the immunogenic peptide (Kalergis et al., 2001) M.M. Davis and colleagues measured the kinetics of TCR-pMHC binding at the cell-cell contact site, by using single-molecule microscopy and fluorescence resonance energy transfer (*FRET*). They showed that, when compared to solution measurements, TCR/pMHC association and dissociation rates are even faster (Huppa et al., 2010). Complementary results were obtained using a different approach by J. Huang et al. (Huang et al., 2010). Together these results underline the extreme rapidity of TCR/pMHC binding at the T cell/APC contact site and suggest that, for sustained signaling in T cells, multiple rounds of TCR/pMHC binding are required (Huang et al., 2010; Huppa et al., 2010).

1.5.2 PROBABILITY OF INTERACTION

Interaction of TCR with pMHC has major constraints. First, although T cells express a significant number of TCRs with the same affinity (30,000-50,000 TCR per cell) for a specific antigen, the APCs present only a small number of pMHC molecules that can be recognized by those TCRs. In fact, most of the pMHC expressed on an APC surface are self-antigens, resulting from the degradation of intra and extracellular proteins. Demotz et al. reported that T cells are activated by APCs that display on their surface as little as 0.03% specific pMHC complexes. Therefore, the probability that a specific pMHC complex is present at the contact area between T cells and APCs during antigen recognition is low. An additional parameter that further reduces the probability of TCR/pMHC interaction is the length of the extracellular domains of TCR and of their ligands when compared to other membrane molecules. Both TCR and pMHC are approximately 7 nm long. Therefore, to allow productive TCR engagement, the membranes of a T cell and an APC should be ~14 nm apart. This scenario is difficult to envisage because of the presence of numerous glycosylated long-ectodomain proteins on the surface of cells that might prevent such proximity.

In spite of those compelling factors, TCR/pMHC interaction is extremely sensitive. Recent studies, demonstrated that a single pMHC is able to induce signaling, as detected by a transient $[Ca^{2+}]i$ increase in mouse

$CD4^+$ T cells and that by maintaining a sustained $[Ca^{2+}]i$ increase in T cells, TCR recognition of only 10-15 pMHC complexes is strong enough to induce T cell activation (Irvine et al., 2002; Purbhoo et al., 2004). Likewise, CTLs were capable of killing target cells expressing only 1-10 pMHC complexes on their surface (Huse et al., 2007; Jiang et al., 2011; Sykulev et al., 1996).

In the last decades, many studies tried to investigate this intriguing paradox. Three models have been proposed to explain the mechanisms regulating antigen recognition by T cells: the kinetic-segregation model, the kinetic proofreading model, and the serial TCR engagement model.

1.5.3 KINETIC-SEGREGATION MODEL

About 20 years ago, S. Davis and P.A. van der Merwe proposed a model of T cell activation to explain how productive TCR and pMHC interaction might take place at the T cell/APC contact site leading to TCR-coupled signal transduction. The "kinetic-segregation model" of TCR triggering postulates that upon T cell/APC encounter, small areas of close contact between their plasma membranes are formed, which then allow TCR and pMHC to come in contact. The inhibitory CD45 phosphatase, as well as other large-ectodomain tyrosine phosphatases, is excluded from the TCR signaling area. CD45 steric exclusion on the one hand facilitates TCR/pMHC encounters but on the other hand extends signal transduction associated to TCRs by amplifying protein tyrosine kinase signaling. When T cells detach from the APC, the intimate cell-cell contact areas are dissolved and large-ectodomain tyrosine phosphatases are allowed to restore the basal level of signaling (Davis and van der Merwe, 2006). Recent studies have confirmed the importance of local segregation of CD45 tyrosine phosphatase from kinases for the initiation of productive signaling in T cells (Chang et al., 2016; Choudhuri et al., 2005).

1.5.4 KINETIC PROOFREADING MODEL

In 1995, T.W. McKeithan proposed the kinetic proofreading model in which a long enough time of interaction between TCR and pMHC is considered a crucial element for full activation of T cells (McKeithan, 1995). According to this model, there is a lapse of time between the initial TCR and pMHC interaction and signal transduction. The kinetic proofreading model proposes that TCR-coupled signaling consists of a series of intermediate reversible steps leading to full activation of the signaling cascade (Figure 1.10). The model is based on three hypotheses. First, the inactive primary TCR/pMHC complex undergoes a sequence of N modifications (number of possible modifications) leading to an activated state via a series of intermediaries. Even though these modifications have not been described in detail, they can include: phosphorylation in tyrosine within the receptor complex, conformational changes of proteins, generation of second messengers,

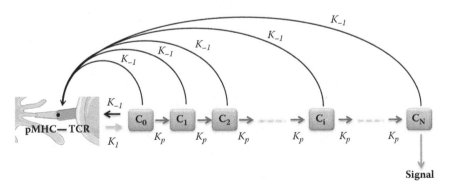

Figure 1.10 Kinetic proofreading model. The kinetic proofreading model suggests that the binding of a TCR to a pMHC to form a TCR/pMHC complex initiates a sequence of signaling events with intermediates (C_1, C_2, ...). This process culminates in the formation of the final signaling product (C_N), which signals to the cell. However, if the TCR/pMHC complex dissociates before the formation of C_N, the signaling fails. The association (k_1) and dissociation (k_{-1}) rate constants for the TCR/pMHC interaction are shown, as are the rate constants of the intermediate pathway (k_p, assumed to be the same for every step). Adapted from A.J. George et al. (2005) "Understanding specificity and sensitivity of T-cell recognition", Trends in Immunology, 26: 653-659, with permission from Elsevier.

or recruitment of scaffolding components to the receptor. Second, dissociation of the interaction leads to the reversion of these modifications. Third, upon interaction between TCR and non-specific pMHC, the rate of dissociation is sufficiently high to avoid formation of productive interactions. This model explains how T cells discriminate among ligands based on kinetic differences in the assembly of the signaling cascade. It also implies that variations of the TCR/pMHC binding kinetics can be amplified by signal transduction in order to maximize minor binding differences and explain the high specificity of TCR/pMHC interactions.

The kinetic proofreading theory revolves around the concept that short-term TCR engagement will induce early signaling events but not late T cell responses, due to the reversibility of early activation steps. The model is supported by measurement of TCR/pMHC binding kinetics in solution showing a correlation between the duration of TCR/ligand binding and the biologic efficacy of this interactions (Davis et al., 1998; Gascoigne et al., 2001; Germain and Stefanova, 1999).

1.5.5 SERIAL TCR ENGAGEMENT

Even though kinetic proofreading can explain the high specificity of T cell activation induced by TCR/pMHC interactions, it does not provide a model to describe the high sensitivity of such interactions with a small number of specific pMHC. It has been previously shown that T cells need to undergo sustained signaling to be activated to cytokine production and that a prolonged TCR engagement with pMHC is required for sustained signaling in T cells (Valitutti et al., 1995). Considering the fact that TCR/pMHC binding has low affinity and rapid off-rate, how can TCR engagement be prolonged?

In 1995, S. Valitutti et al. proposed the serial engagement model in order to explain how sustained TCR signaling might take place during antigen recognition. The authors used TCR internalization as a parameter of TCR/pMHC binding and observed that a few specific pMHC can lead to high levels of TCR internalization, meaning that a small number of pMHC can engage, trigger, and down-regulate a considerable number of TCRs. The model postulates that low affinity TCRs can rapidly and sequentially bind a small number of specific pMHC resulting in a sustained and amplified signaling (Valitutti et al., 1995). The model provides a plausible explanation to the high sensitivity of antigen recognition by T cells equipped with low affinity TCRs (Figure 1.11).

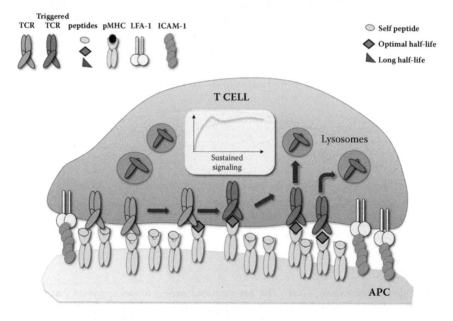

Figure 1.11 The serial TCR engagement model. At the T cell/APC contact site a few specific pMHC (red) sequentially trigger incoming TCR resulting in sustained signaling. Triggered TCR are internalized and targeted to lysosomes for degradation while unbound pMHC bind new TCR. Reproduced from S. Valitutti (2012), The serial engagement model 17 years after: From TCR triggering to immunotherapy, *Frontiers in Immunology* 3, 272.

Measurements of very fast TCR/pMHC binding on- and off-rates at the contact site between T cells and immobilized pMHC (Huang et al., 2010) as well as other experimental and computational studies support serial TCR engagement (Valitutti, 2012). However other observations do not support the model (reviewed in (van der Merwe and Dushek, 2011) and (Valitutti, 2012)).

Kinetic proofreading and serial engagement models might be not mutually exclusive. In fact, on the one hand, the kinetic proofreading explains the specificity of interactions at the molecular level; on the other hand, serial engagement explains the sensitivity of T cells to antigenic stimulation at the cellular level.

1.6 CYTOTOXIC T LYMPHOCYTES/TARGET CELL INTERACTION

In this section, we outline the competitive interaction that takes place during adaptive immune responses between the main killer cells (CTLs) and their target cells (virally infected and tumor cells). The balance between CTL efficacy and target cell resistance can be indeed viewed as a complex predator/prey system in which CTLs act as predators and target cells act as prey undergoing evolution. During the last 20-30 years the synergy between experimental, mathematical, and physical approaches has contributed to the understanding of such complex competitive interaction.

1.6.1 ACTIVATION AND DIFFERENTIATION OF NAIVE CD8+ T CELLS INTO CTLs

Naive CD8+ T cells that have not previously encountered the antigen express neither cytotoxic molecules nor activation markers and are incapable of cell-mediated cytotoxicity. The activation process of the CD8+ T cells starts when naive T cells recognize their specific antigen presented by a DC in the context of MHC Class I molecules. This first encounter between naive CD8+ T cells and a DC occurs in secondary lymphoid organs such as the lymph nodes and the spleen. Antigen recognition by TCR provides a first activation signal and confers specificity to the response. The second signal is provided by the engagement of co-stimulatory molecules of CD8+ T cells such as CD28 with their ligands on the DC surface (CD80 and CD86, Figure 1.5). Contrary to the first signal, this signal is nonspecific, but it is crucial to the development of an effective CD8+ T cell mediated immune response. Absence of the second signal may lead to a sustained state of T cell inactivation, named *T cell anergy*.

Moreover, there is evidence supporting the idea that CD8+ T cell proliferation and differentiation can be influenced by the microenvironment (third signal). This signal is mediated by exogenous inflammatory and antiviral cytokines. It provides the means for a CD8+ T cell that encounters the antigen to determine if there is "danger" present and to respond accordingly. For instance, *in vitro* and *in vivo* experiments identified IL-12 and IFN α/β as predominant sources of signal three for CD8+ T cell responses to a variety of stimuli (Curtsinger and Mescher, 2010).

The combination of these three signals causes clonal expansion of a specific CD8+ T cell population and induces its differentiation into cytotoxic T cells (CTL). While clonal expansion guarantees the presence of a sufficient number of antigen specific T cells for eradication of invading pathogens or cancerous cell, it is also controlled by a contraction phase during which the number of cells declines and only a limited number of memory T cells specific for that given antigen is maintained (Figure 1.3). Memory CD8+ T cells are long-lived antigen specific cells that are ready to respond in a faster and stronger manner upon second encounter with the same antigen. For instance, after the clearing of a skin infection, a stable population of memory T cells continuously patrols skin epithelia in order to rapidly control secondary infections (Ariotti et al., 2012).

1.6.2 CTL EFFECTOR FUNCTION

Within about 5 days after the initial encounter with DCs, naive CD8+ T cells differentiate into effector CTLs equipped with lytic molecules. Upon encounter with cognate target cells, CTLs activate different cytotoxic mechanisms, leading to target cell annihilation. Among those mechanisms, the most rapid and efficient pathway of CTL-mediated cytotoxicity is the release of the pore-forming protein perforin together with granzymes and other proteolytic enzymes (all stored in cytosolic granules, named lytic granules) at the CTL or target cell IS (Bertrand et al., 2013). CTLs can also trigger target cell death by ligation of target cells surface receptors containing cytoplasmic death domains, such as the molecule Fas (Rouvier et al., 1993). Moreover, following their activation, CTLs secrete cytokines such as IFN-γ that contribute to their function in controlling tumorigenesis (Kortylewski et al., 2004).

1.6.3 EFFICACY OF CTL

As mentioned above, CTL are extremely sensitive to antigenic stimulation since they can be activated to secrete their lytic granules by a small number of specific pMHC complexes displayed on the APC surface (Purbhoo et al., 2004; Sykulev et al., 1996; Valitutti et al., 1996). In addition, lytic granule secretion is a very rapid response. Indeed, cytotoxicity occurs within a few minutes or even seconds after the initial contact between CTLs and target cells, independently of the strength of antigenic stimulation (Bertrand et al., 2013; Stinchcombe et al., 2001; Wiedemann et al., 2006). Another distinct feature of CTL biology is that these cells can kill multiple target cells, either simultaneously or serially by bouncing from one target cell to another (Macken and Perelson, 1984; Perelson and Bell, 1982; Poenie et al., 2004; Rothstein et al., 1978; Wiedemann et al., 2006). This property allows each individual CTL to annihilate more than one target cell. Interestingly, in clonal CTL populations, although all CTLs are genetically identical, some of them (super-killers) are much more efficient than others at killing target cells (Vasconcelos et al., 2015). It should be noted that recent *in vitro* and *in vivo* studies redefined the paradigm of CTL efficacy by showing that the number of target cells that an individual CTL can kill is limited to about 12 cells per day (Halle et al., 2016; Vasconcelos et al., 2015).

1.6.4 CTL/TUMOR CELL INTERACTION

The paradigm of exquisitely efficient CTLs does not directly translate into an efficient status of immune surveillance against tumors. Indeed, although tumor-specific CTLs expand at relatively high frequency in cancer patients and infiltrate malignant tissues, the effector function of these naturally occurring CTLs is often insufficient to achieve clinical remission (Gajewski et al., 2007; Romero et al., 2006; Zitvogel et al., 2006). Various immunotherapy strategies are currently being tested in cancer patients in order to potentiate CTL responses against tumor cells. Among those, therapies based on monoclonal antibodies targeting inhibitory surface molecules such as CTLA-4/CD80-CD86 or the PD-1/PD-L1 axis are certainly very promising (Aris and Barrio, 2015; Gajewski et al., 2013; Lindsay et al., 2015); however, they need to be optimized to establish the best compromise between clinical benefits and adverse effects.

Several molecular mechanisms account for tumor escape from CTL-driven immune surveillance (Zitvogel et al., 2006). Effector CTL generation can be impaired by the low immunogenicity of tumor antigens and low expression of co-stimulation signals. Once generated, effector CTLs must overcome additional barriers for successful control of tumor growth. On the one hand, the tumor micro-environment can be enriched in immune-suppressive cytokines and/or metabolic factors (e.g., TGF-β, IL-10, indoleamine 2, 3-dioxygenase, arginase-1, and nitric-oxide synthase 2) (Viola and Bronte, 2007; Zitvogel et al., 2006). On the other hand, tumor cells can modulate the expression of surface molecules to avoid recognition by CTLs (e.g., by downregulating Class I MHC molecules) (Gajewski et al., 2007; Zitvogel et al., 2006). Furthermore, Tregs and other suppressor cells are frequently enriched in tumor infiltrates and can contribute to the inhibition of CTL effector function (Gajewski et al., 2013). An additional level of tumor resistance is based on tumor cell molecules that can "defuse" the lytic potential of CTLs. Among these, granzyme inhibitors of the serpin family have been thoroughly characterized (Medema et al., 1997). We recently showed that, in melanoma cells, CTL attack triggers a rapid lysosome secretory burst at the IS. This leads to degradation of perforin and to sustained melanoma cell resistance to CTL-mediated cytotoxicity (Caramalho et al., 2009; Khazen et al., 2016). All in all, it is now well established that, although CTLs are not the only actors of the anti-tumor immune response (Zitvogel et al., 2006), a global failure in the CTL "effector phase" contributes to the inefficiency of the immune surveillance against tumors (Gajewski et al., 2007).

The description of the complex multitude of escape mechanisms deployed on tumor sites suggests that, under the selective pressure of the immune system, cancer cells can undergo several evolutionary alterations in their molecular expression as well as in their growth behavior in order to subvert such immune responses and finally escape immune surveillance. This concept, named *immunoediting* was put forth by R.D. Schreiber et al. in the early 2000s and has since received substantial experimental support (Schreiber et al., 2011). Our research team has recently started to combine experimental and mathematical approaches to study the dynamic interaction of CTLs with tumor target cells undergoing immunoediting. In an initial study, we developed a computational model that mimics the interaction between CTLs and tumor cell nodules using numerical simulations. The model describes the competition between CTLs and the tumor nodules and allows both temporal and two-dimensional spatial progression. It provides probabilistic estimates of tumor eradication in numerical simulations in which tunable parameters influencing CTL efficacy against the tumor nodule are tested. Our results show that in a context of stochastically occurring mutations leading to tumor immunoediting, CTL attraction towards scout siblings having detected the tumor is a crucial parameter allowing early productive CTL/tumor collisions and therefore tumor eradication (Christophe et al., 2015). This recent study is only one among several computational studies that have addressed the complex issue of CTL target cell interaction. For instance, mathematical studies contributed to shed light on the capacity of CTLs to kill several target cells either sequentially (Macken and Perelson, 1984; Perelson and Bell, 1982) or simultaneously (Gadhamsetty et al., 2014) and on the parameters that influence CTL killing efficacy during 3D CTL/target cell interaction (Graw and Regoes, 2009). Moreover, mathematical modeling has been instrumental to estimate CTL killing efficacy *in vivo* (Yates et al., 2007) and to provide a better understanding of the balance between CTL efficacy and virus escape during infection (Garcia et al., 2015; Garcia et al., 2016).

1.7 OF MICE AND MEN: KEY ISSUES THAT REMAIN TO BE ELUCIDATED

During the writing of this chapter we have deliberately avoided precisely distinguishing between results obtained by using *in vivo* mouse or *in vitro* human models, as this distinction might be confusing for non-expert readers. Results obtained using the two experimental approaches are complementary, yet important differences exist between *in vivo* and *in vitro* protocols and sometimes results diverge. Mouse *in vivo* immunology has been traditionally recognized as the leading immunological science allowing, for obvious ethical reasons, to address questions that could not be addressed in humans and to recapitulate the entire pathophysiology of immune responses. Yet, a recent view, based on major advancement in the experimental tools by which human T cells are interrogated, postulates that human immunology is indeed extremely relevant to the understanding of immune system function in health and disease (Mestas and Huges, 2004; Davis, 2008). The availability of various "humanized mouse" models such as patient derived tumor xenografts (*PDTX*) will be instrumental to address "human immunology" questions within an *in vivo* environment, but will be probably not sufficient to fill the gap between human and mouse immunology.

Today, a major and key opportunity for physicists, mathematicians, and computer scientists interested to immunology is to provide computational tools, data analysis solutions, and mathematical models that might allow the merging of the knowledge derived from *in vivo* studies with the *ex vivo* and *in vitro* results obtained from patients' specimens, thus contributing to a "integrated" view of human immunology.

1.8 CONCLUDING REMARKS

In this short chapter we attempted to offer to non-biologist readers a "flavor" of the fascinating complexity of the immune system. We do not have the ambition to provide an exhaustive survey of such a complex topic. However, we hope to have raised the attention on several aspects of immune system biology that might strongly profit of collaboration between immunologists and mathematicians/physicists. For the sake of clarity and due to length limitation, we could not discuss in depth aspects of immune cell biology that are currently at the leading edge of the research in computational biology, such as cell motility behaviors, gene expression profiles by individual cells, and asymmetric and heterogeneous cellular behaviors. These and additional exciting topics are discussed in dedicated publications.

It is intriguing that immunology is, among life science disciplines, the one that frequently raises interest in epistemologists and computational scientists. The reasons for such an interdisciplinary interest to immunology are manifold and include the complexity of cellular and molecular networks, the high degree of plasticity of immune responses, and even the evolution of a dedicated immunological language and nomenclature that recapitulates immune system complexity. It is important to remember that the immune system, together with the nervous system, is the only multi-cellular apparatus able to keep a memory of previous experiences and to provide adapted responses to challenges. Moreover and intriguingly, both cells of the immune and nervous system have developed synaptic tools for complex intercellular communication.

Deciphering the complexity of the immune system learning mechanisms and adapted responses remains a formidable challenge for both experimental and computational scientists today.

REFERENCES

Abbas, A.K., Litchman, A.H., and S, P. (2015). *Cellular and molecular immunology*. Philadelphia, PA: Elsevier/Saunders.

Alarcon, B., Berkhout, B., Breitmeyer, J., and Terhorst, C. (1988). Assembly of the human T cell receptor-CD3 complex takes place in the endoplasmic reticulum and involves intermediary complexes between the CD3-gamma.delta.epsilon core and single T cell receptor alpha or beta chains. *J Biol Chem 263*, 2953–2961.

Ariotti, S., Beltman, J.B., Chodaczek, G., Hoekstra, M.E., van Beek, A.E., Gomez-Eerland, R., Ritsma, L., van Rheenen, J., Maree, A.F., Zal, T. et al. (2012). Tissue-resident memory CD8+ T cells continuously patrol skin epithelia to quickly recognize local antigen. *Proc Natl Acad Sci U S A 109*, 19739–19744.

Aris, M., and Barrio, M.M. (2015). Combining immunotherapy with oncogene-targeted therapy: A new road for melanoma treatment. *Front Immunol 6*, 46.

Asperti-Boursin, F., Real, E., Bismuth, G., Trautmann, A., and Donnadieu, E. (2007). CCR7 ligands control basal T cell motility within lymph node slices in a phosphoinositide 3-kinase-independent manner. *J Exp Med 204*, 1167–1179.

Benvenuti, F., Lagaudriere-Gesbert, C., Grandjean, I., Jancic, C., Hivroz, C., Trautmann, A., Lantz, O., and Amigorena, S. (2004). Dendritic cell maturation controls adhesion, synapse formation, and the duration of the interactions with naive T lymphocytes. *J Immunol 172*, 292–301.

Bertrand, F., Muller, S., Roh, K.H., Laurent, C., Dupre, L., and Valitutti, S. (2013). An initial and rapid step of lytic granule secretion precedes microtubule organizing center polarization at the cytotoxic T lymphocyte/target cell synapse. *Proc Natl Acad Sci U S A 110*, 6073–6078.

Bousso, P., and Robey, E. (2003). Dynamics of CD8+ T cell priming by dendritic cells in intact lymph nodes. *Nat Immunol 4*, 579–585.

Bouvier, M. (2003). Accessory proteins and the assembly of human class I MHC molecules: A molecular and structural perspective. *Mol Immunol 39*, 697–706.

Caramalho, I., Faroudi, M., Padovan, E., Muller, S., and Valitutti, S. (2009). Visualizing CTL/melanoma cell interactions: Multiple hits must be delivered for tumour cell annihilation. *Journal of Cellular and Molecular Medicine 13*, 3834–3846.

Celli, S., Day, M., Muller, A.J., Molina-Paris, C., Lythe, G., and Bousso, P. (2012). How many dendritic cells are required to initiate a T-cell response? *Blood 120*, 3945–3948.

Chang, V.T., Fernandes, R.A., Ganzinger, K.A., Lee, S.F., Siebold, C., McColl, J., Jonsson, P., Palayret, M., Harlos, K., Coles, C.H. et al. (2016). Initiation of T cell signaling by CD45 segregation at "close contacts." *Nat Immunol 17*, 574–582.

Chothia, C., Boswell, D.R., and Lesk, A.M. (1988). The outline structure of the T-cell alpha beta receptor. *Embo Journal 7*, 3745–3755.

Choudhuri, K., Wiseman, D., Brown, M.H., Gould, K., and van der Merwe, P.A. (2005). T-cell receptor triggering is critically dependent on the dimensions of its peptide-MHC ligand. Nature 436, 578–582.

Christophe, C., Muller, S., Rodrigues, M., Petit, A.E., Cattiaux, P., Dupre, L., Gadat, S., and Valitutti, S. (2015). A biased competition theory of cytotoxic T lymphocyte interaction with tumor nodules. PLoS One 10, e0120053.

Chyi-Song Hsieh, Hyang-Mi Lee1, and Lio, C.-W.J. (2012). Selection of regulatory T cells in the thymus. Nat Rev Immunol 12, 157–167.

Collins, T., Korman, A.J., Wake, C.T., Boss, J.M., Kappes, D.J., Fiers, W., Ault, K.A., Gimbrone, M.A., Jr., Strominger, J.L., and Pober, J.S. (1984). Immune interferon activates multiple class II major histocompatibility complex genes and the associated invariant chain gene in human endothelial cells and dermal fibroblasts. Proc Natl Acad Sci U S A 81, 4917–4921.

Curtsinger, J.M., and Mescher, M.F. (2010). Inflammatory cytokines as a third signal for T cell activation. Curr Opin Immunol 22, 333–340.

Davis, M.M. (2008). A prescription for human immunology. Immunity 29, 835–838.

Davis, M.M., Boniface, J.J., Reich, Z., Lyons, D., Hampl, J., Arden, B., and Chien, Y. (1998). Ligand recognition by alpha beta T cell receptors. Annu Rev Immunol 16, 523–544.

Davis, S.J., and van der Merwe, P.A. (2006). The kinetic-segregation model: TCR triggering and beyond. Nat Immunol 7, 803–809.

Dustin, M.L. (2008). T-cell activation through immunological synapses and kinapses. Immunol Rev 221, 77–89.

Dustin, M.L., Bromley, S.K., Kan, Z., Peterson, D.A., and Unanue, E.R. (1997). Antigen receptor engagement delivers a stop signal to migrating T lymphocytes. Proc Natl Acad Sci U S A 94, 3909–3913.

Faroudi, M., Utzny, C., Salio, M., Cerundolo, V., Guiraud, M., Muller, S., and Valitutti, S. (2003). Lytic versus stimulatory synapse in cytotoxic T lymphocyte/target cell interaction: Manifestation of a dual activation threshold. Proc Natl Acad Sci U S A 100, 14145–14150.

Friedl, P., den Boer, A.T., and Gunzer, M. (2005). Tuning immune responses: Diversity and adaptation of the immunological synapse. Nat Rev Immunol 5, 532–545.

Gadhamsetty, S., Maree, A.F., Beltman, J.B., and de Boer, R.J. (2014). A general functional response of cytotoxic T lymphocyte-mediated killing of target cells. Biophys J 106, 1780–1791.

Gajewski, T.F., Schreiber, H., and Fu, Y.X. (2007). Innate and adaptive immune cells in the tumor microenvironment. Nat Immunol 14, 1014–1022.

Gajewski, T.F., Woo, S.R., Zha, Y.Y., Spaapen, R., Zheng, Y., Corrales, L., and Spranger, S. (2013). Cancer immunotherapy strategies based on overcoming barriers within the tumor microenvironment. Curr Opin Immunol 25, 268–276.

Garcia, K.C., Degano, M., Stanfield, R.L., Brunmark, A., Jackson, M.R., Peterson, P.A., Teyton, L., and Wilson, I.A. (1996). An alphabeta T cell receptor structure at 2.5 A and its orientation in the TCR-MHC complex. Science 274, 209–219.

Garcia, V., Feldman, M.W., and Regoes, R.R. (2015). Investigating the consequences of interference between multiple CD8+ T cell escape mutations in early HIV infection. PLoS Comput Biol 12, e1004721.

Garcia, V., Richter, K., Graw, F., Oxenius, A., and Regoes, R.R. (2016). Estimating the in vivo killing efficacy of cytotoxic T lymphocytes across different peptide-MHC complex densities. PLoS Comput Biol 11, e1004178.

Gascoigne, N.R., Zal, T., and Alam, S.M. (2001). T-cell receptor binding kinetics in T-cell development and activation. Expert Rev Mol Med 2001, 1–17.

Gaudenzio, N., Espagnolle, N., Mars, L.T., Liblau, R., Valitutti, S., and Espinosa, E. (2009). Cell-cell cooperation at the T helper cell/mast cell immunological synapse. Blood 114, 4979–4988.

George, A.J., Stark, J., and Chan, C. (2005). Understanding specificity and sensitivity of T-cell recognition. Trends Immunol 26, 653–659.

Germain, R.N., and Stefanova, I. (1999). The dynamics of T cell receptor signaling: Complex orchestration and the key roles of tempo and cooperation. Annu Rev Immunol 17, 467–522.

Grakoui, A., Bromley, S.K., Sumen, C., Davis, M.M., Shaw, A.S., Allen, P.M., and Dustin, M.L. (1999). The immunological synapse: A molecular machine controlling T cell activation. Science 285, 221–227.

Graw, F., and Regoes, R.R. (2009). Investigating CTL mediated killing with a 3D cellular automaton. *PLoS Comput Biol 5*, e1000466.

Gunzer, M., Schafer, A., Borgmann, S., Grabbe, S., Zanker, K.S., Brocker, E.B., Kampgen, E., and Friedl, P. (2000). Antigen presentation in extracellular matrix: Interactions of T cells with dendritic cells are dynamic, short lived, and sequential. *Immunity 13*, 323–332.

Halle, S., Keyser, K.A., Stahl, F.R., Busche, A., Marquardt, A., Zheng, X., Galla, M., Heissmeyer, V., Heller, K., Boelter, J. et al. (2016). In vivo killing capacity of cytotoxic T cells is limited and involves dynamic interactions and T cell cooperativity. *Immunity 44*, 233–245.

Hauss, P., Selz, F., Cavazzana-Calvo, M., and Fischer, A. (1995). Characteristics of antigen-independent and antigen-dependent interaction of dendritic cells with CD4+ T cells. *Eur J Immunol 25*, 2285–2294.

Huang, J., Zarnitsyna, V.I., Liu, B., Edwards, L.J., Jiang, N., Evavold, B.D., and Zhu, C. (2010). The kinetics of two-dimensional TCR and pMHC interactions determine T-cell responsiveness. *Nature 464*, 932–936.

Hugues, S., Fetler, L., Bonifaz, L., Helft, J., Amblard, F., and Amigorena, S. (2004). Distinct T cell dynamics in lymph nodes during the induction of tolerance and immunity. *Nat Immunol 5*, 1235–1242.

Huppa, J.B., Axmann, M., Mortelmaier, M.A., Lillemeier, B.F., Newell, E.W., Brameshuber, M., Klein, L.O., Schutz, G.J., and Davis, M.M. (2010). TCR-peptide-MHC interactions in situ show accelerated kinetics and increased affinity. *Nature 463*, 963–967.

Huppa, J.B., Gleimer, M., Sumen, C., and Davis, M.M. (2003). Continuous T cell receptor signaling required for synapse maintenance and full effector potential. *Nat Immunol 4*, 749–755.

Huse, M., Klein, L.O., Girvin, A.T., Faraj, J.M., Li, Q.J., Kuhns, M.S., and Davis, M.M. (2007). Spatial and temporal dynamics of T cell receptor signaling with a photoactivatable agonist. *Immunity 27*, 76–88.

Iezzi, G., Karjalainen, K., and Lanzavecchia, A. (1998). The duration of antigenic stimulation determines the fate of naive and effector T cells. *Immunity 8*, 89–95.

Irvine, D.J., Purbhoo, M.A., Krogsgaard, M., and Davis, M.M. (2002). Direct observation of ligand recognition by T cells. *Nature 419*, 845–849.

Jiang, N., Huang, J., Edwards, L.J., Liu, B., Zhang, Y., Beal, C.D., Evavold, B.D., and Zhu, C. (2011). Two-stage cooperative T cell receptor-peptide major histocompatibility complex-CD8 trimolecular interactions amplify antigen discrimination. *Immunity 34*, 13–23.

Jorgensen, J.L., Esser, U., Fazekas de St Groth, B., Reay, P.A., and Davis, M.M. (1992). Mapping T-cell receptor-peptide contacts by variant peptide immunization of single-chain transgenics. *Nature 355*, 224–230.

Kalergis, A.M., Boucheron, N., Doucey, M.A., Palmieri, E., Goyarts, E.C., Vegh, Z., Luescher, I.F., and Nathenson, S.G. (2001). Efficient T cell activation requires an optimal dwell-time of interaction between the TCR and the pMHC complex. *Nat Immunol 2*, 229–234.

Khazen, R., Muller, S., Gaudenzio, N., Espinosa, E., Puissegur, M.P., and Valitutti, S. (2016). Melanoma cell lysosome secretory burst neutralizes the CTL-mediated cytotoxicity at the lytic synapse. *Nat Commun 7*, 10823.

Klein, L.O., B, K., Allen, P.M., and A, H.K. (2014). Positive and negative selection of the T cell repertoire: What thymocytes see (and don't see). *Nature Rev Immunol 14*, 377–339.

Kortylewski, M., Komyod, W., Kauffmann, M.E., Bosserhoff, A., Heinrich, P.C., and Behrmann, I. (2004). Interferon-gamma-mediated growth regulation of melanoma cells: Involvement of STAT1-dependent and STAT1-independent signals. *J Invest Dermatol 122*, 414–422.

Lindquist, R.L., Shakhar, G., Dudziak, D., Wardemann, H., Eisenreich, T., Dustin, M.L., and Nussenzweig, M.C. (2004). Visualizing dendritic cell networks in vivo. *Nat Immunol 5*, 1243–1250.

Lindsay, C.R., Spiliopoulou, P., and Waterston, A. (2015). Blinded by the light: Why the treatment of metastatic melanoma has created a new paradigm for the management of cancer. *Therapeutic Advances in Medical Oncology 7*, 107–121.

Macken, C.A., and Perelson, A.S. (1984). A multistage model for the action of cytotoxic T lymphocytes in multicellular conjugates. *J Immunol 132*, 1614–1624.

Matsui, K., Boniface, J.J., Reay, P.A., Schild, H., Fazekas de St Groth, B., and Davis, M.M. (1991). Low affinity interaction of peptide-MHC complexes with T cell receptors. *Science 254*, 1788–1791.

McKeithan, T.W. (1995). Kinetic proofreading in T-cell receptor signal transduction. *Proc Natl Acad Sci U S A 92*, 5042–5046.

Medema, J.P., Toes, R.E., Scaffidi, C., Zheng, T.S., Flavell, R.A., Melief, C.J., Peter, M.E., Offringa, R., and Krammer, P.H. (1997). Cleavage of FLICE (caspase-8) by granzyme B during cytotoxic T lymphocyte-induced apoptosis. *Eur J Immunol 27*, 3492–3498.

Mempel, T.R., Henrickson, S.E., and Von Andrian, U.H. (2004). T-cell priming by dendritic cells in lymph nodes occurs in three distinct phases. *Nature 427*, 154–159.

Mestas, J., and Hughes, C.C. (2004). Of mice and not men: Differences between mouse and human immunology. *J Immunol 172*, 2731–2738.

Miller, M.J., Hejazi, A.S., Wei, S.H., Cahalan, M.D., and Parker, I. (2004). T cell repertoire scanning is promoted by dynamic dendritic cell behavior and random T cell motility in the lymph node. *Proc Natl Acad Sci U S A 101*, 998–1003.

Miller, M.J., Wei, S.H., Cahalan, M.D., and Parker, I. (2003). Autonomous T cell trafficking examined in vivo with intravital two-photon microscopy. *Proc Natl Acad Sci U S A 100*, 2604–2609.

Miller, M.J., Wei, S.H., Parker, I., and Cahalan, M.D. (2002). Two-photon imaging of lymphocyte motility and antigen response in intact lymph node. *Science 296*, 1869–1873.

Mombaerts, P., Iacomini, J., Johnson, R.S., Herrup, K., Tonegawa, S., and Papaioannou, V.E. (1992). RAG-1-deficient mice have no mature B and T lymphocytes. *Cell 68*, 869–877.

Monks, C.R., Freiberg, B.A., Kupfer, H., Sciaky, N., and Kupfer, A. (1998). Three-dimensional segregation of supramolecular activation clusters in T cells. *Nature 395*, 82–86.

Moreau, H.D., Lemaitre, F., Garrod, K.R., Garcia, Z., Lennon-Dumenil, A.M., and Bousso, P. (2015). Signal strength regulates antigen-mediated T-cell deceleration by distinct mechanisms to promote local exploration or arrest. *Proc Natl Acad Sci U S A 112*, 12151–12156.

Murphy, K.M., Travers, P., Walport, M. (2012). *Janeway's immunobiology*. London: Garland Science.

Nikolich-Zugich, J., Slifka, M.K., and Messaoudi, I. (2004). The many important facets of T-cell repertoire diversity. *Nat Rev Immunol 4*, 123–132.

Okada, T., and Cyster, J.G. (2007). CC chemokine receptor 7 contributes to Gi-dependent T cell motility in the lymph node. *J Immunol 178*, 2973–2978.

Okada, T., Miller, M.J., Parker, I., Krummel, M.F., Neighbors, M., Hartley, S.B., O'Garra, A., Cahalan, M.D., and Cyster, J.G. (2005). Antigen-engaged B cells undergo chemotaxis toward the T zone and form motile conjugates with helper T cells. *PLoS Biol 3*, e150.

Paul, W.E. (2013). *Fundamental immunology*. Philadelphia : Wolters Kluwer Health/Lippincott Williams & Wilkins.

Perelson, A.S., and Bell, G.I. (1982). Delivery of lethal hits by cytotoxic T lymphocytes in multicellular conjugates occurs sequentially but at random times. *J Immunol 129*, 2796–2801.

Perrigoue, J.G., Saenz, S.A., Siracusa, M.C., Allenspach, E.J., Taylor, B.C., Giacomin, P.R., Nair, M.G., Du, Y., Zaph, C., van Rooijen, N. et al. (2009). MHC class II-dependent basophil-CD4+ T cell interactions promote T(H)2 cytokine-dependent immunity. *Nat Immunol 10*, 697–705.

Pieters, J. (2000). MHC class II-restricted antigen processing and presentation. *Adv Immunol 75*, 159–208.

Poenie, M., Kuhn, J., and Combs, J. (2004). Real-time visualization of the cytoskeleton and effector functions in T cells. *Curr Opin Immunol 16*, 428–438.

Purbhoo, M.A., Irvine, D.J., Huppa, J.B., and Davis, M.M. (2004). T cell killing does not require the formation of a stable mature immunological synapse. *Nat Immunol 5*, 524–530.

Romero, P., Cerottini, J.C., and Speiser, D.E. (2006). The human T cell response to melanoma antigens. *Adv Immunol 92*, 187–224.

Rothstein, T.L., Mage, M., Jones, G., and McHugh, L.L. (1978). Cytotoxic T lymphocyte sequential killing of immobilized allogeneic tumor target cells measured by time-lapse microcinematography. *J Immunol 121*, 1652–1656.

Rouvier, E., Luciani, M.F., and Golstein, P. (1993). Fas involvement in Ca(2+)-independent T cell-mediated cytotoxicity. *J Exp Med 177*, 195–200.

Rudolph, M.G., Stanfield, R.L., and Wilson, I.A. (2006). How TCRs bind MHCs, peptides, and coreceptors. *Annu Rev Immunol 24*, 419–466.

Sant'Angelo, D.B., Waterbury, G., Preston-Hurlburt, P., Yoon, S.T., Medzhitov, R., Hong, S.C., and Janeway, C.A., Jr. (1996). The specificity and orientation of a TCR to its peptide-MHC class II ligands. *Immunity 4*, 367–376.

Schreiber, R.D., Old, L.J., and Smyth, M.J. (2011). Cancer immunoediting: Integrating immunity's roles in cancer suppression and promotion. *Science 331*, 1565–1570.

Schumacher, T.N. (2002). T-cell-receptor gene therapy. Nat Rev Immunol 2, 512–519.

Shinkai, Y., Koyasu, S., Nakayama, K., Murphy, K.M., Loh, D.Y., Reinherz, E.L., and Alt, F.W. (1993). RestoMOM. *Science 259*, 822–825.

Skokos, D., Shakhar, G., Varma, R., Waite, J.C., Cameron, T.O., Lindquist, R.L., Schwickert, T., Nussenzweig, M.C., and Dustin, M.L. (2007). Peptide-MHC potency governs dynamic interactions between T cells and dendritic cells in lymph nodes. *Nat Immunol 8*, 835–844.

Sokol, C.L., Chu, N.Q., Yu, S., Nish, S.A., Laufer, T.M., and Medzhitov, R. (2009). Basophils function as antigen-presenting cells for an allergen-induced T helper type 2 response. *Nat Immunol 10*, 713–720.

Stinchcombe, J.C., Bossi, G., Booth, S., and Griffiths, G.M. (2001). The immunological synapse of CTL contains a secretory domain and membrane bridges. *Immunity 15*, 751–761.

Stoll, S., Delon, J., Brotz, T.M., and Germain, R.N. (2002). Dynamic imaging of T cell-dendritic cell interactions in lymph nodes. *Science 296*, 1873–1876.

Sykulev, Y., Joo, M., Vturina, I., Tsomides, T.J., and Eisen, H.N. (1996). Evidence that a single peptide-MHC complex on a target cell can elicit a cytolytic T cell response. *Immunity 4*, 565–571.

Tadokoro, C.E., Shakhar, G., Shen, S., Ding, Y., Lino, A.C., Maraver, A., Lafaille, J.J., and Dustin, M.L. (2006). Regulatory T cells inhibit stable contacts between CD4+ T cells and dendritic cells in vivo. *J Exp Med 203*, 505–511.

Trautmann, A., and Valitutti, S. (2003). The diversity of immunological synapses. *Curr Opin Immunol 15*, 249–254.

Valitutti, S. (2012). The serial engagement model 17 years after: From TCR triggering to immunotherapy. *Front Immunol 3*, 272.

Valitutti, S., Dessing, M., Aktories, K., Gallati, H., and Lanzavecchia, A. (1995). Sustained signaling leading to T cell activation results from prolonged T cell receptor occupancy. Role of T cell actin cytoskeleton. *J Exp Med 181*, 577–584.

Valitutti, S., Muller, S., Dessing, M., and Lanzavecchia, A. (1996). Different responses are elicited in cytotoxic T lymphocytes by different levels of T cell receptor occupancy. *J Exp Med 183*, 1917–1921.

van der Merwe, P.A., and Dushek, O. (2011). Mechanisms for T cell receptor triggering. *Nat Rev Immunol 11*, 47–55.

Vasconcelos, Z., Muller, S., Guipouy, D., Yu, W., Christophe, C., Gadat, S., Valitutti, S., and Dupre, L. (2015). Individual human cytotoxic T lymphocytes exhibit intraclonal heterogeneity during sustained killing. *Cell Rep 11*, 1474–1485.

Viola, A., and Bronte, V. (2007). Metabolic mechanisms of cancer-induced inhibition of immune responses. *Semin Cancer Biol 17*, 309–316.

von Boehmer, H., Teh, H.S., and Kisielow, P. (1989). The thymus selects the useful, neglects the useless and destroys the harmful. *Immunol Today 10*, 57–61.

Weber, S., Traunecker, A., Oliveri, F., Gerhard, W., and Karjalainen, K. (1992). Specific low-affinity recognition of major histocompatibility complex plus peptide by soluble T-cell receptor. *Nature 356*, 793–796.

Wiedemann, A., Depoil, D., Faroudi, M., and Valitutti, S. (2006). Cytotoxic T lymphocytes kill multiple targets simultaneously via spatiotemporal uncoupling of lytic and stimulatory synapses. *Proc Natl Acad Sci U S A 103*, 10985–10990.

Woolf, E., Grigorova, I., Sagiv, A., Grabovsky, V., Feigelson, S.W., Shulman, Z., Hartmann, T., Sixt, M., Cyster, J.G., and Alon, R. (2007). Lymph node chemokines promote sustained T lymphocyte motility without triggering stable integrin adhesiveness in the absence of shear forces. *Nat Immunol 8*, 1076–1085.

Worbs, T., Mempel, T.R., Bolter, J., von Andrian, U.H., and Forster, R. (2007). CCR7 ligands stimulate the intranodal motility of T lymphocytes in vivo. *J Exp Med 204*, 489–495.

Yates, A., Graw, F., Barber, D.L., Ahmed, R., Regoes, R.R., and Antia, R. (2007). Revisiting estimates of CTL killing rates in vivo. *PLoS One 2*, e1301.

Yoshimoto, T., Yasuda, K., Tanaka, H., Nakahira, M., Imai, Y., Fujimori, Y., and Nakanishi, K. (2009). Basophils contribute to T(H)2-IgE responses in vivo via IL-4 production and presentation of peptide-MHC class II complexes to CD4+ T cells. *Nat Immunol 10*, 706–712.

Zitvogel, L., Tesniere, A., and Kroemer, G. (2006). Cancer despite immunosurveillance: Immunoselection and immunosubversion. *Nat Rev Immunol 6*, 715–727.

Overview of mechanistic modeling
Techniques, approximations, and assumptions

STEVEN M. ABEL

2.1 INTRODUCTION

The immune system consists of many interacting components that collectively identify and respond to a multitude of pathogens. Importantly, a well-functioning immune system eliminates pathogens while avoiding a response against cells and tissues of the host organism. The components that comprise an immune system are numerous, ranging from molecular players such as cytokines and antibodies to cells such as T and B cells of the adaptive immune system. Because the immune system utilizes processes ranging from the molecular to the organismal level, many different time and length scales are relevant. Additionally, immune responses are governed by networks of interactions, including feedback among the various scales.

Due to the complicated, multiscale nature of the immune system, mathematical and computational modeling has emerged as an important tool in understanding immune responses [1–5]. It is often difficult to understand immune responses by intuition alone, and experiments frequently produce confounding results whose mechanistic underpinnings are most readily teased apart by mechanistic modeling. Mechanistic modeling represents underlying biological processes in a mathematical framework. Mathematical and computational analysis can then be used to investigate the behavior of the model. The usefulness of the model is gauged by its consistency with existing experiments and its ability to predict or explain new behavior (for example, behavior under different experimental conditions). This can provide mechanistic insight, and the model can be used to test new hypotheses.

In this chapter, we provide an overview of modeling techniques that are commonly used to study the immune system on a systems level. For a given biological question, one must decide which methods are most appropriate in order to gain mechanistic insight. We also highlight assumptions and approximations that underlie the various modeling approaches, which can help guide decisions about which methods to use. Throughout, we use T cells as an example by which to explore various modeling techniques, relevant scales, and underlying approximations and assumptions.

2.1.1 T CELLS: AN ILLUSTRATIVE EXAMPLE

T cells play a key role in adaptive immunity, coordinating the immune response against pathogens and directly killing infected cells. T cells vividly illustrate the varied scales relevant to an immune response: They translate information about receptor binding into a cellular response that leads to altered gene transcription, cell proliferation, and effector functions such as the secretion of cytokines that influence the behavior of other cells. Thus, understanding T cell immunology requires understanding processes ranging from individual protein-protein interactions to cell proliferation and ultimately host-pathogen dynamics (including pathogen evolution). We present here a short description of relevant T cell biology to provide context for the remainder of the chapter. Many excellent reviews can be found on T cell signaling and the role of T cells in immune response [6–10].

T cells physically interact with other cells, which they monitor for molecular signatures of pathogens. They do this using the T cell receptor (TCR) complex, which binds to major histocompatibility complex proteins (MHCs) on other cells that present short peptide fragments derived from either self or non-self proteins. Each T cell expresses many copies of a distinct TCR and functions as a specific and sensitive detector of antigenic peptides. Different T cells have different specificity.

How T cells reliably translate information about TCR binding into a functional response remains an important open question in immunology. Most of the key proteins involved in transducing the signal are likely known. These range from transmembrane coreceptors and phosphatases to proteins involved in the intracellular signaling cascade. The earliest events in T cell activation involve TCR binding, which occurs on the time scale of seconds. T cell activation is strongly correlated with the average binding time of a TCR to a particular peptide-MHC (pMHC) [11,12]. Early intracellular signatures of T cell activation (such as calcium flux) can be seen on a time scale of ~15 s [13]; over minutes to hours, proteins at the cell-cell junction reorganize to form a micron-scale immunological synapse [9]. Upon activation, T cells proliferate, differentiating into both short-lived effector T cells and long-lived memory T cells (these quickly expand in number upon re-exposure to the stimulating antigen). The effector T cell populations contribute to the immune response by influencing the behavior of other immune cells or by killing infected cells directly. Multiple antigenic peptide fragments may be present during an infection, leading to the expansion of multiple T cell lines with different specificity. Once the infection is cleared, the immune system must return to a quiescent state, so as to avoid long-term damage brought about by persistent immune activity.

2.2 TECHNIQUES

The goal of computational modeling in systems immunology is to provide mechanistic insight into biological processes underlying immune responses. In this section, we provide an overview of the most common modeling techniques used. The overview of techniques here is not exhaustive, and variants of the methods, various combinations of the methods, and other modeling frameworks can be found in the literature. For each modeling technique, we provide illustrative examples in which the formalism was applied to aspects of T cell biology.

The starting point for modeling is typically an experimentally motivated network of interactions. For example, for signal transduction, one would start with the relevant proteins and their fundamental interactions such as binding, unbinding, and enzymatic activity leading to post-translational modification (e.g., protein phosphorylation). Experiments ideally help to parameterize the various kinetic rates associated with the relevant processes such as protein-protein binding. The methods below focus on the systems level, with details relevant at finer scales (such as molecular details of proteins) reflected in the kinetic parameters.

2.2.1 ORDINARY DIFFERENTIAL EQUATION (ODE) MODELS

One of the most common modeling approaches in systems immunology uses ordinary differential equations (ODEs) to describe the dynamics of specific components that interact through a network of well-defined interactions. The dynamical variables are continuous and typically represent quantities like the concentration of a protein in a cell or the concentration (or number) of a cell type in blood. The differential equations describe the time evolution of the dynamical variables and are parameterized by kinetic rates such as the binding and dissociation rates of two proteins that physically interact.

ODE models provide a deterministic description of the dynamics without consideration of spatial variation. They describe the dynamics of average concentrations and are often referred to as well-mixed. Although molecules and cells are discrete entities, when the total number of each species is large, it is often a reasonable approximation to assume that they vary continuously. Having on order of hundreds of proteins, for example, is often enough to justify this approximation, although details of the specific system matter in assessing whether this is the case.

The use of ODE models relies on the assumption that fluctuations and spatial heterogeneity are not important features of the dynamics being studied. These types of models have been used widely to study signal transduction networks, gene regulatory networks, and cell populations. Models of the TCR signaling network have ranged from variations of the kinetic proofreading model to detailed models involving hundreds of biochemical components [13,14]. Below, we provide an example of a relatively simple model that produces a sharp response threshold as a function of the TCR-pMHC dissociation rate. Models of gene regulatory networks have included work investigating effective network topologies underlying lineage commitment as T cells differentiate from a naïve state to an effector state [15]. ODE models have also been used to understand T cell population dynamics, including the division, differentiation, and maturation of immature T cells in the thymus and the response of T cell populations to HIV infection [16,17].

2.2.1.1 EXAMPLE: EARLY TCR SIGNALING NETWORK

To illustrate the use of ODE-based modeling, we consider the phosphorylation of residues within immunoreceptor tyrosine-based activation motifs (ITAMs) on the intracellular portion of the TCR complex. Phosphorylation of these residues is a key initial step in T cell signaling and activation. This example involves TCRs, pMHCs, and coreceptors, which are the individual components depicted in Figure 2.1(a).

Coreceptors are transmembrane proteins at the T cell surface that can bind to a conserved region on the extracellular part of MHC proteins. The intracellular portion of coreceptors can also bind to the tyrosine kinase Lck, which is responsible for phosphorylating residues within ITAMs on the TCR complex. Because it interacts with both the TCR complex and coreceptors, Lck indirectly couples the TCR and coreceptor. The model we consider here is restricted to two phosphorylation sites on the TCR complex (corresponding to a single ITAM region). Each of the three individual components depicted in Figure 2.1(a) can bind with the other two, leading to binary and ternary complexes. With the three different phosphorylation states of the TCR, there are a total of 24 distinct species to track over time. The time dependence of each species is described by mass-action kinetics, resulting in a system of 24 coupled ODEs governed by eight kinetic rates. The ODE describing the concentration of unbound, unphosphorylated TCRs is given in Figure 2.1(b). The full set of ODEs is described in detail in reference [18].

This network has been studied using ODE models [18] as well as stochastic, particle-based simulations (see below for a discussion of these methods) [19,20]. As mentioned above, the TCR-pMHC dissociation rate

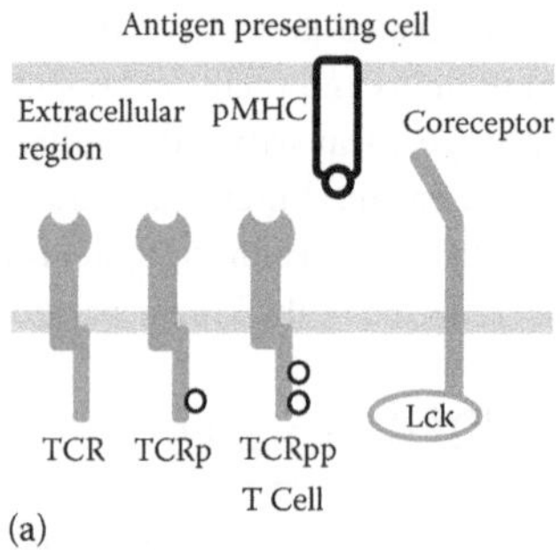

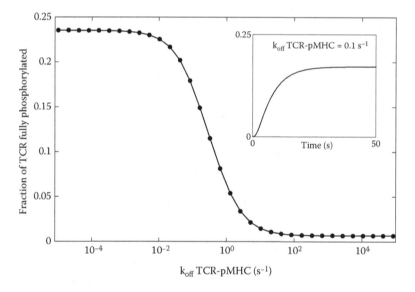

Figure 2.1 (a) Schematic view of the individual components of the model. Each component (TCR, pMHC, and coreceptor) can bind to each of the other two. Ignoring the phosphorylation state of the TCR, there are three distinct binary complexes and four distinct ternary complexes that can form. **(b)** Representative ODE describing the concentration of unbound, unphosphorylated TCRs. The concentrations of other species are described by analogous ODEs, leading to a set of 24 coupled, nonlinear ODEs. Square brackets denote concentrations, which are time dependent. Coreceptors are denoted by CD in the equation.

Figure 2.2 The fraction of TCRs that are fully phosphorylated at steady state as a function of the TCR-pMHC dissociation rate. As the binding time increases (decreasing dissociation rate), there is an increase from low to high levels of fully phosphorylated TCRs. This represents a transition from an inactive to an active signaling state. Inset: Time-dependent response of the fraction of TCRs that are fully phosphorylated for a specific value of the TCR-pMHC dissociation rate.

is strongly correlated with T cell activation. In Figure 2.2, we see that this relatively simple network produces results consistent with experimental trends: There is a sharp transition from low to high TCR phosphorylation levels around a threshold value of the dissociation rate. The system of ODEs was solved using the numerical solver ode23s in MATLAB (all files are available upon request).

2.2.2 Partial Differential Equation (PDE) Models

Partial differential equation (PDE) models are typically used as an extension of ODE models when spatial degrees of freedom are important. For example, they may describe both reactions and the diffusion of proteins in a signal transduction network. As in ODE models, dynamical variables are continuous and the time evolution is deterministic. The PDEs describe the time evolution of each dynamical variable in both time and space. PDE models also ignore fluctuations and are useful when the number of each component is large.

PDE models are computationally more expensive than corresponding ODE models, but spatial details are important in some cases. For example, upon stimulation, T cells eventually form an immunological synapse in which surface proteins are segregated into distinct spatial regions [9]. The size of the immunological synapse is several microns in diameter and proteins are present in large numbers, making the synapse a candidate for PDE models that describe the motion and reactions of proteins. In a study using both experiments and computation, Cemerski *et al.* observed that a weak agonist peptide could stimulate greater T cell proliferation than a strong agonist [21]. Using drift-diffusion PDEs that incorporated relevant signaling reactions, the authors showed that an inability to form part of the immunological synapse could promote the ability of the weak agonist to stimulate proliferation. This highlighted that nontrivial spatial effects could impact the efficacy of agonist peptides in stimulating T cells to proliferate.

2.2.3 Particle-based Stochastic Models

Many processes associated with an immune response are inherently stochastic. For example, T cell activation can be initiated by even a single antigenic pMHC on the surface of another cell [22–24]. When such small numbers of molecules play an important role, fluctuations can have significant effects.

Particle-based stochastic models treat the components of the model as discrete objects (often referred to as particles or individuals) rather than as continuous variables. For example, the abundance of a particular protein is measured by the integer number of that type of protein. The dynamics of the system are governed by a Markov process that is formally described by the chemical master equation. The master equation expresses the time dependence of the probability of each possible state of the system in terms of a differential equation. Such systems of equations are usually difficult or impossible to solve analytically. However, computer simulations can be used to generate stochastic trajectories consistent with the underlying probability distribution. These methods are known as kinetic Monte Carlo simulations and are commonly carried out using the well-known Gillespie algorithm [25,26]. Stochastic simulations are computationally more demanding than the ODE and PDE models described above, and hence can limit the size and scope of the networks considered.

Particle-based stochastic simulations can be well-mixed or spatially resolved. Spatially resolved simulations often discretize space into a lattice, with particles that can transition from one lattice site to another (typically a neighboring site). Since one must keep track of the number of each type of particle, as well as where each particle is in space, this leads to a much larger state space. Additionally, the spatial motion of the particles leads to much larger computational costs. Stochastic effects can be incorporated into other modeling formalisms as well. One approach is to use stochastic differential equations (SDEs) to describe the stochastic evolution of chemical concentrations. Under certain conditions, one can derive SDEs (Langevin equations) starting from the particle-based chemical master equation [27].

TCR signaling is initiated by potentially small numbers of molecules in a noisy environment. It remains unclear how T cells make fast and reliable decisions in the presence of fluctuations. Many cells, including T cells, utilize networks that give rise to bistability—the ability of the network to stably reside in one of two steady states. Bistable networks can be used by cells to make binary (on or off) decisions in response to a graded stimulus. Das *et al.* used well-mixed stochastic simulations in an extensive study showing that the protein Ras can be activated in a bistable manner [28]. Ras, a small GTPase, can exist in an inactive or active form. It is a key signaling protein in T cells and many other cell types. The authors showed that the bistability arose due to positive feedback through SOS, a guanine nucleotide exchange factor that activates Ras and is allosterically controlled by binding to Ras. The stochastic simulations provided insight into populations of lymphocytes that, in response to a given stimulus, had both active and inactive subpopulations.

Spatially resolved stochastic simulations, while computationally more expensive, can give insight when spatiotemporal correlations are important. For example, they helped to elucidate the role of coreceptors in the earliest stages of T cell activation [19,20], and they have been used to model populations of migrating cells in the lymph node [29].

2.2.4 LOGIC MODELS

For many problems of interest, there is a paucity of experimental results by which to parameterize the rates of a kinetic model like the ODE, PDE, and stochastic models described above. Systematically characterizing the behavior of the kinetic model and conducting parameter sensitivity analysis can be prohibitively time consuming and may not lead to mechanistic insight. A class of models known as logic models can be useful in such situations. While they lack detail about kinetics of interactions and absolute concentrations of species, they capture significant relationships between components and are relatively efficient to simulate. The basic idea is that variables are restricted to a small number of possible values (e.g., on or off) and the network of interactions is translated into update rules based on logical rules. As the system evolves in time, given the current state of the system, the next state is determined by evaluating the logical rules (e.g., if proteins A and B are active ("on"), then C is "on" after the update occurs).

A logic model incorporating many components of the TCR signaling network was used recently to investigate fate determination in naïve T cells [30]. The model, constructed by systematic comparison with experiments, was used to identify key proteins in the signaling network and to make experimentally confirmed predictions about the effects of transient TCR stimulation and altered cytokine milieu. The computationally efficient nature of such models allows rapid feedback between changing the model and comparison with experimental results. This can provide important mechanistic insight even though the underlying kinetic parameters are largely ignored.

2.3 ASSUMPTIONS AND APPROXIMATIONS

In this section, we provide an overview of some of the common assumptions and approximations made when developing mechanistic models. To set the stage, we start with an aphorism attributed to the statistician George Box [31]: "All models are wrong but some are useful." The immune system operates over multiple scales with nontrivial networks of interactions that control immune responses. As such, mathematical modeling is essential for understanding and predicting its behavior, but the complex nature of the immune system also means that approximations and assumptions must be made. A primary challenge of modeling is constructing models that are both tractable and useful, meaning that they provide biological insight. Each subsection below describes an assumption that is commonly used when developing models. We illustrate cases in which the assumption is inadequate or an altered or more nuanced model is required.

2.3.1 ASSUMPTION 1: RELEVANT COMPONENTS AND INTERACTIONS ARE KNOWN (OR HYPOTHESIZED)

The starting point for any model is a list of components relevant to the biological process of interest. Depending on what is known experimentally and what level of detail is desired in the model, this may involve few to many components. Once the components are enumerated, the interactions between them must be identified to define a network. The most important step in developing a model is defining the network topology, as all subsequent results depend on the interactions defined. Missing components, interactions, or even entire pathways may lead to results that are inconsistent with experiments. While this may seem disheartening, it can lead to insight, as failed models often suggest places to look for missing components and interactions [32].

2.3.2 ASSUMPTION 2: KINETICS ARE WELL DEFINED

It is often difficult to construct computational models because the individual kinetic parameters governing the dynamics are largely unknown. In some cases, the rates may be measured explicitly or have some constraints placed on their value. However, as we discuss here, even "known" quantities may depend strongly on the method used to measure them.

Binding kinetics *in situ*. The kinetics of TCR-pMHC binding are often measured using surface plasmon resonance techniques in which soluble TCRs in solution bind with pMHCs immobilized on a surface [33]. However, this is a much different situation than the one encountered *in situ*, in which both TCRs and pMHCs are associated with flexible membranes that contain many proteins and are coupled to the cytoskeleton and cytoplasmic processes.

Measuring and understanding TCR binding kinetics *in situ* is an exciting and challenging area from both experimental and computational perspectives. Two pioneering works first demonstrated that the binding kinetics *in situ* vary significantly compared with traditionally measured values [34,35]. Huppa *et al.* used FRET (fluorescence resonance energy transfer) between TCRs and pMHCs to show that the unbinding rate and the binding rate both increased significantly *in situ* [35]. The effect was shown to depend on the actin cytoskeleton. Huang *et al.* used mechanical assays to probe TCR-pMHC binding kinetics when both were in a membrane environment [34]. They also discovered strongly altered binding kinetics when compared with solution measurements, with a broader range of affinities measured *in situ* for a panel of different pMHCs.

Force-dependent binding kinetics. A recent study by Liu *et al.* utilized a biomembrane force probe to analyze the kinetics of TCR-pMHC interactions *in situ* with various forces applied to the TCR-pMHC bond [36]. Their measurements produced a counterintuitive result: At zero applied force, stimulatory pMHCs had shorter lifetimes than non-stimulatory pMHCs when bound to TCRs. However, the trend was reversed when TCR-pMHC lifetimes were characterized with 10 pN of applied tensile force. Hence, T cell receptors exhibit nontrivial binding kinetics under the application of force and, upon encountering stimulatory ligands, exhibit the characteristics of what are commonly called catch bonds [36–38]. This is an important observation, since TCRs likely experience a variety of forces at cell-cell interfaces. Understanding the force-dependence of binding kinetics is likely to influence our understanding of the mechanisms of T cell activation and will likely influence systems approaches to modeling T cell signal transduction [39,40].

Allosteric control of catalytic fluctuations. We previously described positive feedback in the activation of the small GTPase Ras by SOS [28]. A recent study provided additional insight by quantifying the rate of Ras activation by single SOS molecules [41]. Surprisingly, it was observed that individual SOS molecules sample a broad range of Ras activation rates and that the SOS molecules stochastically transitioned between long-lived catalytic states. The average lifetime of a state was on the order of 100 s. It was further observed that transitions between catalytic states were subject to allosteric regulation: Longer-lived, highly active states of SOS were promoted when active Ras was bound allosterically. This suggests a potential regulatory mechanism in which allosteric control of rare high-activity states controls the activation of Ras. Stochastic computational models incorporating these effects demonstrated the possibility of catalytic fluctuations serving as a regulatory mechanism. It remains to develop a better understanding of the functional role of fluctuations between different states in individual molecules.

2.3.3 ASSUMPTION 3: THE IMPORTANCE OF FLUCTUATIONS IS KNOWN

As discussed previously, different modeling frameworks make different assumptions about stochasticity. For example, ODE and PDE models do not account for fluctuations. Given a set of initial conditions, the models evolve in time deterministically. Particle-based models, in contrast, incorporate the effects of fluctuations but are computationally more expensive. It can be difficult to know *a priori* which type of modeling framework to use. In some cases, certain components (key protein or cellular players, for example) are present in small numbers. This often indicates that stochastic effects may be important, and hence a particle-based method is most appropriate.

At other times, it is less clear whether stochastic fluctuations may play an important role. For example, the presence of positive feedback can lead to bistability, as was seen in the Ras activation network [28]. Due to spontaneous fluctuations, it is possible to stochastically switch from one state to another, although the chance of switching becomes vanishingly small as the system size increases in the well-mixed limit. In this regime, an ODE model may seemingly provide an adequate description. However, when space is considered, localized fluctuations involving much smaller numbers of particles—even in an initially homogeneous system—can lead to stochastic switching that would be highly unlikely in the well-mixed limit [42]. The switching occurs by a nucleation and growth mechanism, in which an active domain forms in a localized region and then grows by positive-feedback induced spreading [43]. This mechanism is influenced by the mobility of particles and the geometry of the system (e.g., membrane versus cytoplasm). This highlights a case in which a potentially unknown and nonobvious mechanism like the localized fluctuation-induced nucleation of an active domain can dramatically influence the emergent behavior of a network. Simple models that capture key biological features can provide insight into unexpected fluctuation-dependent phenomena.

2.3.4 ASSUMPTION 4: SPATIALLY HOMOGENEOUS SYSTEMS CAN BE TREATED AS WELL-MIXED

In the previous assumption, we highlighted a mechanism by which an initially homogeneous system can spontaneously form localized domains. This suggests that spatial degrees of freedom can influence the dynamics of initially homogeneous systems in a manner that cannot be captured in well-mixed simulations. Most proteins in the cytoplasm or at the plasma membrane are mobile, with diffusion coefficients that depend on the local environment [44]. It is often assumed that a spatially homogeneous system can be regarded as well-mixed (either ODE or stochastic), with effects of diffusion incorporated into effective, diffusion-influenced kinetic parameters. There are cases in which this assumption works well. For example, Dushek *et al.* studied rebinding of kinases to the TCR and explicitly checked that an ODE model using diffusion-influenced parameters was consistent with a stochastic, spatially resolved simulation [14]. However, it is often difficult to capture the effects of space and diffusion in effective well-mixed models [45]. Calculating diffusion-influenced parameters is a difficult theoretical task, and it has been done only for simple reaction schemes in infinite domains. Application to finite systems with arbitrary geometries and network structures remains an open problem.

In addition to theoretical challenges in calculating effective rate parameters, spatiotemporal correlations between particles can influence network behavior in nontrivial ways. A striking example is seen in a kinase-phosphatase reaction network in which a substrate protein can be phosphorylated at two sites. This network is a caricature of early TCR signaling, in which the cytoplasmic tail of the TCR is phosphorylated by the kinase Lck. The toy network can exhibit bistability in some parameter regimes. Takahashi *et al.* showed that spatiotemporal correlations between substrate molecules and the modifying enzymes could suppress bistability in a way that was not captured by well-mixed models with modified rates [46]. The reason was that after dissociation, rebinding between the two molecules could occur much faster than in a well-mixed system. Other studies further investigated the role of crowding and dimensionality on rebinding, showing that the effects of rebinding were enhanced in crowded environments and at the membrane [45,47].

2.3.5 ASSUMPTION 5: THE CELL HAS A SIMPLE SHAPE AND ORGANIZATION

The cell environment is complex, and most modeling approaches make significant approximations when treating spatial aspects of biological processes. For example, the membrane and cytoplasm are spatially heterogeneous, crowded, and dynamic [44]. The cytoskeleton influences membrane shape, contributes to non-diffusive transport through the cell, and can locally trap molecules in "corrals" at the plasma membrane. Additionally, the cortical actin cytoskeleton modulates TCR binding kinetics and contributes to synapse formation [48,49]. Most models are formulated with simple geometries that lack many of the structural features (organelles, crowding molecules, etc.) of real systems.

In many cases, it is likely a good approximation to assume the complicating features of cell geometry and organization are captured by effective diffusion coefficients and kinetic parameters [44]. However, as experimental techniques allow finer-resolution imaging of cells, spatial heterogeneity is emerging as a potentially important regulatory mechanism [50,51]. For example, Lillemeier *et al.* studied the spatial distribution of TCRs and a membrane-associated scaffold protein, Linker for Activation of T cells (LAT). LAT recruits a number of key signaling proteins upon its phosphorylation. Before T cell stimulation, TCR and LAT appear to reside in separate clusters that then come together after stimulation [52]. Interestingly, subsequent studies identified a separate pool of LAT that resides on vesicles near the membrane [53,54]. These studies indicate that surface-bound LAT plays a minor role in T cell signaling compared with the intracellular pool. This highlights an example in which initial assumptions about spatial organization are influenced by higher-resolution experiments. Formulating models that account for spatially heterogeneous distributions of molecules may provide more insight into mechanisms associated with the spatial organization.

Additional features that are emerging as regulators of cell responses include compartmentalization of network components, spatial confinement within regions of the cell, and membrane curvature. Compartmentalization within a cell can lead to separate populations of proteins that interact only when they are exchanged through boundaries between the compartments. For example, the cytosol and nucleus can have different populations of proteins that are exchanged by an active transport process across the nuclear membrane. In such a case, each compartment might be regarded as well-mixed, but coupling between the compartments would occur through boundary conditions. Theoretical work has shown that when compartmentalized, protein populations can transmit larger amounts of information to the nucleus [55]. Physical confinement of networks can also influence responses. For example, in a computational study of B cell activation, displacing the nucleus so that is was close to the plasma membrane on one side of the cell was sufficient to initiate B cell activation [56]. The confined region promoted the nucleation of an active domain that spread throughout the cell.

Biophysical features of membranes are emerging as important regulators of T cell activation [57]. Membrane curvature can affect the organization of proteins and lipids, and hence cellular responses [58–60]. Additionally, forces generated by the membrane and cytoskeleton may play important roles in antigen discrimination [39,61,62] and can potentiate killing of other cells by cytotoxic T cells [63]. Such problems highlight interesting areas for hybrid computational models that account for both physical features of the cellular environment and the signaling networks they influence.

2.3.6 Assumption 6: Many (most) kinetic parameters are "sloppy"

We conclude this section on a positive note. While some modeling approaches (like logic models) allow one to avoid choosing detailed kinetic parameters, other modeling approaches require parameters to be defined. These parameters can be experimentally measured, estimated based on other rates, trained on experimental data sets, or, as often is the case, chosen (somewhat) arbitrarily [64]. It appears that a commonly valid assumption is that the specific value of many kinetic parameters is not important for understanding overall network behavior [32]. Such parameters have been termed "sloppy" in the literature [65,66]. In some cases, parameters can be changed by orders of magnitude without significantly affecting the system behavior. This flexibility in parameter values often allows mechanistic models to provide insight even when some parameter values are not known explicitly. On a cautionary note, it is desirable to show that results obtained with a certain set of parameters are robust to changes in the parameters, as this strengthens claims made based on the model.

2.4 FUTURE DIRECTIONS

The main challenge of systems immunology is to develop multiscale understanding of immunological responses. This requires approaches that span scales and methodologies. For example, in this chapter, we outlined methods to analyze networks of interacting components. Most modeling studies focus on a particular level of modeling, such as a signal transduction network, a gene regulatory network, etc. Coupling models of cell regulatory networks with population models will be an interesting future direction that will capture potentially important interplay between cellular decisions and the population responses that they influence. It will also be useful to incorporate additional molecular-level information, for example, from experiments or molecular dynamics simulations, into network-level models. For example, one could ask how immune responses are influenced by a mutation in a protein or by a drug-protein interaction.

Another important direction for systems immunology is to couple high-throughput and information-rich experimental data sets with molecular modeling. The data sets can be used to generate and parameterize networks, suggest biological mechanisms, etc. Data mining and experimentally-motivated model construction are likely to provide a productive avenue that can be coupled with model analysis to gain additional mechanistic insight into the biological processes underlying immune responses.

REFERENCES

1. Chakraborty, A.K., and Das, J. (2010). Pairing computation with experimentation: A powerful coupling for understanding T cell signalling. *Nat Rev Immunol 10*, 59–71.
2. Germain, R.N., Meier-Schellersheim, M., Nita-Lazar, A., and Fraser, I.D.C. (2011). Systems biology in immunology: A computational modeling perspective. *Annu Rev Immunol 29*, 527–585.
3. Goldstein, B., Faeder, J.R., and Hlavacek, W.S. (2004). Mathematical and computational models of immune-receptor signalling. *Nat Rev Immunol 4*, 445–456.
4. Morel, P.A., Faeder, J.R., Hawse, W.F., and Miskov-Zivanov, N. (2014). Modeling the T cell immune response: A fascinating challenge. *J Pharmacokinet Phar 41*, 401–413.
5. Narang, V. *et al.* (2012). Systems immunology: A survey of modeling formalisms, applications and simulation tools. *Immunol Res 53*, 251–265.
6. Brownlie, R.J., and Zamoyska, R. (2013). T cell receptor signalling networks: Branched, diversified and bounded. *Nat Rev Immunol 13*, 257–269.
7. van der Merwe, P.A., and Dushek, O. (2011). Mechanisms for T cell receptor triggering. *Nat Rev Immunol 11*, 47–55.
8. Chakraborty, A.K., and Weiss, A. (2014). Insights into the initiation of TCR signaling. *Nat Immunol 15*, 798–807.
9. Fooksman, D.R. *et al.* (2010). Functional anatomy of T cell activation and synapse formation. *Annu Rev Immunol 28*, 79–105.
10. Masopust, D., and Schenkel, J.M. (2013). The integration of T cell migration, differentiation and function. *Nat Rev Immunol 13*, 309–320.
11. Lever, M., Maini, P.K., van der Merwe, P.A., and Dushek, O. (2014). Phenotypic models of T cell activation. *Nat Rev Immunol 14*, 619–629.
12. Zhu, C., Jiang, N., Huang, J., Zarnitsyna, V.I., and Evavold, B.D. (2013). Insights from *in situ* analysis of TCR-pMHC recognition: Response of an interaction network. *Immunol Rev 251*, 49–64.
13. Altan-Bonnet, G., and Germain, R.N. (2005). Modeling T cell antigen discrimination based on feedback control of digital ERK responses. *PLoS Biol 3*, 1925–1938.
14. Dushek, O., Das, R., and Coombs, D. (2009). A role for rebinding in rapid and reliable T cell responses to antigen. *PLoS Comput Biol 5*, e1000578.
15. Hong, T., Xing, J.H., Li, L.W., and Tyson, J.J. (2011). A mathematical model for the reciprocal differentiation of T helper 17 cells and induced regulatory T cells. *PLoS Comput Biol 7*, e1002122.
16. Mehr, R., Globerson, A., and Perelson, A.S. (1995). Modeling positive and negative selection and differentiation processes in the thymus. *J Theor Biol 175*, 103–126.
17. Perelson, A.S., Kirschner, D.E., and de Boer, R. (1993). Dynamics of HIV-infection of CD4+ T-cells. *Math Biosci 114*, 81–125.
18. Prescott, A.M., and Abel, S.M. (2016). Combining in silico evolution and nonlinear dimensionality reduction to redesign responses of signaling networks. *Phys Biol 13*, 066015.
19. Artyomov, M.N., Lis, M., Devadas, S., Davis, M.M., and Chakraborty, A.K. (2010). CD4 and CD8 binding to MHC molecules primarily acts to enhance Lck delivery. *Proc Natl Acad Sci USA 107*, 16916–16921.
20. Hoerter, J.A.H. *et al.* (2013). Coreceptor affinity for MHC defines peptide specificity requirements for TCR interaction with coagonist peptide-MHC. *J Exp Med 210*, 1807–1821.
21. Cemerski, S. *et al.* (2007). The stimulatory potency of T cell antigens is influenced by the formation of the immunological synapse. *Immunity 26*, 345–355.

22. Irvine, D.J., Purbhoo, M.A., Krogsgaard, M., and Davis, M.M. (2002). Direct observation of ligand recognition by T cells. *Nature 419*, 845–849.

23. Huang, J. *et al.* (2013). A single peptide-Major Histocompatibility Complex ligand triggers digital cytokine secretion in CD4+ T cells. *Immunity 39*, 846–857.

24. Sykulev, Y., Joo, M., Vturina, I., Tsomides, T.J., and Eisen, H.N. (1996). Evidence that a single peptide-MHC complex on a target cell can elicit a cytolytic T cell response. *Immunity 4*, 565–571.

25. Gillespie, D.T. (1977). Exact stochastic simulation of coupled chemical reactions. *J Phys Chem 81*, 2340–2361.

26. Gillespie, D.T. (2007). Stochastic simulation of chemical kinetics. *Annu Rev Phys Chem 58*, 35–55.

27. Gillespie, D.T. (2000). The chemical Langevin equation. *J Chem Phys 113*, 297–306.

28. Das, J. *et al.* (2009). Digital signaling and hysteresis characterize Ras activation in lymphoid cells. *Cell 136*, 337–351.

29. Gong, C. *et al.* (2013). Predicting lymph node output efficiency using systems biology. *J Theor Biol 335*, 169–184.

30. Miskov-Zivanov, N., Turner, M.S., Kane, L.P., Morel, P.A., and Faeder, J.R. (2013). The duration of T cell stimulation is a critical determinant of cell fate and plasticity. *Sci Signal 6*, ra97.

31. Box, G.E.P. (1976). Science and Statistics. *J Am Stat Assoc 71*, 791–799.

32. Janes, K.A., and Lauffenburger, D.A. (2013). Models of signalling networks - what cell biologists can gain from them and give to them. *J Cell Sci 126*, 1913–1921.

33. Wu, L.C., Tuot, D.S., Lyons, D.S., Garcia, K.C., and Davis, M.M. (2002). Two-step binding mechanism for T-cell receptor recognition of peptide-MHC. *Nature 418*, 552–556.

34. Huang, J. *et al.* (2010). The kinetics of two-dimensional TCR and pMHC interactions determine T-cell responsiveness. *Nature 464*, 932–936.

35. Huppa, J.B. *et al.* (2010). TCR-peptide-MHC interactions *in situ* show accelerated kinetics and increased affinity. *Nature 463*, 963–967.

36. Liu, B.Y., Chen, W., Evavold, B.D., and Zhu, C. (2014). Accumulation of dynamic catch bonds between TCR and agonist peptide-MHC triggers T cell signaling. *Cell 157*, 357–368.

37. Das, D.K. *et al.* (2015). Force-dependent transition in the T-cell receptor beta-subunit allosterically regulates peptide discrimination and pMHC bond lifetime. *Proc Natl Acad Sci USA 112*, 1517–1522.

38. Hong, J. *et al.* (2015). Force-regulated *in situ* TCR-peptide-bound MHC class II kinetics determine functions of CD4+ T cells. *J Immunol 195*, 3557–3564.

39. Depoil, D., and Dustin, M.L. (2014). Force and affinity in ligand discrimintion by the TCR. *Trends Immunol 35*, 597–603.

40. Pullen, R.H., III and Abel, S.M. (2017). Catch bonds at T cell interfaces: Impact of surface reorganization and membrane fluctuations. *Biophys J 113*, 120–131.

41. Iversen, L. *et al.* (2014). Ras activation by SOS: Allosteric regulation by altered fluctuation dynamics. *Science 345*, 50–54.

42. Mlynarczyk, P.J., Pullen, R.H., and Abel, S.M. (2016). Confinement and diffusion modulate bistability and stochastic switching in a reaction network with positive feedback. *J Chem Phys 144*, 015102.

43. Das, J., Kardar, M., and Chakraborty, A.K. (2009). Positive feedback regulation results in spatial clustering and fast spreading of active signaling molecules on a cell membrane. *J Chem Phys 130*, 245102.

44. Luby-Phelps, K. (2000). Cytoarchitecture and physical properties of cytoplasm: Volume, viscosity, diffusion, intracellular surface area. *Int Rev Cytol 192*, 189–221.

45. Abel, S.M., Roose, J.P., Groves, J.T., Weiss, A., and Chakraborty, A.K. (2012). The membrane environment can promote or suppress bistability in cell signaling networks. *J Phys Chem B 116*, 3630–3640.

46. Takahashi, K., Tanase-Nicola, S., and ten Wolde, P.R. (2010). Spatio-temporal correlations can drastically change the response of a MAPK pathway. *Proc Natl Acad Sci USA 107*, 2473–2478.

47. Aoki, K., Yamada, M., Kunida, K., Yasuda, S., and Matsuda, M. (2011). Processive phosphorylation of ERK MAP kinase in mammalian cells. *Proc Natl Acad Sci USA 108*, 12675–12680.

48. Yu, Y., Smoligovets, A.A., and Groves, J.T. (2013). Modulation of T cell signaling by the actin cytoskeleton. *J Cell Sci 126*, 1049–1058.

49. Billadeau, D.D., Nolz, J.C., and Gomez, T.S. (2007). Regulation of T-cell activation by the cytoskeleton. *Nat Rev Immunol 7*, 131–143.

50. Groves, J.T., and Kuriyan, J. (2010). Molecular mechanisms in signal transduction at the membrane. *Nat Struct Mol Biol 17*, 659–665.

51. Manz, B.N., and Groves, J.T. (2010). Spatial organization and signal transduction at intercellular junctions. *Nat Rev Mol Cell Bio 11*, 342–352.

52. Lillemeier, B.F. *et al.* (2010). TCR and Lat are expressed on separate protein islands on T cell membranes and concatenate during activation. *Nat Immunol 11*, 543–543.

53. Larghi, P. *et al.* (2013). VAMP7 controls T cell activation by regulating the recruitment and phosphorylation of vesicular Lat at TCR-activation sites. *Nat Immunol 14*, 723.

54. Williamson, D.J. *et al.* (2011). Pre-existing clusters of the adaptor Lat do not participate in early T cell signaling events. *Nat Immunol 12*, 655–662.

55. Harrington, H.A., Feliu, E., Wiuf, C., and Stumpf, M.P.H. (2013). Cellular compartments cause multistability and allow cells to process more information. *Biophys J 104*, 1824–1831.

56. Hat, B., Kazmierczak, B., and Lipniacki, T. (2011). B cell activation triggered by the formation of the small receptor cluster: A computational study. *PLoS Comput Biol 7*, e1002197.

57. Hivroz, C., and Saitakis, M. (2016). Biophysical aspects of T lymphocyte activation at the immune synapse. *Front Immunol 7*, 1–12.

58. He, H.T., and Bongrand, P. (2012). Membrane dynamics shape TCR-generated signaling. *Front Immunol 3*, 90.

59. McMahon, H.T., and Gallop, J.L. (2005). Membrane curvature and mechanisms of dynamic cell membrane remodelling. *Nature 438*, 590–596.

60. Vogel, V., and Sheetz, M. (2006). Local force and geometry sensing regulate cell functions. *Nat Rev Mol Cell Bio 7*, 265–275.

61. Upadhyaya, A. (2017). Mechanosensing in the immune response. *Semin Cell Dev Biol 71*, 137–145.

62. Liu, Y. et al. (2016). DNA-based nanoparticle tension sensors reveal that T-cell receptors transmit defined pN forces to their antigens for enhanced fidelity. *Proc Natl Acad Sci USA 113*, 5610–5615.

63. Basu, R. *et al.* (2016). Cytotoxic T cells use mechanical force to potentiate target cell killing. *Cell 165*, 100–110.

64. Sun, J.Y., Garibaldi, J.M., and Hodgman, C. (2012). Parameter estimation using metaheuristics in systems biology: A comprehensive review. *IEEE/ACM Trans Comput Biol Bioinf 9*, 185–202.

65. Gutenkunst, R.N. *et al.* (2007). Universally sloppy parameter sensitivities in systems biology models. *PLoS Comput Biol 3*, 1871–1878.

66. Transtrum, M.K. *et al.* (2015). Perspective: Sloppiness and emergent theories in physics, biology, and beyond. *J Chem Phys 143*, 010901.

The fundamentals of statistical data analysis

WILLIAM C. L. STEWART

3.1 INTRODUCTION

Statistical data analysis is an integral part of scientific research. It provides acceptably *fuzzy* answers to questions that are difficult to answer exactly. For example, "What is the average height of humans?" or "Are men taller on average than women?" Obtaining exact answers to these questions is impractical, as it would require the measurement of every living human being! On the other hand, obtaining acceptably *fuzzy* answers through the statistical analysis of real data, despite its caveats,[1] is fairly routine. For example, the first question is often answered by a parameter estimate and its corresponding confidence interval, while the second typically involves a hypothesis test and a suitable statistic. This chapter explains some of the essential aspects of parameter estimation and hypothesis testing, without abandoning the statistical analysis of data. A brief description of the interplay between estimation and testing, and its corresponding practical implication, are also given. Throughout, I will assume that a well-defined question already exists and that appropriate levels of planning and diligence have been given to the design and execution of each experiment or study. Therefore, the only thing left to discuss is the statistical data analysis itself.

3.2 STATISTICS PRIMER

Before I begin, it is important that a number of elementary terms are well understood. Advanced readers may prefer to skip this section and start immediately with likelihoods—the topic of Section 3.3.

Typically, an algebraic variable (denoted x) is an unknown number, and it is only after solving some equation of interest that we come to know *which* number. For example, the equation $x + 3 = 5$ implies that the variable x is the number 2. By contrast, a random variable is a collection of numbers, and each number in the collection occurs with a certain probability whenever an experiment (or study) is performed. For example, if we define the random variable X to be the integers 1 through 6 with each number having probability 1/6 of being observed, then X corresponds to the roll of a fair (six-sided) die. The probability assigned to each outcome is called the *distribution* of X, and these probabilities can be estimated from a number of rolls. For example, an excellent estimator of p_j—the probability that $X = j$ for each possible outcome $j \in \{1,..., 6\}$ is n_j/N, where n_j is the number of times that j was rolled, and N is the total number of rolls. Note that p_j is more similar to an algebraic variable than is the random variable X; however, in Statistics p_j is typically called a parameter, not a variable.

Now, let's suppose that after 100 rolls, our estimate of the distribution of X is (0.16, 0.13, 0.19, 0.19, 0.18, 0.15). Intuitively, these numbers appear to be *close* to $0.16\overline{6}$, but is the die fair? Answering this seemingly simple question is complicated because two experimenters using the same die will almost certainly arrive at different estimates, and because, irrespective of the number of replicates, the estimate will never be exactly $(0.16\overline{6},...,0.16\overline{6})$. Therefore, we shall decide the fairness of the die on the basis of a test statistic and its p-value. Let's define an intuitively appealing test statistic (denoted T) to be the Euclidean distance between our estimate of the distribution and $(0.16\overline{6},...,0.16\overline{6})$. As such, large values of T suggest that the die is not fair, but "How do we know if T is large?" In Statistics, we agree that T is large when the chance (i.e., the probability) of seeing something *"more extreme"* with a fair die is rare [i.e. less than α, for some $\alpha \in (0,1)$ that the experimenter selects before the die is rolled]. This probability is called the p-value, the number α is the false positive rate (i.e., the chance of falsely concluding that a fair die is unfair), the parameter vector $(0.16\overline{6},...,0.16\overline{6})$ is the quantification of the null hypothesis that the die is fair, and the entire decision-making procedure is an example of a hypothesis test.

It is also useful at this time to review a couple of basic ideas in probability theory. In keeping with our six-sided die example, a useful concept in probability theory is the idea of expectation—that is, "What do we expect to see on average over a large number of independent rolls?" The expectation of the random variable X (denoted $\mathbf{E}X$) is the weighted average of the outcomes of X. The weights depend on the parameters $(p_1,..., p_5)$ through the probability of each outcome. Hence, the expectation of X is defined as $\sum j \cdot Pr(X = j)$, which comes to 3.5 for a fair die. Note that the expected value of X (i.e., the average value across an infinite number of rolls) need not be an observable outcome of X (e.g., $\mathbf{E}X \notin \{1,...,6\}$). Another useful quantity that summarizes the degree to which the distribution of X concentrates around $\mathbf{E}X$ is the variance, defined as $Var(X) \equiv \mathbf{E}(X - \mathbf{E}X)^2$.

3.3 LIKELIHOODS

The likelihood function is the backbone of any statistical data analysis that posits a parametric model for the data. The likelihood function, or "the likelihood" as it is more commonly called was invented by Fisher [1] and is defined as

$$L(\theta, \mathbf{R}) \equiv P_\theta(\mathbf{R}) \tag{3.1}$$

Thus, the likelihood is a real-valued function of a finite-dimensional parameter θ that depends on observed (i.e., real) data $\mathbf{R}$ through $P_\theta(\mathbf{R})$—the probability of the data given the model specified by θ. Many commonly used statistical techniques in data analysis including (but not limited to) linear models, analysis of variance, z-tests, t-tests, and contingency tables, arise quite naturally from likelihood theory [2]. This is also true for several less common statistical techniques including (but not limited to) Markov models, hidden Markov models, autoregressive models, and models for the multilocus inheritance of genetic material across generations [3,4].

For large samples, likelihoods have a host of extremely useful statistical properties, provided that a certain set of mild "regularity conditions" [5] are met. In order to understand these properties, let's define the maximum likelihood estimator (MLE) (denoted $\hat{\theta}$) as the value of θ that maximizes the likelihood in Eq. (3.1).

Note that $\hat{\theta}$ also maximizes any non-negative function that is proportional to $P_\theta(\mathbf{R})$, irrespective of sample size. However, for large samples the following statements are also true:

1. The distribution of $\hat{\theta}$ is approximately normal.
2. $\hat{\theta}$ approaches the true value of θ.
3. The variance of $\hat{\theta}$ can be estimated from the curvature of the log-likelihood, and approaches the Cramér-Rao lower bound [6].
4. MLE's are approximately best unbiased estimators of the true value of θ.
5. Using the method of test inversion [6], certain null hypotheses can be tested (see Section 3.4 for details).

These statistical properties of MLEs are seminal, but they only represent a small fraction of the intellectual treasures that lie deep within the likelihood coffer. Although the following concepts are beyond the scope of this chapter, the highly motivated student may be interested to know that the asymptotic distribution of twice the log-likelihood ratio (described in Section 3.8) is essentially completely characterized under the null hypothesis (and to some extent, under various alternative hypotheses as well) for tests involving composite nulls, nuisance parameters, and null hypotheses on the boundary of the parameter space [7]. Furthermore, because of various maximization algorithms, such as Newton-Raphson [8], expectation-maximization (EM) [9], stochastic approximation [10,11], and simulated annealing [12], efficient parameter estimation is possible in the presence of missing data. In addition, robust parameter estimation in the presence of model misspecification is often achievable through sandwich estimators and influence functions [13,14]. Lastly, many of the aforementioned results continue to hold even when the so-called "regularity conditions" are relaxed. In particular, it is not necessary for all observations to be identically distributed, nor is it necessary for all observations to be independent [15].

To give a numerical example illustrating the importance and generality of likelihoods, consider the following: Suppose we have CD4 T-cell count data (see Table 3.1) on 12 mice at day 30 post influenza infection (Group A) and 10 mice at day 35 (Group B). Further, let's suppose that we are interested in testing the null hypothesis of equal means between the groups, that is $H_0 : \mu_A = \mu_B$. The scatter plot of the data along with the best fit from a simple linear regression (Figure 3.1) shows that the sample mean of Group A (1077.7) is larger than the sample mean of Group B (1070.1). However, because two random continuous outcomes will never be the same, we must ask ourselves, "How likely are we to see a difference this large (or larger) simply by chance?", or put another way, "Would a difference of this magnitude be *rare*, if the null hypothesis were true?" This question is answered by the p-value, and when the p-value is sufficiently small (say $p < 0.05$), we are

Table 3.1 Data pictured in Figure 3.1

Group A	Group B
1092	1074
1088	1062
1080	1059
1067	1067
1072	1078
1093	1070
1078	1082
1066	1065
1075	1063
1084	1081
1074	
1063	

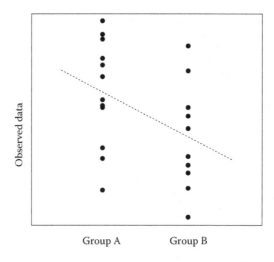

Figure 3.1 Scatter plot of the data in Table 3.1 along with its corresponding regression line.

obliged to reject the null hypothesis in favor of the alternative hypothesis that the group means are different (i.e., $H_I : \mu_A \neq \mu_B$).

The *p-value* from the simple linear regression is 0.07145, so a difference of this magnitude (or larger) occurs by chance about 7% of the time. This result is suggestive but not statistically significant at the 5% level, so we do not have sufficient evidence in these data to reject $H_0 : \mu_A = \mu_B$ (i.e., the null hypothesis that the average count of CD4 T-cells is the same across groups). However, a more interesting point is that the two-sample t-test, which is the scaled difference between group means, yields the same *p-value*: 0.07145 as a simple linear regression. To understand why, let's take a closer look at the two-sample t-test:

$$T \equiv \frac{\overline{G}_a - \overline{G}_b}{S_p\sqrt{1/n + 1/m}}, \tag{3.2}$$

where $n = 12$, $m = 10$, $\overline{G}_a$ is the sample mean of Group A, and $\overline{G}_b$ is the sample mean of Group B. Here,

$$S_p \equiv \sqrt{\frac{(n-1)S_a^2 + (m-1)S_b^2}{n+m-2}}, \tag{3.3}$$

where S_a^2 and S_b^2 are the usual unbiased estimators of variance for groups A and B, respectively. Surprisingly, with a little algebra, one can show that the likelihood ratio test statistic (i.e., twice the log-likelihood ratio) can be rewritten in terms of the expression on the righthand side of Eq. (3.2) [6]. Thus, three seemingly unrelated statistical tests are in fact the same. Moreover, many commonly used tests are either equivalent or closely related to a test within the likelihood umbrella [2].

3.4 PARAMETER ESTIMATION AND HYPOTHESIS TESTING

In the previous section, I tried to convey a basic and rudimentary understanding of the importance and generality of likelihoods, without paying too much attention to Eq. (3.1). Now, I will peel back the thinnest layer of likelihood theory to illustrate its importance and generality in a quantitative sense, using symbolic abstraction, calculus, and set theoretic arguments along the way.

For ease of exposition, let us begin by assuming that the data $\mathbf{R} \equiv \{R_1, R_2, \ldots, R_n\}$ are *iid* (independent and identically distributed) according to $P_\theta(\mathbf{R})$, and that the likelihood in Eq. (3.1) satisfies the aforementioned "regularity conditions." For a concrete example, let's assume that the data $\{R_1, R_2, \ldots, R_n\}$ are the heights of n randomly sampled adult individuals,[2] and let's assume that the data are normally distributed with unknown mean μ and known variance σ^2. For technical reasons that are beyond the scope of this chapter, we equate the likelihood to the probability density function whenever the data are continuous[3] (as opposed to the *actual* probability when the data are discrete). Furthermore, recall that the probability of two independent events in succession is the product of their individual probabilities. Therefore, given the independence across individuals, the likelihood of μ is:

$$L(\mu;\mathbf{R}) \equiv f(r_1;\mu) \times \cdots \times f(r_n;\mu) \tag{3.4}$$

$$= \prod_{i=1}^{n} f(r_i;\mu)$$

$$= \prod_{i=1}^{n} \frac{1}{\sqrt{2\pi}\sigma} e^{-(r_i-\mu)^2/(2\sigma^2)} \tag{3.5}$$

Note that each $f(\cdot)$ in Eq. (3.4) has the same characteristic "bell-shaped" curve centered around μ, and that the likelihood only depends on μ, because σ^2 is assumed to be known.

An excellent estimator of μ is the argument that maximizes Eq. (3.5): this estimator is called the maximum likelihood estimator (MLE) of μ (denoted $\hat{\mu}$). Since $g(t) = \log(t)$ is increasing on $(0,\infty)$, $\log L(\mu;\mathbf{R})$ is maximized at the same location as $L(\mu; \mathbf{R})$. Hence, we can compute $\hat{\mu}$ by taking the first derivative of $\log L(\mu; \mathbf{R})$:

$$\frac{d\log L(\mu;\mathbf{R})}{d\mu} = \frac{d}{d\mu}\left[\frac{n}{2}\log\left(\frac{1}{2\pi\sigma}\right) + \sum_{i=1}^{n}\log e^{-(r_i-\mu)^2/(2\sigma^2)}\right]$$

$$= \frac{-d}{d\mu}\sum_{i=1}^{n}(r_i-\mu)^2/(2\sigma^2)$$

$$= \frac{-1}{2\sigma^2}\sum_{i=1}^{n}\frac{d}{d\mu}(r_i-\mu)^2 \tag{3.6}$$

$$= \frac{1}{\sigma^2}\sum_{i=1}^{n}(r_i-\mu)$$

setting it to zero, and solving for μ:

$$\frac{1}{\sigma^2}\sum_{i=1}^{n}(r_i-\mu) = 0$$

$$\sum_{i=1}^{n} r_i = n\mu \tag{3.7}$$

$$\hat{\mu} \equiv \frac{1}{n}\sum_{i=1}^{n} r_i$$

Thus, in the case of *iid* normal data, the MLE(μ) is the sample mean, and because σ^2 is assumed known, a 95% confidence interval for the unknown μ is: $\left(\hat{\mu} \pm 1.96 \dfrac{\sigma}{\sqrt{n}} \right)$. Moreover, for any parametric probability model satisfying the "regularity conditions," the difference between $Var(\hat{\mu})$ and $-\mathbf{E}\left[\dfrac{d^2 \log L(\mu; \mathbf{R})}{d\mu^2} \right]^{-1}$ goes to zero as the sample size goes to infinity, which means that the latter is an excellent estimator of the former. Here, in the special case of *iid* normal data, $-\mathbf{E}\left[\dfrac{d^2 \log L(\mu; \mathbf{R})}{d\mu^2} \right]^{-1} = \dfrac{\sigma^2}{n}$, which of course is exact. The entire theory of maximum likelihood (ML) estimation extends to higher dimensions, where ordinary derivatives are replaced by partial derivatives, and to more complicated models and data structures, where the equation: $\dfrac{d \log L(\mu; \mathbf{R})}{d\mu} = 0$ may not have a closed form solution.

There is a rather interesting connection between parameter estimation and hypothesis testing when one is interested in testing whether the true (but unknown) value of the parameter is equal to a specific value of interest (e.g., a simple null hypothesis). To see how these two concepts are connected, let's suppose that instead of an estimate of μ, we now want to test $H_0 : \mu = \mu_0$ at a fixed false positive rate of 5%. As in Section (3.2), we could form a test statistic, compute its p-value, and decide to reject (accept) H_0 if the p-value is less than or equal to (greater than) 5%. However, an equivalent procedure called *test inversion* states that we can decide to reject (accept) H_0 if μ_0 falls outside (inside) the 95% confidence interval (CI). Recall that a 95% CI for μ is a random interval that depends on the observed data $\mathbf{r}$ and has probability 95% of covering μ. The test inversion procedure hinges on the following tautology:

$$\mu \in C(\mathbf{r}) \Leftrightarrow \mathbf{r} \in A(\mu),$$

where $C(\mathbf{r})$ is a confidence set containing plausible values of μ, and $A(\mu)$ is a set of outcomes (i.e., hypothetical observations), such that for each outcome in the set, one would *accept* H_0 if the hypothesized value were μ and the false positive rate were α. With this tautology, one can show that $C(\mathbf{r})$ is a (1-α) CI for μ, and that for any point μ^* outside of $C(\mathbf{r})$, the observed data $\mathbf{r}$ is sufficient evidence to reject the simple null hypothesis that μ equals μ^* [6]. In practice, testing a simple null hypothesis indirectly through ML estimation and test inversion is sometimes preferable to the direct approach outlined in Section (3.2).

Nevertheless, despite this fairly amazing relationship between estimation and testing, the test inversion method of Section (3.2) can be quite cumbersome when testing more complicated hypotheses, such as composite null hypotheses (e.g., $H_0 : \mu_A - \mu_B = 0$) or simple null hypotheses in the presence of nuisance parameters (e.g., $H_0 : \mu = \mu_0$ with σ^2 unknown), or null hypotheses with vector valued parameters (e.g., $H_0 : \mu = \mu_0, \sigma^2 = \sigma_0^2$). A more elegant and general approach that can handle all of these cases (and many more) is the method of likelihood ratio tests (LRTs).

The theory behind LRTs is extensive, and much of it is too advanced to discuss in this introductory chapter. However, one result is so important and fundamental to hypothesis testing and data analysis that I will state it here, and in defense of the underlying rationale, I will give a simple heuristic argument that might appeal to the reader's intuition.

Recall that the MLE is the value of the parameter that makes the observed data most probable. Thus, the likelihood is greater at the $\text{MLE} \equiv \hat{\theta}$ than it is at any other possible value of θ. Let's suppose that we are interested in testing some other value of θ (e.g., $H_0 : \theta = \theta^\dagger$). Because $\hat{\theta}$ is the MLE, the data must be more probable at $\hat{\theta}$ than at $\theta^\dagger$, and so the likelihood ratio (LR): $L(\hat{\theta}) / L(\theta^\dagger))$ must be greater than 1. Moreover, large values of the LR suggest that the null hypothesis: $H_0 : \theta = \theta^\dagger$ is false. This overarching idea is formalized in the LR testing procedure. Specifically, let the parameter space (denoted Ω) be a Euclidean space of dimension u (e.g., the real line), and let ω be a *nested* subspace of Ω with dimension v (e.g., a single point), and let $\theta^\dagger$ be the *constrained* MLE (i.e., the MLE subject to $\theta \in \omega$;). Then, when $H_0 : \theta = \theta^\dagger$ is true, the following is also true:

$$2\log \frac{L(\hat{\theta}; \mathbf{R})}{L(\theta^\dagger; \mathbf{R})} \to \chi_k^2 \text{ as } n \to \infty, \tag{3.8}$$

where n denotes the sample size with respect to independent realizations $\mathbf{R} = (R_1, R_2, \ldots, R_n)$, and the integer $k = u - v$ is the difference between the dimensionality of Ω and ω. Therefore, for large samples, the null distribution of any LRT is approximately χ^2 with k degrees of freedom.

3.5 MAXIMUM ENTROPY

Although the likelihood approach to statistical inference (e.g., ML estimation or LRTs of simple or composite nested hypotheses) is used extensively, there are other alternative approaches as well. In the fields of Statistical Mechanics and Information Theory for example, probability distributions are routinely estimated from empirical data in accordance with the principle of maximum entropy, not maximum likelihood. One issue with the ML approach in this setting (i.e., when an aggregate measure of the entire sample is observed, instead of a collection of measurements from n individuals or experimental units) is that there can be an infinite number of solutions. Another issue (albeit philosophical) is that ML yields the distribution that makes the observed data *most probable*, whereas maximizing the entropy, which is the tendency of an ordered system to become disordered over time, yields the *most disordered* (i.e., completely random) distribution subject to constraints imposed by the data.

To better understand the maximum entropy (ME) approach, let's revisit our discrete random variable X from Section 3.2 (i.e., the roll of a six-sided die). The entropy of the distribution of X is defined as

$$H(\mathbf{p}) \equiv -\sum p_i \log p_i,$$

where the summation is taken over the set of possible outcomes $i \in \{1, \ldots, 6\}$, and $\mathbf{p}$ is the parameter vector $\{p_i\}$. Now, one could imagine that a newly manufactured set of low-quality dice might for example favor the value 6 because this face has the most material removed and presumably is the lightest. However, we suspect that the real-world effects of wear and tear from successive rolls will increase the entropy over time, and that after a certain number of rolls each future outcome will essentially be equally likely. Let's suppose that we observe a mean of 3.9 from 100 rolls, and that we want to estimate $\mathbf{p}$ subject to constraints imposed by the observed data, and in accordance with our belief that entropy is always increasing. This is a standard Lagrange multiplier problem [8] with a criterion function $H(\mathbf{p})$ and two constraints: $\mathbf{E}X = 3.9$ and $\sum_j p_j = 1$. The maximum entropy (ME) estimate of $\mathbf{p}$ is the argument that maximizes

$$Q(\mathbf{p}; \lambda, \phi) = -\sum_j p_j \log p_j + \lambda \left(\sum_j p_j - 1 \right) + \phi \left(\sum_j j p_j - 3.9 \right), \tag{3.9}$$

where λ and ϕ are the Lagrange multipliers, one for each constraint. To maximize (3.8), we set its partial derivative to zero and solve for p_j

$$\frac{\partial Q(\mathbf{p}; \lambda, \phi)}{\partial p_j} = -[1 + \log p_j] + \lambda + \phi j$$

$$0 = \lambda + \phi j - 1 - \log P_j$$

$$\log p_j = \lambda + \phi j - 1 \tag{3.10}$$

$$p_j = \exp(\lambda + \phi j - 1)$$

$$p_j = \exp(\lambda + \phi j - 1)$$

Since the p_j's sum to 1, Eq. (3.9) implies that $\exp(\lambda - 1 / \sum \exp(\phi j)$. Therefore, $p_j = \exp(\phi j) / \sum \exp(\phi j)$. Furthermore, because $\sum j p_j = 3.9$, we can use the Newton-Raphson algorithm to solve for ϕ. Starting with an initial guess of 0, which corresponds to a $\mathbf{p}$ of (1/6, …, 1/6), the algorithm converges after four iterations to $\phi \approx 0.1387638$. Hence the maximum entropy (ME) estimate of $\mathbf{p}$ is (0.1146, 0.1316, 0.1512, 0.1737, 0.1996, 0.2293), and indeed, the probabilities are increasing in j.

Note that the ME approach is quite general, and in addition to discrete distributions over finite sample spaces, there are ME distributions for discrete distributions over unbounded supports and for continuous distributions defined on (a,b), for real numbers a and b with $b > a$. For a list of commonly used ME distributions see [16].

3.6 CONCLUDING REMARKS

Throughout this chapter, I have focused on parameter estimation and hypothesis testing, with several illustrative examples of relevant data analyses. More formally, given a family of probability distributions $P_\theta(\cdot)$ indexed by a parameter θ, I have addressed two main questions: "Which distribution is best supported by the data?" and "How well do the data support this distribution over a competing hypothesis of lower dimension?" Becoming proficient at answering these two questions is invaluable; but proficiency is really just the beginning. In addition to parametric estimation and testing, there is also the class of nonparametric statistics to consider. These statistics do not assume a parametric model. They are often criticized for being less powerful than their parametric counterparts when the parametric model is correctly specified, but they are also praised for being more robust when the parametric model is mis-specified. Two other important areas of interest are imputation and classification. Although, these terms are often used interchangeably with estimation and testing, respectively, the former pertains to unobserved random variables, whereas the latter pertains to unknown (but fixed) parameters.

In any event, strategic decisions will have to be made when choosing the type of statistical analysis. Typically, these decisions will depend on the scientific questions of interest, the complexity of the data, and the experience of the analyst. Then, in implementing this overall strategic plan, a myriad of smaller decisions will usually have to be made along the way. Often, there will not be a *right* or *wrong* decision *per se*, but one hopes that every decision will be justified in some way. The prudent data analyst is reminded to remain passionate about the analysis, but indifferent about the results! This will give the data a better chance to tell *their* story, and in hearing it, Science will have a better chance to advance.

ENDNOTES

1. The statistical analysis of real data has hidden costs that include, but are not limited to, the identification and management of any number of the following: data processing errors, outliers, misinformation, and incoherent data points.
2. Because the genes that influence growth are under selective evolutionary pressure, most humans do not continue to grow into adulthood.
3. For a continuous random variable Z with density $f(z|\theta)$, the $Pr_\theta(a < Z < a+h) = \int_a^{a+h} f(z|\theta)dz$ for $h > 0$.

   If θ^* denotes the value of θ that maximizes $f(z|\theta)$, then it can be shown that θ^* also maximizes $\lim_{h\to 0} Pr\theta(a < Z < a + h)$; and intuitively, this final expression is $L(\theta; z)$.

REFERENCES

1. Fisher, R.A. (1922). On the mathematical foundations of theoretical statistics. *Philosophical Transactions of the Royal Society Series A 222*, 309–368.
2. Hogg, R.V., and Tanis, E.A. (1997). *Probability and statistical inference.* Upper Saddle River, NJ: Prentice Hall.
3. Guttorp, P. (1995). *Stochastic modeling of scientific data.* London, UK: Chapman & Hall.
4. Thompson, E.A. (2000). Statistical Inferences from Genetic Data on Pedigrees. *NSF-CBMS Regional Conference Series in Probability and Statistics* Vol. 6. Beachwood, OH: Institute of Mathematical Statistics.
5. Wald, A. (1949). Note on the consistency of the maximum likelihood estimate. *Annals of Mathematical Statistics 20*, 595–601.
6. Casella, G., and Berger, R.L. (1990). *Statistical inference.* Belmont, CA: Wadsworth, Inc.
7. Self, S.G., and Liang, K-Y. (1987). Asymptotic properties of maximum likelihood estimators and likelihood ratio tests under non-standard conditions. *Journal of the American Statistical Association 82*, 605–610.
8. Edwards, Jr., C.H., and Penney, D.E. (1986). *Calculus and Analytic Geometry* (2d ed.). Englewood Cliffs, NJ: Prentice-Hall.
9. Dempster, A.P., Laird, N.M., and Rubin, D.B. (1977). Maximum likelihood from incomplete data via the EM algorithm (with discussion). *Journal of the Royal Statistical Society, Series B 39*, 1–37.
10. Robbins, H. and Monro, S. (1951). A stochastic approximation method. *Annals of Mathematical Statistics 22*, 400–407.
11. Stewart, W.C.L., and Thompson, E.A. (2006). Improving estimates of genetic maps: A maximum likelihood approach. *Biometrics 62*, 1–8.
12. Ewens, W.J., and Grant, G.R. (2001). *Statistical methods in bioinformatics.* New York, NY: Springer-Verlag.
13. Van Der Vaart, A.W. (1998). *Asymptotic Statistics.* Cambridge, UK: Cambridge University Press.
14. Hampel, F.R., Ronchetti, E.M., Rousseeuw, P.J., and Stahel, W.A. (1986). *Robust statistics.* New York, NY: John Wiley & Sons.
15. Ferguson, T.S. (1996). *A course in large sample theory.* Boca Raton, FL: Chapman & Hall.
16. Lisman, J.H.C., and van Zuylen, M.C.A. (1972). Note on the generation of most probable frequency distributions. *Statistica neerlandica 26*, 19–23.

Using data to guide model construction
Application of principal component analysis and related methods in immunology research

KATHRYN MILLER-JENSEN AND KELLY B. ARNOLD

4.1 INTRODUCTION

Recent technological advances such as bead-based multiplexed cytokine screening, RNA deep sequencing, and mass cytometry have significantly expanded the number of multiplexed measurements that can be collected from the same biological sample and from single cells. However, acquiring these data sets is far from the end of the experiment. One major challenge is how to derive meaning from these hundreds or thousands of measurements.

A useful approach to analyzing large data sets is to use the data to guide model construction without making any prior assumptions about underlying mechanisms. Given the biological complexity of the immune system, there are few cases in which mechanisms are known in enough detail to fit experimental data to a preexisting model of biological interactions. However, **data-driven models** allow the user to more intuitively understand the biological information contained within large, multivariate data sets and often reveal new biological insights. For example, data-driven models may identify critical protein species that need to be included in future mechanistic models, they might suggest new hypotheses for future experimental studies, or they might provide clinically relevant diagnostic models that lead to predictive tests of some disease conditions.

There are many data-driven modeling approaches to choose from, some of which are covered in later chapters. In this chapter, we introduce **principal component analysis (PCA)**, one of the most established data-driven modeling methods, and one that has been used to gain novel biological insights from large immunological data sets. In addition, we will also discuss two useful variations of PCA, **partial least squares discriminant analysis (PLSDA)** and **partial least squares regression (PLSR)**. PLSDA and PLSR not only aid in condensing and visualizing large data sets, but also allow for data prediction.

4.2 PRINCIPAL COMPONENT ANALYSIS: AN OVERVIEW

4.2.1 GRAPHICAL ILLUSTRATION

PCA is a linear regression method that takes a set of experimental observations for which a large number of variables have been measured (referred to as the data matrix **X**) and identifies new "super" variables called principal components. Principal components allow the user to view the entire data space in two or three dimensions that capture the most important information in the original measurements. This **dimensionality reduction** (reducing a high number of axes, or dimensions, to just two or three) is accomplished mathematically by analyzing how each variable changes with every other variable in the data set. PCA places high weight on those variables that change together and deemphasizes those that show little covariation with other variables. The principal component coordinates are weighted linear combinations of the original variables, allowing users to see how each measured variable relates to other variables in the data set and how all variables contribute to the observed differences among the biological samples.

To understand PCA conceptually, we will provide an example drawn from the immunology literature involving T cell phenotype classification. T cells play a central role in cell-mediated immunity. In the example study, researchers were interested in quantifying the range of functions that are exhibited by CD8+ cytotoxic T cells. CD8+ T cells, similar to other cells of the immune system, differentiate into distinct subsets based on their exposure to antigens. The subsets are traditionally classified based on surface marker expression into naïve, central memory (T_{CM}), or effector memory (T_{EM}) cell groups. Although it is thought that these subsets have distinct functions (e.g., secretion and cytotoxic potential), little is known about which functions are associated with each group. To explore the variability in these classifications and functions at the single-cell level, mass cytometry was used to measure 25 functional and phenotypic cellular markers for single CD8+ T cells following activation with phorbol myristate acetate-ionomycin (PMA/I) [1]. PCA was then used to understand how these markers varied by subsets classified by traditional surface marker staining.

We will use this example to provide a graphical illustration of PCA. Imagine a simplified mass cytometry experiment as described above but with only two functional readouts for each single CD8+ T cell: the level of intracellular cytokine staining for tumor necrosis factor-α (TNF-α) and macrophage inflammatory protein-1β (MIP-1β). In this case, our data matrix contains a different single cell in each row and each cell is described by two variables, TNF-α and MIP-1β level, arranged into columns (Figure 4.1a). Thus, it is possible to plot each cell in two-dimensional space based on the level of these functional markers (Figure 4.1b). To demonstrate the classification capability of PCA, we have labeled each cell as naïve, T_{CM}, or T_{EM} based on surface marker expression that was measured at the same time as cytokine production (Figure 4.1c).

We are now ready to perform PCA on this simplified data set. As described above, the first principal component (PC1) is directed along the axis that captures the most co-variation among the measured variables. It is possible to visually see this axis (Figure 4.1c), which corresponds to a positive covariation in production of TNF-α and MIP-1β. After the direction of PC1 is identified, the data are rotated (i.e., transformed) and the remaining variation is subtracted, such that each cell is described by a single coordinate on PC1 (Figure 4.1d). This PC1 coordinate effectively classifies naïve versus differentiated T cells by a single coordinate along PC 1, which is a combination of the original TNF-α and MIP-1β coordinates. This illustrates how PCA can be used to find a new axis that captures important information about the data.

However, we can see that PC1 alone cannot distinguish between T_{CM} and T_{EM} cells. To distinguish between these cells, we can draw a second line that is orthogonal to PC1 that captures the negative covariation in TNF-α and MIP-1β (Figure 4.1e). This is the second principal component (PC2). By rotating the data and plotting them on PC1 versus PC2, it is now possible to classify the cells into naïve, T_{CM}, and T_{EM} groups, albeit with some error (Figure 4.1f).

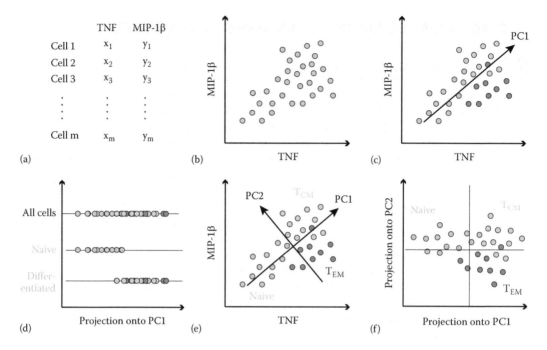

Figure 4.1 Graphical illustration of principal component analysis (PCA) for a mass cytometry data set. **(a)** Measurements of TNF and MIP-1β are recorded for m cells to form an m × 2 data matrix. **(b)** Cells can be plotted as points in the TNF- MIP-1β data space. **(c)** PCA identifies the direction along which the data has the largest variance (PC1). By classifying the cells based on surface marker expression (measured separately), it is possible to see that the variation captures systematic differences between the cells. **(d)** Samples plotted in one dimension using the PC1 coordinate, which effectively separates naïve versus differentiated CD8+ T cells. **(e)** PCA also identifies an orthogonal direction that captures the second largest variance in the data (PC2) and separates T_{CM} and T_{EM} cells. **(f)** Projections along PC1 and PC2 partition the different cell states but do not identify three separate clusters. (Adapted from Ringer, M., *Nat Biotechnol*, 26, 303–304, 2008.)

4.2.2 Mathematical explanation

Now we can return to the real biological problem for which 25 variables describe each sample (i.e., single cell). In this case, the axes in data space are highly multi-dimensional and thus it would be difficult to visualize the direction that captures the most variation on a two-dimensional page. Mathematically, however, the process is the same regardless of the number of variables. The direction of maximum variation in the data can be identified by calculating the covariance matrix, a matrix of values that describe the covariation between each variable and every other measured variable in the data set. Thus for a data matrix of m observations and three variables (x, y, and z), the data matrix $\mathbf{X}$ is defined as

$$\mathbf{X} = \begin{bmatrix} a_1 & b_1 & c_1 \\ \vdots & \vdots & \vdots \\ a_m & b_m & c_m \end{bmatrix}$$

where each row contains the measurements associated with one biological sample. The covariance matrix $\mathbf{C}$ of $\mathbf{X}$ is defined as

$$\mathbf{C} = \begin{bmatrix} cov\,(\boldsymbol{a},\boldsymbol{a}) & cov\,(\boldsymbol{a},\boldsymbol{b}) & cov\,(\boldsymbol{a},\boldsymbol{c}) \\ cov\,(\boldsymbol{b},\boldsymbol{a}) & cov\,(\boldsymbol{b},\boldsymbol{b}) & cov\,(\boldsymbol{b},\boldsymbol{c}) \\ cov\,(\boldsymbol{c},\boldsymbol{a}) & cov\,(\boldsymbol{c},\boldsymbol{b}) & cov\,(\boldsymbol{c},\boldsymbol{c}) \end{bmatrix}$$

The covariance matrix $\mathbf{C}$ is a square matrix (i.e., it has an equal number of rows and columns). Square matrices have special vectors associated with them called eigenvectors, for which multiplication by $\mathbf{C}$ maps the eigenvector to a multiple of itself:

$$\mathbf{C}\mathbf{z} = \lambda\mathbf{z}$$

The eigenvector $\mathbf{z}$ has a corresponding eigenvalue λ, and the total number of eigenvectors is equal to the dimensions of $\mathbf{C}$. The eigenvector with the highest value of λ identifies the direction in data space that will capture the most variation in the original measurements of the data matrix $\mathbf{X}$, the eigenvector with the second highest value of λ identifies the direction of the second highest variation in the data set, and so on. The eigenvectors of the covariance matrix are identified and rearranged in order from highest to lowest. This creates a new square matrix that is used to do a coordinate transformation on the original data set.

Following transformation of the data matrix into a new coordinate space, each sample in the data set is expressed as a linear combination of the original variables. However, due to the arrangement of the eigenvectors in order of decreasing eigenvalue, the first vector in the new coordinate system is optimized to capture the most variation in the original data set. The reduction in data dimensionality is achieved because typically only the two to three eigenvectors with the highest eigenvalues are retained prior to the data transformation. Dropping the remaining eigenvectors effectively emphasizes the directions (axes) that capture the most variation in the data set and eliminates those that capture little variation. The underlying assumption is that systematic variation contains information that is biologically relevant and lack of systematic variation is noise. In summary, the eigenvectors of $\mathbf{C}$ arranged from high to low values of λ mathematically identify the principal components of the data set.

For an in-depth discussion of the linear algebra and data matrix manipulations that underlie PCA, we refer our readers to other resources at the end of the chapter. In the remainder of the chapter, we will focus on the practical steps of PCA implementation and how these steps change for variations on PCA, including PLSDA and PLSR. We further provide the reader with a framework for analyzing different types of data sets using PCA (Example 1), PLSDA (Example 2), and PLSR (Example 3) that are drawn from the immunology literature.

4.3 PCA: IMPLEMENTATION

4.3.1 THE DATA MATRIX

PCA is performed on a data matrix ($\mathbf{X}$) that is arranged by placing the experimental samples (observations) in rows and the measurements (variables) in columns. For example, measurements of secretion of 10 cytokines at three time points for samples from three donors separately treated with four different stimuli would result in a data matrix of 12 rows (samples: three donors by four treatments) by 30 columns (three time point entries for 10 cytokines).

The PCA algorithm is not sensitive to the order of the observations or variables in the data matrix, even if the variables represent measurements over time, because PCA does not incorporate any a priori information about the data. One way to incorporate additional information from a time course of measurements is to calculate metrics from the time course. These could include mean values, maximum values, slopes between time points, and area under the curve [2].

4.3.2 PREPROCESSING THE DATA

PCA derives principal components by capturing variation directly from the input data set. In most cases, it is important to perform data pre-processing on the data matrix prior to performing PCA to avoid emphasizing variations in the data that are not necessarily related to information content. Without preprocessing, PCA will overemphasize variables that have high mean values and that vary over a large range and will deemphasize variables that have low mean values and vary over a more limited range. In many biological examples, the absolute value of the measurement is not indicative of the importance of that variable. For example, the range of measurement intensity values for a protein detected with a fluorescently conjugated antibody will be affected by the background intensity or specificity of the antibody used for detection, and therefore the relative differences between measurements of two different proteins within a single sample are not meaningful. Data preprocessing avoids the pitfall of assigning meaning to these experimental measurement artifacts.

Data are commonly standardized by "mean centering" the data by subtracting the mean of a given measurement across all the observations (i.e., subtracting the mean from the column). The data are further "variance scaled" by dividing by the square root of the variance of the measurement (i.e., dividing by the standard deviation of the column):

$$x_{scaled} = \frac{x_{i,raw} - \overline{x_{i,raw}}}{\sqrt{var(x_{i,raw} - \overline{x_{i,raw}})}}$$

Variance scaling has the added benefit of making the variables non-dimensional in the data matrix. Thus, preprocessing is especially important when measurements from different experimental assays that have different units and data ranges are combined in the same data matrix. While mean centering and variance scaling tends to be the most common approach for preprocessing biological data, there are other approaches available that may be more appropriate for specific implementations of PCA.

4.3.3 SCORES AND LOADINGS

As described above, the eigenvectors of the covariance matrix $\mathbf{C}$ form the mathematical basis of PCA. However, most practical applications of PCA identify principal components by decomposing (or factoring) the data matrix into a structure part and a noise part:

$$X = TP^T + E$$

The structured part is a sum of vector products that recapitulate the eigenvectors. The vectors that are multiplied together are called the **scores** vectors of the matrix $\mathbf{T}$ and the **loadings** vectors of the matrix $\mathbf{P}^T$. The vector products are the principal components. The **residuals** (or the data variability that is not captured by the factorization into the principal components) are collected in the matrix $\mathbf{E}$. The matrix algebra can be visualized graphically as:

$$\boxed{X} = \boxed{t_1}\overline{\boxed{p_1^T}} + \boxed{t_2}\overline{\boxed{p_2^T}} + \dots + \boxed{E}$$

Typically we are only interested in the first two or three principal components (i.e., the first two or three vector products), which means that the unaccounted for variability in the data that is collected in the residual matrix $\mathbf{E}$ will be disregarded. Although at first this might seem undesirable, this so-called data reduction is one of the advantages of PCA because we assume that the information contained in the residuals is "noise" and thus not biologically relevant. By eliminating that noise, it is easier to interpret the data. The maximum number of scores and loadings vectors is equivalent to either the number of total observations in the data matrix or the total number of variables, whichever is fewer. If all principal components are included, then the residuals matrix $\mathbf{E}$ will be 0 because all of the information in the original data set is retained.

The scores matrix ($\mathbf{T}$) contains the projection (or coordinates) for each observation in the data matrix along each principal component. The first vector of the scores matrix ($\mathbf{t_1}$) contains the coordinates on principal component 1, the second scores vector ($\mathbf{t_2}$) contains the coordinates on principal component 2, and so on.

Table 4.1 Useful software for PCA, PLSR, and PLSDA implementation

Software	Analysis	Variable selection
Matlab (Mathworks)	PCA, PLSR	LASSO, VIP
Eigenvector Solo (Eigenvector Research)	PCA, PLSR, PLSDA	VIP
Eigenvector PLS_Toolbox extension for Matlab (Eigenvector Research)	PCA, PLSR, PLSDA	VIP
SIMPCA (Umetrics)	PCA, PLSR, PLSDA	VIP

By replotting the samples using these coordinates, it is possible to see how the different samples relate to each other in principal component space. The distance between samples is directly related to their similarity: samples that map closely together are more similar than samples that are far apart.

The loadings matrix (**P**) contains loadings vectors that are linear combinations of the weights (or influence) of each of the original variables that define the principal component. The loadings can be plotted in a lower dimensional space (i.e., principal component 1 versus principal component 2), depending on the number of components used in the model. This is sometimes referred to as a map of variables. Importantly, by plotting the scores and loadings together in principal component space, it is possible to see how they relate to each other.

Scores and loadings vectors are calculated iteratively using a search algorithm. There are several software programs available (Table 4.1) that will implement PCA and most of them use the Nonlinear Iterative Partial Least Squares (NIPALS) algorithm to calculate principal components. Briefly, the algorithm iteratively searches for a direction in the data space that captures the maximal variance for all the variables in the starting data set, which is the first loadings vector. Once the first loadings vector is identified, the corresponding scores vector is calculated by projecting the data set onto the loadings vector. The result is that each observation in the data matrix is now represented by a single value on principal component 1, providing a one-dimensional approximation of the data matrix. Together, the first scores–loadings vector pair identifies the first principal component and is equivalent to selecting the eigenvector with the largest eigenvalue in the covariance matrix.

Eigenvectors must be orthogonal to each other, meaning that the second eigenvector is linearly independent of the first. The same constraint is placed on the second loadings vector, such that no information about the data is captured in more than one principal component. This is done mathematically by subtracting out the variance that was captured in the first principal component, which is equivalent to considering the residuals matrix **E**. The search for the second loadings vector starts with the "leftover" variance contained in **E** and identifies the direction that captures the maximum variance contained in this residual data set.

4.3.4 Variance explained and choosing principal components

By definition, the first principal component will capture the highest fraction of variance in the data set, and each subsequent principal component will capture a smaller fraction of the variance. Principal components can be iteratively calculated up to the number of observations or variables in the data set (whichever is smaller) until 100% of the variance is accounted for. However, one of the advantages of PCA is the ability to discard information in the data set that is not meaningful. For biological data matrices, the residual information captured by principal components usually drops off quickly, and often only the first two to three principal components are retained.

One approach to objectively identify which principal components likely contain meaningful information is to use a resampling technique called cross validation, in which the data are separated into a **training set** (the data set used to build or train the model) and a **test set** (data that was withheld when training the model that can be used to test the model). In this method, PCA is performed on a data matrix in which a single experimental sample (row) or a subset of samples of the original data set has been removed (i.e., the training set). The resulting PCA model is then used to estimate the values of the independent variables in the excluded sample(s) (i.e., the test set). A popular version of cross validation is the jackknife (also referred to as "leave one out" cross validation). In this cross-validation technique, each sample is dropped from the full data set in turn, with the remaining observations used to build the PCA model, until all combinations have been performed. The predicted observations are stored in a test matrix, $\mathbf{X}^{test}$.

It is possible to evaluate the quality of the PCA model by comparing the original data matrix $\mathbf{X}$ to the test matrix $\mathbf{X}^{test}$. A common metric used to make this evaluation is the predicted residual sum of squares (PRESS):

$$PRESS\ (m) = \sum_{i=1}^{k} \sum_{j=1}^{l} (x_{ij} - x_{ij}^{test})^2$$

for a data matrix with k independent variables (columns) and l samples (rows) and for a PCA model with m principal components retained. A smaller PRESS value indicates a better quality model for the estimation of new data.

Although adding a principal component will always increase the total amount of variance captured by the model for the entire data set, adding a principal component will not always improve the cross-validation predictions. Thus, principal components can be retained until they start to increase error in the predictions (e.g., increase the PRESS value). The simplest approach is to stop adding components when the PRESS values starts to increase.

The appropriate size of the data subset to remove during cross validation is dependent on the number of samples available and organization of the data. For a small number of samples, the jackknife cross-validation technique described above may be most appropriate. In larger data sets, it is usually recommended to exclude larger subsets during cross validation to get a more thorough understanding of model performance on unknown data.

In the text that follows we continue with a practical discussion of PCA implemented on immune data, using the CD8+ T cell study we began with above.

4.4 EXAMPLE 1: PCA TO DISCOVER COMBINATORIAL PROTEIN RESSION THAT DISTINGUISHES CD8+ T CELL PHENOTYPES [1]

4.4.1 BIOLOGICAL QUESTION

CD8+ T cells can be classified into distinct differentiation states based on the presence and/or absence of surface markers, but little is known about the functions associated with each state (e.g., which cytokines they can produce or their potential for cytotoxicity). This study used mass cytometry (also called cytometry by time-of-flight, or CyTOF) to measure functional and phenotypic markers simultaneously on single cells. The researchers used a PCA model to determine if different stages of CD8+ T cell differentiation could be classified based on combinations of phenotypic and functional markers. They further asked if antigen-specific cells occupy T cell niches that can be defined based on combinations of phenotypic and functional markers.

4.4.2 DATA ORGANIZATION

The data were collected by CyTOF. The data set consisted of 25 phenotypic and functional markers measured in single CD8+ T cells isolated from human PBMCs and stimulated with PMA+ionomycin for three hours. The data matrix X was an $m \times n$ matrix of m cells (>1000 "observations") and $n = 25$ functional and phenotypic markers. The functional and phenotypic markers were given binary classifications of "on" ($x_n = 1$) or "off" ($x_n = 0$) based on background thresholds so that the final matrix contained only ones and zeros.

4.4.3 PREPROCESSING

Because the data were given binary classifications, all the variables had the same dynamic range and therefore data preprocessing was not necessary.

4.4.4 MODEL REFINEMENT

The first two principal components accounted for 50% of the variation in the single-cell data; the third component covered an additional 10% (for 60% cumulative variance explained). The authors chose to include only the first three principal components based on the qualitative judgment that the remaining principal components did not show any informative biological patterns.

4.4.5 CROSS VALIDATION

No formal cross validation was performed in this study.

4.4.6 INTERPRETATION OF RESULTS

The principal components were able to classify CD8+ T cells based on differentiation state. PC1 classified naïve versus differentiated T cells. PC2 tracked differentiated state (from T_{CM} to T_{EM} to T_{SLEC}). PC3 further segregated variation within the central memory compartment. Interestingly, the distribution of cells within the principal component space was the same across patients, suggesting that the pattern of functional and phenotypic markers used to classify the cells were conserved across individuals.

The conserved pattern in principal component space allowed the researchers to additionally label virus-specific tetramers to visualize the location of virus-specific cells within the continuum of CD8+ T cell compartments. They found that T cells specific for cytomegalovirus (CMV), Epstein-Barr virus (EBV), and influenza occupied distinct phenotypic and functional niches. The authors note that the different phenotypes likely reflect characteristics of the pathogen. Influenza infections are episodic, and were associated with T_{CM}-like phenotypes. In contrast EBV and CMV are chronic infections and thus occupy more T_{EM}-like phenotypes and late state effect (T_{SLE})-like phenotypes, respectively.

4.4.7 LIMITATIONS

The PCA results were benchmarked against standard surface marker classification of the CD8+ T cell differentiation states. This type of verification is useful but will not always be possible with biological data sets. A limitation of this verification was the fact that it was made using markers that were also included in the PCA model. It would have been interesting to see, for example, to what extent functional markers alone could differentiate between CD8+ T cell differentiation states. By repeating PCA with subsets of the original data set, it would be possible to identify minimal requirements for CD8+ T cell classification that did not include the classical surface markers.

4.5 EXTENSIONS OF PCA: PLSDA AND PLSR – AN OVERVIEW

Partial least squares discriminant analysis (**PLSDA**) and partial least squares regression (**PLSR**) can be considered extensions of PCA because they identify variation or "super" variables (principal components) in the data matrix (**X**, described above). However, in contrast to PCA, which identifies principal components in an **unsupervised** manner (i.e., no expected output is specified), PLSDA and PLSR are **supervised** methods that identify principal components from a proposed relationship. Both methods require defining a dependent output or response variable block (**Y**), and then finding the principal components that relate the variation in the independent matrix of variables (**X**) to the dependent variables (**Y**). For this reason PLSR and PLSDA can be especially useful for hypothesis-driven biological research, as the result is linear combinations of experimental measurements associated with a known biological function or state. For example, PLSR or PLSDA could be used to identify multivariate combinations of cytokines, antibodies, or transcriptional events ($\mathbf{X}$) associated with a known cell type or disease state ($\mathbf{Y}$).

All information presented above about PCA also applies to PLSDA and PLSR. The added extension is that PLSDA and PLSR provide information about the relationship between the data matrix $\mathbf{X}$ and a known label or response vector, $\mathbf{Y}$. For PLSDA, $\mathbf{Y}$ contains known class or label information for each sample, which corresponds to each row in the data matrix $\mathbf{X}$. For PLSR, $\mathbf{Y}$ contains additional biological measurements that are hypothesized to depend on the variables in the data matrix $\mathbf{X}$. $\mathbf{Y}$ is often a single column vector (i.e., only one response variable), but it can also be a matrix (with multiple columns) in situations for which there are several response variables of interest. The most important difference between PLSDA and PLSR can be summarized as follows: for PLSDA, $\mathbf{Y}$ is a discrete class; for PLSR, $\mathbf{Y}$ is a continuous variable.

4.6 PLSR AND PLSDA: IMPLEMENTATION

4.6.1 THE DATA MATRIX: DEFINING DEPENDENT AND INDEPENDENT BLOCKS

Both PLSR and PLSDA are performed on two data matrices: an independent data matrix $\mathbf{X}$ and a dependent data matrix $\mathbf{Y}$. As in PCA, $\mathbf{X}$ contains the experimental observations in rows and the variables in columns. For example, identical to PCA implementation described above, consider a data matrix of 12 rows (samples: three donors by four treatments) by 30 columns (three time point entries for 10 cytokines). Implementation of PLSDA requires an additional response vector ($\mathbf{Y}$) that includes the treatment class for each sample (12 rows and 1 column). The exact input format for $\mathbf{Y}$ may depend on the software used to perform the analysis. In some cases, $\mathbf{Y}$ input may be accepted as a text label, or in some cases a vector of discrete numbers may be required. Implementation of PLSR requires a response vector or matrix $\mathbf{Y}$ that contains continuous cell measurements. For example, if quantitative measures of cell migration and cell proliferation are hypothesized to be dependent on the independent variables and thus are recorded at a single time point for all samples, then the independent $\mathbf{Y}$ matrix would consist of 24 data points (12 samples by two response measurements).

4.6.2 PREPROCESSING THE DATA

It is important to preprocess the $\mathbf{X}$ data matrix for PLSR and PLSDA for the same reasons as described above for PCA in Section 4.3.2. If $\mathbf{Y}$ is a single column vector, it often does not need pre-processing, especially in the case of PLSDA, where $\mathbf{Y}$ is a discrete class. However when $\mathbf{Y}$ is a matrix containing multiple responses, preprocessing is usually necessary and can be performed similarly as is on the $\mathbf{X}$ data matrix.

4.6.3 SCORES AND LOADINGS

Above we described how PCA identifies principal components by decomposing (or factoring) the independent data matrix $\mathbf{X}$ into a structure part and a noise part:

$$X = TP^T + E$$

$\mathbf{T}$ is the matrix of scores for the observations in $\mathbf{X}$ and $\mathbf{P^T}$ is the matrix of loadings for the variables in $\mathbf{X}$. Similarly, the dependent data matrix $\mathbf{Y}$ is factored in an analogous manner:

$$Y = UQ^T + F$$

U contains the scores for the observations in **Y**, and $\mathbf{Q}^\mathrm{T}$ contains the loadings for the variables in **Y**. To enforce the linear relationship between the independent and dependent blocks, the **Y** factorization is forced to use a multiple of the scores vector of **X**. The scores vectors for principal components are related by:

$$\mathbf{U} = \mathbf{BT}$$

The scores matrix for **Y** can now be expressed as a multiple of the scores matrix of **X**:

$$Y = TBQ^T + F$$

The scores and loadings for **X** and **Y** are calculated using an iterative algorithm similar to that described above for PCA. However, rather than calculating the scores and loadings vectors independently for **X** and **Y**, the scores vectors are exchanged within the algorithm to strengthen the relationship between the **X** scores matrix **U** and the **Y** scores matrix **T**. As a result, the loadings vectors capture the covariance between **X** and **Y** rather than the overall variance in **X**. The identification of principal components that predict a relationship between **X** and **Y** is the key difference between PLSDA and PLSR as compared to PCA. To emphasize this important difference, the "super" variables identified by PLSR and PLSDA are sometimes referred to as latent variables rather than principal components. Similar to PCA, we are typically only interested in the first two or three score–loading vector pairs because these usually capture most of the covariance between **X** and **Y**. The remaining information collected in the residuals matrices (**E** and **F**) is typically experimental or biological noise. How to quantitatively determine the appropriate number of latent variables to use in a PLS model is described in the next section.

One of the most important advantages of PLS models is that they can be used to predict dependent response variables from the independent variables in **X**, including responses that were not included in the original training set (i.e., the data set that was used to build the model). Predictions are made using the proposed relationship between **X** and **Y**:

$$Y = XB_{PLS} + F$$

The matrix of regression coefficients $\mathbf{B}_{\mathrm{PLS}}$ is estimated as a function of $\mathbf{P}^\mathrm{T}$ (loadings of **X**) and $\mathbf{Q}^\mathrm{T}$ (loadings of **Y**).

4.6.4 Choosing latent variables and assessment of model quality

By definition, the first latent variable in PLS models will capture the variance that best relates **X** and **Y**, the second latent variable will capture the second most variance, etc. As in PCA, latent variables can be iteratively calculated up to the number of variables in the data set, at which point 100% of the relationship between **X** and **Y** will be captured. However, usually the goal is to limit the number of latent variables used in order to improve predictive power of the model and minimize the contribution of noise. Just as in PCA, one approach to objectively identify which latent variables contain meaningful information is to use cross validation.

Cross validation for PLSDA and PLSR can be performed by iteratively splitting data into training sets and test sets as described above for PCA. Model predictions of the dependent variables ($\mathbf{Y}^{\text{Predicted}}$) are then compared to actual values of the dependent variables in **Y**. The ability to predict **Y** for training data and test data is often reported as the **calibration error** and **cross-validation error**, respectively. For PLSDA models, these errors are calculated as the fraction of samples that were incorrectly predicted by the model during training and testing. Analogous measures of model predictive ability for PLSR models are R^2, which indicates how well the model is able to reproduce the training data set, and Q^2, which indicates how well the model can reproduce the test data set. R^2 is computed based on the residual sum of squares (RSS) of $\mathbf{Y}^{\text{Predicted}}$

for the training data and the total sum of squares (SS_{tot}) (proportional to the total variance of the training data):

$$R^2 = 1 - \frac{RSS}{SS_{tot}} \text{ (training data)}$$

Q^2 is computed from the PRESS (predicted residual sum of squares) described above in Section 4.3.4 for PCA that is obtained during cross validation using a method such as jackknifing:

$$Q^2 = 1 - \frac{PRESS}{SS_{tot}} \text{ (test data)}$$

An R^2 close to 1 indicates that a PLSR model fits the existing data well, while a Q^2 value close to 1 indicates that the model is expected to perform well on unknown data. Although adding latent variables will always increase the calibration accuracy (R^2) of the model, adding latent variables will not always improve the cross-validation predictions (Q^2). The reason for this minimum is that some of the information contained in the data set is noise (i.e., not correlated to the dependent block) and therefore by excluding this information, the predictive capability of the model is improved. The optimal number of latent variables to include in a PLSR or PLSDA model can be determined by plotting calibration and cross-validation error (or $1 - R^2$ and $1 - Q^2$) for each model as latent variables are added, and selecting the model that minimizes cross-validation error (Figure 4.2).

For binary classification (a PLSDA model with only two classes), a receiver operating characteristic (ROC) curve could additionally be used to assess predictive performance of the model. An ROC curve is created by plotting the true positive rate (sensitivity) against the false positive rate (1-specificity). For example, if a PLSDA model is being used to predict the presence of an infection (Y = "infected" or "not infected"), "true positives" would be samples that are correctly predicted by the model as "infected". The true positive rate (specificity) is then computed as the total number of true positives divided by the total number of infected individuals. "Uninfected" individuals who were incorrectly predicted to be "infected" would be considered

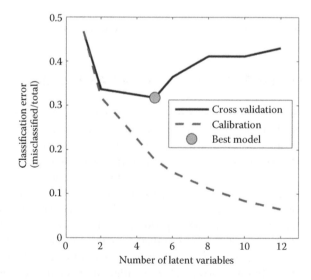

Figure 4.2 Graphical illustration of how calibration and cross validation may be used to select the appropriate number of latent variables for a PLSDA model. In this example, a model with five latent variables had the lowest cross-validation and calibration error (circle), and represents the model with the best expected predictive power. A similar figure with R^2 and Q^2 values plotted on the Y axis could be used to select the number of latent variables to be used in a PLSR model.

"false positives". The false positive rate is then computed as the total number of false positives divided by the total number of uninfected individuals (1-specificity).

4.6.5 MODEL REFINEMENT AND VARIABLE SELECTION METHODS

Even when calibration and cross validation are used to select the appropriate number of latent variables for a PLSDA or PLSR model, a large difference in calibration and cross-validation error (or R^2 and Q^2 values) may still remain. This indicates a model is "over-fit" (see Figure 4.2 above) and some independent variables should be removed to eliminate noise and improve cross-validation accuracy. There are several variable selection methods that can be used to eliminate variables that are not useful in a PLSR or PLSDA model. One commonly used approach computes a Variable Importance Projection (VIP) score for each variable. Variables with VIP scores less than 1 can be considered less important and removed from the model. Another method for variable selection is the least absolute shrinkage and selection operator (LASSO) method, which is especially useful for situations with hundreds or thousands of independent variables. Variable selection can greatly improve cross-validation accuracy (Q^2) while maintaining calibration accuracy (R^2). Both VIP variable selection and LASSO can be implemented using software packages that perform PLSDA and PLSR (Table 4.1). Detailed mathematical descriptions of each method can be found elsewhere [3].

In the text that follows we include a practical discussion of published studies that used PLSDA and PLSR to gain new insight into immune processes.

4.7 EXAMPLE 2: PLSDA TO IDENTIFY CYTOKINE-CHEMOKINE NETWORK CHANGES IN THE IMMUNE RESPONSES OF HIV-INFECTED INDIVIDUALS [4]

4.7.1 BIOLOGICAL QUESTION

In this example, PLSDA was used to gain new mechanistic insight into altered cytokine communication networks in HIV-infected individuals. Susceptibility to opportunistic infection and cancer indicates that the immune response of HIV-infected individuals is clearly impaired, but it has been difficult to assess the relative importance of many different immune cell alterations that have been reported. This study used a PLSDA model to determine how cytokine response profiles differed in HIV-infected individuals compared to healthy individuals, and which alterations could be explained by the loss of CD4+ T cell numbers that occurs during HIV infection.

4.7.2 DATA ORGANIZATION

Cytokine responses of cultured, peripheral blood mononuclear cells (PBMCs) were compared between seven HIV-infected donors, five healthy donors, and five healthy donors for which CD4+ T cells had been depleted to match levels in the HIV-infected group, for a total of 17 samples distributed among three classifications. The measured variables included 16 cytokines measured at 6 and 72 hours in the supernatant from cultured PBMCs following stimulation with LPS, R848, or anti CD3/28 beads. Three different PLSDA models (one for each stimulus) were created to compare changes in networks of HIV infected individuals to those in healthy individuals and in healthy individuals where CD4+ T cells were depleted experimentally.

Independent Data Matrix X: 32 cytokine measurements (16 measured at two time points), measured from PBMCs from healthy individuals, HIV-infected individuals, and from healthy individuals in which CD4+ T cells had been depleted experimentally. The resulting X data matrix was 17 rows by 32 columns because each stimulation was analyzed separately.

Dependent Variable Y: Each sample was labelled according to class: HIV, CD4+ T cell depleted, or healthy. The result was a 17 x 1 matrix. Three separate models were made, one for each stimulus (LPS, R848, and CD3/28).

4.7.3 PREPROCESSING

In this model it was important to normalize the data to account for: (1) cytokines with absolute concentrations that were higher than other cytokines and (2) cytokines with a greater range of concentration values than other cytokines. In this case mean centering (subtracting the mean) was used to address (1) and variance scaling (dividing by the standard deviation) was used to address (2).

4.7.4 CROSS VALIDATION

Cross validation was performed by excluding ~20% of the data during model training, and then testing the model on the excluded data. This was done iteratively until each sample was excluded at least once, although some samples were excluded more than once. Finally, cross-validation error was computed by averaging the error computed for the test data predictions from all iterations of model training.

4.7.5 MODEL REFINEMENT AND FEATURE SELECTION

After cross validation and calibration were performed, it was noted that cross-validation error was high, while calibration error was low. This indicated that some of the cytokine measurements in the PLSDA models did not contribute to classification, and models were over-fit. Variable Importance Projection (VIP) scores computed for each cytokine measurement were used to determine which cytokines were most useful for differentiating the classes of each PLSDA model. Cytokine measurements were eliminated from the model if they had a VIP Score less than one. New models created using only VIP cytokines had much lower cross-validation error, and were therefore more likely to perform well on unknown data. A final model with two latent variables was selected as these had the lowest calibration and cross-validation errors.

4.7.6 INTERPRETATION OF RESULTS

Model results indicated that the immune response of HIV-infected individuals to a T cell stimulus were more similar to healthy responses than to responses from PBMCs where CD4+ T cells had been depleted experimentally. Loadings on the critical latent variable in this model showed that PBMCs with CD4+ T cells depleted lost secretion of many adaptive cytokines (including IL-2, IFN-γ, and IL-4), whereas HIV-infected individuals were able to maintain secretion of these cytokines (even though CD4+ T cell numbers were matched between HIV and CD4+ depleted samples). Overall this suggested that the remaining T cells in HIV-infected individuals were be able to compensate for the lost T cells by compensatory secretion of adaptive cytokines. This was confirmed using additional analytical methods and follow-up flow cytometry experiments guided by model results. In contrast to adaptive responses, the PLSDA models of innate stimuli indicated that innate immune responses of HIV-infected individuals were different than both healthy and CD4+ depleted responses and loadings on latent variable 1 indicated this difference was characterized by lower secretion of a number of cytokines, including IFN-γ secretion at six hours. Additional computational and experimental analyses motivated by the PLSDA model results led to the discovery that NK-cells were responsible for this critical loss.

4.7.7 VARIATIONS ON THE PLSDA MODEL

With the large amount of data collected, it is often possible to ask additional questions by rearranging which data are included in the independent and dependent blocks. With the data collected in this study, the authors also considered how early alterations in cytokine secretion from HIV-infected individuals influence cytokine secretion at later time points. To do this, the independent data matrix (X) was limited to the 16 cytokine measurements measured at the late time point (72 hours) across the three donor groups. The dependent matrix (Y) of class labels remained the same (HIV-infected, CD4+ T cell-depleted, or healthy). The PLSDA models of the innate immune response indicated that HIV responses were different from healthy and CD4+ T cell-depleted responses at 72 hours. Combined with the main results described above, this observation supported the hypothesis that IFN-γ secretion by NK cells, a major early alteration in HIV, could be responsible for changes in the cytokine secretion profiles at 72 hours. In support of this hypothesis, there was a significant Pearson correlation between 6 h IFN-γ secretion and scores on LV1 in the model built from only the 72-hour data. Follow-up experiments confirmed that blocking IFN-γ secretion for six hours in healthy PBMCs altered cytokine secretion profiles at 72 hours to more closely resemble HIV-infected cytokine secretion profiles at that time point.

4.7.8 LIMITATIONS

A limitation of this study was the small sample size (n = 5 healthy, n = 5 CD4+ dep, n = 7 HIV), which resulted from difficulty obtaining PBMCs from HIV-infected individuals and the cost of multiplex cytokine measurements. While the small sample size precluded development of a predictive or diagnostic model based on these data, results still provided new insights into cytokine network alterations in a disease state.

4.8 EXAMPLE 3: PLSR TO PREDICT CYTOTOXIC T CELL AGE FROM STATIC AND DYNAMIC BIOMARKERS [5]

4.8.1 BIOLOGICAL QUESTION

Adoptive T cell therapy for cancer patients involves *ex vivo* expansion of autologous CD8+ T cells for tumor recognition. One major hurdle in this process is *ex vivo* generation of high-quality T cell clones without senescence and loss of function. This study built a PLSR model from high-throughput measurements of cell surface markers and dynamic signaling events to determine if these multivariate biomarkers could be used to predict T cell age and senescence.

4.8.2 DATA ORGANIZATION

CD8+ T cells were isolated from PBMCs collected from four different donors and maintained in culture for different lengths of time (four to five experiments for each donor) for a total of 18 observations (rows). The following data were collected for each observation:

- Flow cytometry measurements, including surface markers, measurements of cell morphology, and signaling proteins. Data included mean intensity, coefficient of variation, and fraction (50 data points).
- Dynamic signaling measurements, including phosphorylation status of six signaling proteins at eight time points measured via a Luminex assay (48 data points).
- Derivatives of the signaling dynamics, calculated by taking the slopes of the dynamic phosphorylation measurements between each time point (42 data points). This is an example of how additional independent variables can be generated from raw data.
- Number of days in culture and population doubling times for each sample.

Independent Data Matrix (X): 18 observations (rows) of 140 independent variables (columns) in CD8+ T cells, including surface markers, cell morphology, intracellular signaling proteins, and derivatives of the signaling dynamics.

Dependent Variable (Y): Number of days in cell culture or number of population doublings for each observation.

4.8.3 PREPROCESSING

Preprocessing of data in this study was especially important because different types of data, from different experimental assays were combined in the data matrix X. Here mean centering and variance scaling were used in each of the models to normalize absolute abundance and variance range, respectively.

4.8.4 MODEL REFINEMENT AND CROSS VALIDATION

Variable Importance Projection (VIP) scores were used to eliminate variables that did not contribute to the model or had high variability. Overall this resulted in pruning 69 of the original variables, for a final data set with 71 variables. A three-component model had minimum R^2 and Q^2 values of 0.96 and 0.78, respectively, and was chosen as the best model to fit the data.

4.8.5 INTERPRETATION OF RESULTS

A three-component PLSR model was able to predict CD8+ T days in culture and population doublings with high accuracy. Individual independent variables and hierarchical clustering approaches were not useful for differentiating cells based on age. Overall, this result suggests that a PLSR model could be valuable for predicting CD8+ T cell age in adoptive T cell therapy applications.

4.8.6 VARIATIONS ON THE PLSR MODEL

The authors of this study asked an additional question by rearranging the data in the independent and dependent blocks. Specifically, they considered if dynamic signaling events could predict cell surface marker expression by dividing the independent data matrix X into independent and dependent blocks and posing a new hypothetical relationship. In this PLSR model, the independent data matrix X consisted of only dynamic signaling events. The dependent matrix Y included CD27 and CD28 surface marker expression, measurements that were originally included in the X matrix but were now considered to be the response variable. This PLSR model using only signaling measurements was able to predict CD27 and CD28 surface marker expression with R^2 values ranging from 0.74 to 0.91. In contrast, a PLSR model built to predict signaling phosphorylation measurements from surface receptor expression data performed poorly ($R^2 = 0.27$ and $Q^2 = 0.1$). This suggested that signaling information may be predictive, or upstream of surface marker expression in CD8+ T cells, but surface marker expression is not directly correlated to T cell receptor signaling.

4.8.7 COMMON PITFALLS FOR APPLYING PLSR METHODS

While PLS methods are useful tools for analyzing large data sets, there are several misconceptions and pitfalls associated with their use. One common pitfall is to over fit PLS models, where low calibration error (or high R^2 values) could misleadingly indicate clear differences between groups and adequate predictive power. This pitfall can be avoided by assessing model performance with cross validation, or (preferably) on new, unknown samples. If cross-validation performance is poor, feature selection techniques discussed above can aid in removing noisy parameters to improve Q^2 and cross-validation accuracy.

Another important consideration is the organization of data for cross validation, especially with smaller sample sizes. The organization of **cross-validation folds**, or how samples are assigned to training sets versus test sets, can lead to large changes in model predictions in some cases and thus affect the estimation of predictive capabilities. In this case a PLS model trained on one subset of the data could generate considerably different R^2 and Q^2 values than a PLS model trained with another subset of the same data. This problem can be addressed by (1) verifying that samples are equally represented in cross-validation folds and (2) obtaining an average Q^2 value from iterative cross validation performed after reorganization of training and test set folds.

As discussed above, appropriate data preprocessing and normalization prior to analysis is also necessary, especially when using PLS methods where both normalization of the independent data matrix (X) and the dependent matrix (Y) must be considered. Finally, in using and interpreting PLS results, it is imperative to remember that PLS and similar methods only identify statistically significant associations between measured parameters. While these relationships are valuable for generating new hypotheses for biological mechanisms, causative relationships can only be confirmed through follow-up experiments. Likewise true diagnostic power can only be assessed by using the PLS model to make predictions about new, unknown samples coupled with an independent evaluation of the accuracy of the model predictions.

4.9 DISADVANTAGES OF PCA AND PLS AND ALTERNATIVE STRATEGIES

There are a number of critical assumptions underlying PCA and PLS that do not always apply to biological data. The most critical assumption is that the independent variables are linearly related to each other and, in the case of PLSDA and PLSR, to the dependent response variables. There are many known biological relationships that are non-linear and these relationships may be poorly represented by linear dimensionality reduction. Another problem related to the linearity assumption is that PCA is not good at identifying and preserving nonlinear local structures in the data in the low-dimensional space. For example, imagine that over time, a biological temporal gene expression pattern follows a spiral structure. If PCA is applied to this sample, the temporal "order" of these points along the spiral (and therefore important biological information) will be lost.

A very simple way of incorporating nonlinear relationships between independent and dependent variables into PLSDA and PLSR is to calculate nonlinear forms of the original measurements (squared terms, logarithms of terms, etc.) and add these to the data matrix of independent variables [6]. If higher-order relationships exist between the independent and dependent variables, then these nonlinear terms will be relatively important in the loadings vector.

There are also many nonlinear dimensionality reduction techniques that have been developed. One example is a technique called diffusion maps [7]. Diffusion maps use a "random-walk" approach in which the algorithm randomly explores directions in the high-dimensional Euclidean space to find all possible paths between any pair of samples. Using this approach it is possible to discover complex, nonlinear geometric structures and construct coordinates called **diffusion maps** that efficient represent these structures in a lower dimensional space. Diffusion maps built from multi-dimensional single-cell data have been used to identify the known stages of T-cell development in the thymus, including a non-linear bifurcation point that is associated with two different developmental pathways [8].

Another population nonlinear dimensionality reduction is t-distributed stochastic neighbor embedding (t-SNE) [9]. Again starting from the coordinates of samples in high-dimensional space, t-SNE uses the Euclidean distance between points to calculate the probability that these points are neighbors, and then these neighbor relationships are preserved in the low-dimensional space. t-SNE can identify both global structures, such as clusters, and local structures in the data matrix. Unlike PCA, t-SNE does not produce a model that can predict the coordinates of new data points in the low-dimensional space and is thus is only a visualization technique. t-SNE is a very popular technique for visualizing structures in high-dimensional single-cell transcriptomic and proteomic data [10].

4.10 DISCUSSION AND FUTURE DIRECTIONS

As illustrated in this chapter, PCA and associated data-driven modeling methods provide a means to infer systems-level interactions from high-throughput, multiplexed experimental data sets that are increasingly common in immunology research. PCA and PLS methods are well established, but discovering novel ways to use them to link disparate immunology data sets across temporal and physiological scales presents exciting opportunities for discovery. In closing, we discuss several distinct advantages of PCA, PLSR, and PLSDA that are especially relevant to immunology research, and briefly highlight studies that illustrate each advantage.

4.10.1 LINKING BIOLOGICAL EVENTS ACROSS PHYSIOLOGICAL SCALES

One advantage of data-driven modeling is that these approaches can associate molecular events to tissue-level phenotypes or cell behaviors. It is now clear that immune behavior and disease pathogenesis usually arise from complex networks of molecular and cellular interactions, rather than simple changes in individual protein levels or states. This presents two challenges to immunology research: (1) identifying key changes in complex networks of molecular and cellular interactions and (2) linking these multivariate interactions to events at different physiological scales (i.e., tissue-level behavior that directly contributes to disease states). PLSR and PLSDA models have the ability to address both of these challenges by identifying critical network-level events in large data matrices (X), and then linking these events to important disease-relevant behavior at another physiological scale (Y). One example study used PLSDA models to find molecular signaling events underlying *in vivo* tissue phenotypes in an animal model of inflammatory bowel disease [11]. Results identified a signature of proteins in the ERK signaling pathway as key regulators of spatial and temporal differences in TNF-induced apoptosis. In this case the PLSDA approach was necessary to identify multivariate relationships between ERK signaling events and also to link them to *in vivo* tissue phenotypes of apoptosis and proliferation.

4.10.2 IMPROVED DIAGNOSIS OR CLASSIFICATION OF IMMUNE DISEASE STATES

The assessment of immune disease state or progression is critical for effective health care, but accurate assessments have been difficult to attain using individual immune parameters. PCA and other data-driven modeling approaches address this limitation by using multivariate parameter profiles, rather than individual parameters, to more accurately differentiate between disease progression states. Such a clinical classification can be useful even without providing insight into the underlying mechanisms. The PLSR example reviewed in this text is an illustration of this application [5]. A PLSR model to predict CD8+ T cell age from intracellular signaling measurements is of high value for clinical applications of cell selection for adoptive T cell therapy, even though mechanistic insight was not the focus of the study.

4.10.3 CONNECTING IMMUNE SIGNALING EVENTS OVER TIME

Molecular and protein signaling events in immune cells evolve dynamically to produce cell and tissue phenotypes and disease-related changes. Given experimental data from multiple time points, it is often difficult to identify dynamic network-level changes that are related to each other in time. PCA, PLSR, and PLSDA provide a means to do this by integrating data across time points that best differentiate based on disease state or treatment. One illustration of this is the PLSDA example outlined in this chapter, in which alterations in cytokine communication networks of HIV-infected individual were linked to each other in time to identify events that were especially important to development of the altered dynamic immune response [4].

4.10.4 ABILITY TO INTEGRATE DIVERSE DATA SETS

Given the wide range of high-throughput experimental assays now available to measure immune parameters, it is often difficult to relate measurements made in one assay to those of another assay. PCA and associated approaches can be used to identify multivariate relationships between immune parameters measured in different experimental assays. For example, antibody titers and neutralization measurements have traditionally been used to identify successful vaccines, however neither has been useful in developing an effective HIV vaccine, or in differentiating HIV vaccine regimens. One example study found that a PLSDA model of combined measurements of antibody titer, neutralization, and other Fc-mediated activity assay measurements was able to differentiate four HIV vaccine regimens with high accuracy, and additionally pinpointed critical relationships between antibody properties measured in different assays that were associated with different regimens and correlative of protection [12]. Previous studies that compartmentalized evaluations of antibody measurements made in different experimental assays were unable to make this advance.

REFERENCES

1. Newell, E.W., Sigal, N., Bendall, S.C., Nolan, G.P., and Davis M.M. (2012). Cytometry by time-of-flight shows combinatorial cytokine expression and virus-specific cell niches within a continuum of CD8+ T cell phenotypes. *Immunity 36*, 142-152.

2. Janes, K.A., Kelly, J.R., Gaudet, S., Albeck, J.G., Sorger, P.K., and Lauffenburger, D.A. (2004). Cue-signal-response analysis of TNF-induced apoptosis by partial least squares regression of dynamic multivariate data. *J Comput Biol 11*, 544-561.

3. Tibshirani, R. (1996). Regression shrinkage and selection via the lasso. *Journal of the Royal Statistical Society. Series B (Methodological) 58*, 267-288.

4. Arnold, K.B., Szeto, G.L., Alter, G., Irvine, D.J., and Lauffenburger, D.A. (2015). CD4+ T cell-dependent and CD4+ T cell-independent cytokine-chemokine network changes in the immune responses of HIV-infected individuals. *Science Signaling 8*, ra104.

5. Rivet, C.A., Hill, A.S., Lu, H., and Kemp, M.L. (2011). Predicting cytotoxic T-cell age from multivariate analysis of static and dynamic biomarkers. *Mol Cell Proteomics 10*, M110 003921.

6. Martens, H., and Martens, M. (2001). *Multivariate Analysis of Quality: An Introduction*. John Wiley & Sons.

7. Coifman, R.R., and Lafon, S. (2006). Diffusion maps. *Appl Comput Harmon A 21*, 5-30.

8. Setty, M., Tadmor, M.D., Reich-Zeliger, S., Angel, O., Salame, T.M., Kathail, P., Choi, K., Bendall, S., Friedman, N., Pe'er, D. (2016). Wishbone identifies bifurcating developmental trajectories from single-cell data. *Nat Biotechnol 34*, 637-645.

9. van der Maaten, L., and Hinton, G. (2008). Visualizing Data using t-SNE. *J Mach Learn Res 9*, 2579-2605.

10. Amir el, A.D., Davis, K.L., Tadmor, M.D., Simonds, E.F., Levine, J.H., Bendall, S.C., Shenfeld, D.K., Krishnaswamy, S., Nolan, G.P., and Pe'er, D. (2013). viSNE enables visualization of high dimensional single-cell data and reveals phenotypic heterogeneity of leukemia. *Nat Biotechnol 31*, 545-552.

11. Lau, K.S., Cortez-Retamozo, V., Philips, S.R., Pittet, M.J., Lauffenburger, D.A., and Haigis, K.M. (2012). Multi-scale in vivo systems analysis reveals the influence of immune cells on TNF-alpha-induced apoptosis in the intestinal epithelium. *PLoS Biol 10*, e1001393.

12. Chung, A.W., Kumar, M.P., Arnold, K.B., Yu, W.H., Schoen, M.K., Dunphy, L.J., Suscovich, T.J., Frahm, N., Linde, C., Mahan, A.E., Hoffner, M., Streeck, H., Ackerman, M.E., McElrath, M.J., Schuitemaker, H., Pau, M.G., Baden, L.R., Kim, J.H., Michael, N.L., Barouch, D.H., Lauffenburger, D.A., and Alter, G. (2015). Dissecting polyclonal vaccine-induced humoral immunity against HIV using systems serology. *Cell 163*, 988-998.

FURTHER READING

Martens, H. and Martens, M. (2001). *Multivariate Analysis of Quality: An Introduction*. John Wiley & Sons.

Eriksson, L., Byrne, T., Johansson, E., Trygg, J., and Vikström, C. (2013). *Multi- and Megavariate Data Analysis: Basic Principles and Applications* (3rd Revised ed.). Umetrics Academy.

Geladi, P. (1986). Partial Least-squares regression: A tutorial. *Analytica Chimica Acta 185*, 1-17.

An introduction to rule-based modeling of immune receptor signaling

JOHN A.P. SEKAR AND JAMES R. FAEDER

5.1 INTRODUCTION

It is well known that cells process external and internal signals through chemical interactions (Lodish et al., 2008; Nelson and Cox, 2013). Cells that constitute the immune system can be of many different types, such as antigen presenting cell, T-cell, B-cell, mast cell, etc. Each of these cells can have different functions, such as adaptive memory or inflammatory response, and the type and functionality of the cell is largely determined by the type and number of receptor molecules on the cell surface and the specific intracellular signaling pathways activated by those receptors (Owen et al., 2013). Given a particular biochemical signaling system in a particular immune cell, explicitly modeling and simulating kinetic interactions between molecules allows us to pose questions about system dynamics under various conditions (Aldridge et al., 2006). A model that recapitulates current experimental data can then be used to predict the results of future experiments and perturbations, and this cycle of model prediction and verification can lead to a better understanding of the system and potential clinical applications (Kitano, 2002). The promise of a mechanistic understanding has led to the enthusiastic application of chemical kinetics to biochemical signaling systems, but it has been limited by the complexity of the systems under consideration (Hlavacek et al., 2003; Borisov et al., 2005). Rule-based modeling is an approach to building and simulating chemical kinetic models that addresses this complexity (Sekar and Faeder, 2012; Chylek et al., 2013). BioNetGen (Hlavacek et al., 2006; Faeder et al., 2009), Kappa (Danos et al., 2007a, 2007b), and Simmune (Meier-Schellersheim et al., 2006; Zhang et al., 2013) are some of the more widely-used rule based frameworks. PySB provides a Python framework for rule-based modeling that uses BioNetGen or Kappa to generate models (Lopez et al., 2013). In this chapter, we will explore the origins of complexity in macromolecular interactions, show how rule-based modeling can be used to address complexity, and demonstrate the construction of a model in the BioNetGen framework. Open source BioNetGen software and documentation are available at http://bionetgen.org. We highly recommend that users start with RuleBender (Smith et al., 2012), which is a graphical user interface for BioNetGen that has text highlighting and syntax checking as well as interactive visualization and simulation capabilities.

5.2 ORIGINS OF COMPLEXITY

For this chapter, we will consider a model of signaling from the FcεRI receptor present in mast cells (Faeder et al., 2003), which we will refer to as "the FcεRI model." Degranulation of mast cells and basophils plays an important role in allergic immune response and this is initiated by signaling from FcεRI receptors on those cells. These receptors recognize the Fc portion of IgE antibodies whose Fab portion binds antigens. The activating ligand molecule is a single antigen bound to multiple antibodies, thereby providing multiple Fc sites to bind FcεRI receptors. When two or more receptors are crosslinked by a ligand, a sequence of binding and phosphorylation events on the cytoplasmic side lead to activation of Syk kinase, which subsequently promotes the degranulation response (Siraganian et al., 2010). Faeder et al. (2003) examined the dose response of Syk activation to ligand concentration and use four molecule types: a ligand, the FcεRI receptor, Lyn kinase, and Syk kinase.

The structural assumptions underlying the FcεRI model are summarized in Figure 5.1a. The model considers a bivalent ligand, i.e., one with two Fc sites for the FcεRI receptor. The receptor itself is made up of three chains: the α subunit capable of binding ligand, the β subunit capable of binding Lyn, and the γ subunit capable of binding Syk. The β and γ subunits have phosphorylation sites present on them, and we assume that the functional states for the subunits are "phosphorylated" and "unphosphorylated." On Lyn kinase, we consider two domains: a unique domain U capable of binding unphosphorylated β subunit of receptor weakly and an SH2 domain that binds the phosphorylated β subunit strongly. On Syk kinase, we consider three domains: a tSH2 domain that binds phosphorylated γ subunit of receptor, a group of phosphorylation motifs on the activation loop of the Syk kinase, and another group of phosphorylation motifs present in a linker region on Syk. Activation loop phosphorylation is known to activate the kinase activity of Syk, whereas linker phosphorylation is presumed to have a modulatory effect. Syk phosphorylated on activation loop can be considered the output of this system.

The reaction mechanisms in the model are summarized in Figure 5.1b. A dimer is formed by the bivalent ligand crosslinking two receptors. Lyn binds weakly using the U domain, and in the dimer form, it phosphorylates the β and γ subunits of the adjacent receptor. The phosphorylated β domain can bind Lyn strongly via its SH2 domain, which leads to increased Lyn-dependent phosphorylation. The phosphorylated γ domain recruits Syk, and recruited Syk is phosphorylated in two ways: on the activation loop by Lyn recruited to the adjacent receptor and on the linker region by Syk recruited to the adjacent receptor. The model makes conservative assumptions about how binding processes influence each other, i.e., it assumes that ligand-binding, Lyn-binding, and Syk-binding events can happen independent of each other as long as the receptor they bind to has the necessary binding site exposed. Similarly, it assumes that Syk binding to receptor happens independent of its phosphorylation status. Given additional information, it is possible to modify these assumptions in the rule-based model and add context to binding events, but we will use the originally published assumptions (Faeder et al., 2003) for the purposes of this chapter.

The independence assumptions lead to many valid combinations of molecules, states, and bonds that can coexist, and this leads to a large state space of chemical species, i.e., a large number of unique molecules and complexes. This phenomenon is called combinatorial complexity (Hlavacek et al., 2003), and Figure 5.2 shows an accounting of the possible species that can form in the FcεRI model given the interactions in the model. There are four variants of the free Syk molecule not bound to anything else because of two phosphorylation motifs on Syk that can each be phosphorylated or unphosphorylated (2x2). Similarly, there are four variants of

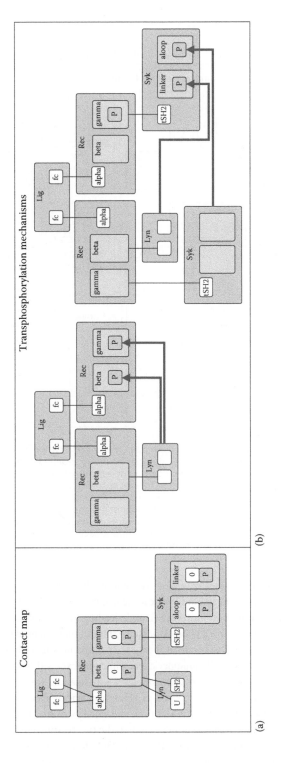

Figure 5.1 Overview of the FcɛRI model. **(a)** Contact Map. This diagram summarizes the molecules, sites, and binding interactions in the system. The ligand has two identical sites named fc that bind the receptor. The receptor has alpha, beta, and gamma subunits, each modeled as a site of the receptor. The alpha subunit is used to bind the ligand, the beta subunit to bind Lyn kinase, and gamma subunit to bind Syk kinase. beta and gamma subunit have phosphorylated (P) and unphosphorylated (0) states available to them. Lyn can bind receptor either through its U domain or its SH2 domain. Syk binds receptor through its tSH2 domain. Syk has two groups of phosphorylation sites, titled aloop and linker respectively which take unphosphorylated and phosphorylated states. **(b)** Transphosphorylation mechanisms. Receptors can be crosslinked to form dimers by the bivalent ligand. Lyn bound on one receptor can phosphorylate beta and gamma subunits on the adjacent (trans) receptor. Similarly, Syk bound to one receptor is phosphorylated by Lyn and Syk bound to the other.

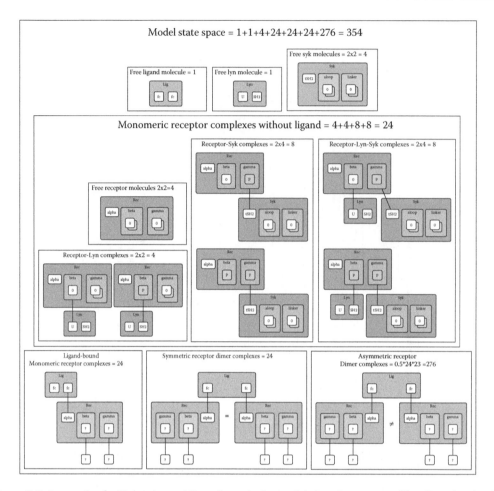

Figure 5.2 Accounting for Molecules and Complexes. In the model, there is one type of free ligand molecule, and one type of free Lyn molecule respectively. Because sites can be independently phosphorylated, there are four types of free Syk molecules and four types of free receptor molecules respectively. Lyn binding to free receptor gives rise to four Rec-Lyn complexes. Syk binding to free receptor leads to eight Rec-Syk complexes. Syk binding to Rec-Lyn leads to eight Rec-Lyn-Syk complexes. In total, there are 24 complexes that have one receptor to which no ligand is bound, called 24 monomeric receptor complexes. When free ligand binds, this leads to 24 ligand-bound monomers. On crosslinked dimers, symmetry between the two recruited monomeric receptors leads to 24 symmetric dimers. When the recruited monomeric receptors are asymmetric, there are 276 combinations that are possible, leading to 276 asymmetric dimers.

free receptor molecule not bound to anything else because of two subunits that can each be phosphorylated or unphosphorylated (2x2). All four free receptors can bind Lyn, leading to four receptor-Lyn complexes. Two free receptors are γ-phosphorylated and can bind four forms of Syk each, leading to eight receptor-Syk complexes (2x4). Similarly, two receptor-Lyn complexes have a phosphorylated γ subunit that can bind four forms of Syk, leading to eight receptor-Lyn-Syk complexes (2x4). In total there are 24 different complexes in which there is exactly one receptor and zero ligand, which we call monomeric receptor complexes without ligand. By binding a free ligand to each of these, we get 24 monomeric receptor complexes with ligand. Dimers, which are formed by a ligand crosslinking two monomeric receptor complexes, can be symmetric or asymmetric. On the symmetric dimer, the two recruited monomeric receptors are identical, and since there are 24 monomeric receptor types, there are also 24 symmetric dimers. On the asymmetric dimer, the two recruited monomeric receptors are dissimilar, and there are 276 such dissimilar pairs available (24x23/2), leading to 276 asymmetric dimer complexes. In total there are 48 monomeric receptor complexes (24+24) and 300 dimer complexes (24+276). Including free ligand, free Lyn, and four forms of free Syk, there are 354 chemical species in the system.

5.3 MOLECULES IN BIONETGEN ARE STRUCTURED OBJECTS THAT CAN COMBINE TO FORM COMPLEXES

Rule-based models can handle the combinatorics of large chemical state spaces automatically without manual curation. In the standard reaction formalism, each chemical species needs to have a unique label assigned by the modeler, but in the rule-based formalism, each chemical species is a structured graph that can be synthesized by a formal algorithm subject to the rules specified in the model. The structural building blocks for chemical species in a BioNetGen model are molecules, components of molecules, internal states of components, and bonds between pairs of components. The `molecule types` block in a BioNetGen model file specifies the types of molecules, components, and internal states.

```
begin molecule types
        Lig(fc,fc)
        Rec(alpha,beta~0~P,gamma~0~P)
        Lyn(U,SH2)
        Syk(tSH2,linker~0~P,aloop~0~P)
end molecule types
```

Here, `Lig`, `Rec`, `Lyn`, and `Syk` refer to the names of the types of molecules. The number and type of each molecular component is specified within brackets. The ligand `Lig` has two components named `fc` referring to binding sites for receptor. Since both sites are named identically, any attribute applicable to `fc` anywhere in the model will be equivalently applied to both sites on `Lig`. The receptor `Rec` has three components `alpha`, `beta`, and `gamma`, and the `~{string}` notation denotes the internal states available to `beta` and `gamma` components, which are `~0` representing unphosphorylated and `~P` representing phosphorylated respectively. `Lyn` is defined to have two components `U` and `SH2`. `Syk` is defined to have three components `tSH2`, `linker`, and `aloop`, with `linker` and `aloop` being allowed to take unphosphorylated and phosphorylated states.

All molecular variants that exist in the model are derived from permutations of internal states defined in the `molecule types` block. In this case, Lyn has one only one variant, Lyn(U,SH2), whereas the receptor has four possible variants, `Rec(alpha,beta~0,gamma~0)`, `Rec(alpha,beta~0,gamma~P)`, `Rec(alpha,beta~P,gamma~0)`, and `Rec(alpha,beta~P,gamma~P)`. Complexes are synthesized by joining molecules using bonds between pairs of components, which is denoted using the ! symbol followed by a bond index. Shown below are three species of increasing size:

```
Rec(alpha,beta~0,gamma~0)
Rec(alpha,beta~0!1,gamma~0).Lyn(U!1,SH2)
Rec(alpha,beta~0!1,gamma~P!2).Lyn(U!1,SH2).Syk(tSH2!2,aloop~0,linker~0)
```

The first species contains a single `Rec` molecule with nothing bound and all sites unphosphorylated (i.e., with states `~0`). The second species has two molecules `Lyn` and unphosphorylated `Rec`, and these are bound via their respective `U` and `beta` components. The bond label `!1` is placed adjacent to `beta` and `U` components to show that there is a binding interaction between them. The third species has three molecules, `Lyn`, `Syk`, and `Rec`, that are bound together by a bond `!1` between `U` and `beta` components and a bond `!2` between `gamma` and `tSH2` components, with `gamma` phosphorylated as indicated by the state `~P`. Arbitrarily large complexes can be constructed in this manner and the process can be automated as discussed below.

5.4 PATTERNS SELECT SPECIES WITH SHARED FEATURES

The advantage of using a structured graph specification for chemical species such as molecules and complexes is that it is possible to refer to multiple species by specifying a shared subgraph. Such a subgraph is called a **pattern** in BioNetGen and serves as a tool to partition the state space into matching versus non-matching chemical species without having to enumerate the full state space of species. Because both patterns and chemical species are graphs constructed from the same fundamental elements, one can define patterns to match any set of structural features in any arrangement of molecules within a complex, and the specified pattern may be matched by any number of molecules and complexes.

Shown below is a pattern that selects free ligand, i.e., ligand with both sites unbound.

```
Lig(fc,fc)
```

This pattern matches exactly one chemical species in the model: the free ligand molecule (Figure 5.3a).

```
Lig(fc,fc)
```

Next, we show a pattern that selects receptors with an unbound alpha domain.

```
Rec(alpha)
```

Note that we have omitted the other receptor components beta and gamma, which means that their binding and modification states will not affect selection of matching species. This pattern matches 24 species in the model (unligated monomeric receptor complexes in Figure 5.2), three of which are shown below and also visualized in Figure 5.3b.

```
Rec(alpha,beta~0,gamma~0)
Rec(alpha,beta~0!1,gamma~0).Lyn(U!1,SH2)
Rec(alpha,beta~0!1,gamma~P!2).Lyn(U!1,SH2).Syk(tSH2!2,aloop~0,linker~0)
```

Next, we show a pattern that selects ligand-containing complexes in which one site on the ligand is free, but the other is bound to a receptor:

```
Lig(fc,fc!0).Rec(alpha!0)
```

This pattern matches 24 species in the model (ligand-bound monomeric receptor complexes in Figure 5.2), three of which are shown below and also visualized in Figure 5.3c.

```
Lig(fc,fc!0).Rec(alpha!0,beta~0,gamma~0)
Lig(fc,fc!0).Rec(alpha!0,beta~0!1,gamma~0).Lyn(U!1,SH2)
Lig(fc,fc!0).Rec(alpha!0,beta~0!1,gamma~P!2).Lyn(U!1,SH2).
                            Syk(tSH2!2,aloop~0,linker~0)
```

In the full model, the patterns Rec(alpha) and Lig(fc,fc!0).Rec(alpha!0) will match all 24 monomeric receptor complexes and 24 ligand-bound monomers respectively, whose accounting was performed in Figure 5.2.

The BioNetGen pattern syntax enables flexible selection of different chemical species based on which structural features are specified. As discussed previously, omitting a component implies that neither its binding nor internal states will be used as match criteria. It is also possible to specify the binding state but not the internal state, e.g., Rec(beta) will match complexes with an unbound beta domain, both beta~0 and beta~P. Similarly, it is also possible to specify the internal state if present, but leave the binding state unspecified (!?) or partially specified (!+). Here, !? matches both bound and unbound states of components, and !? matches all bonds with that component type irrespective of binding partner.

5.5 REACTION RULES DEFINE INTERACTIONS BETWEEN MOLECULES AND CAN GENERATE REACTIONS

Reaction mechanisms specified in the BioNetGen language are called **reaction rules**. A reaction rule has five parts: (1) an optional label, (2) patterns specifying the properties reactants must possess to be selected by the

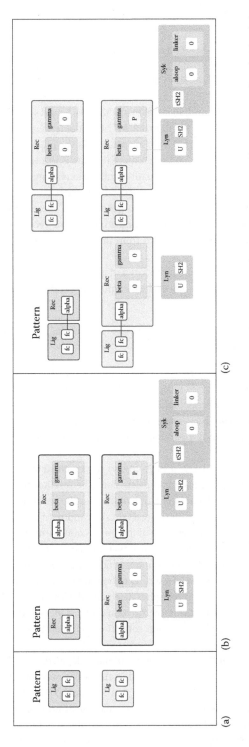

Figure 5.3 Shown are three patterns and how they match various chemical species (molecules and complexes). **(a)** Pattern Lig(fc,fc) specifies that both fc sites are unbound. It matches one species: free ligand. **(b)** Pattern Rec(alpha) specifies that alpha site on receptor is unbound. In the FceRI model, it matches 24 unligated monomeric receptor complexes, three of which are shown here. **(c)** Pattern Lig(fc,fc!0).Rec(alpha!0) specifies that of two fc sites on the ligand; one is unbound and the other is bound to a receptor alpha site. It matches 24 ligand-bound monomeric receptor complexes in the FceRI model, three of which are shown here.

rule, (3) an arrow indicating whether or not the rule is reversible, (4) patterns specifying the products to indicate how reactants are transformed by the rule, and (5) a set of rate laws that govern the kinetics of each reaction generated by the rule. Shown below is a reaction rule involving the three patterns specified above:

```
R1:     Lig(fc,fc) + Rec(alpha) <-> Lig(fc,fc!0).Rec(alpha!0)      kp1,km1
```

The rule is visualized in Figure 5.4a. Here, R1 is the name of the rule. The rule is bidirectional because of the use of the reversible arrow (<->). Lig(fc,fc) and Rec(alpha) are the reactant patterns. Lig(fc,fc) specifies that both sites on ligand are unbound, so it will match the free ligand species. Rec(alpha) matches receptors with an unbound alpha domain, so it will match all 24 monomeric receptor complexes that do not have a bound ligand. The pattern Lig(fc,fc!0).Rec(alpha!0) is the product of the rule. By examining it relative to the reactants, BioNetGen infers that the action of the rule is to add a bond between an available fc site and alpha subunit and can apply the rule to all combinations of matched reactant species. Since Lig(fc,fc) and Rec(alpha) match 1 and 24 species respectively, the reaction rule generates 1×24 ligand-binding reactions. Application of the rule in reverse also generates all corresponding ligand dissociation reactions, i.e., the 24 reactions that result in free ligand and a monomeric receptor complex. kp1 and km1 are the rate constants applicable to reactions generated from the forward and reverse directions of the rule respectively.

Unidirectional rules can be specified by using the forward arrow (->) and specifying only one rate constant. An example of a unidirectional rule is shown below, modeling transphosphorylation of receptor by recruited Lyn:

```
R4:     Lyn(U!1).Rec(beta!1,alpha!2).Lig(fc!2,fc!3).Rec(alpha!3,beta~0)->   \
        Lyn(U!1).Rec(beta!1,alpha!2).Lig(fc!2,fc!3).Rec(alpha!3,beta~P)      pLb
```

The rule named R4 is visualized in Figure 5.4b. Here, the reactant pattern shows four molecules connected by three bonds: a ligand bound to two receptors and Lyn bound to one of the receptors. The other receptor is phosphorylated on the free beta component, i.e., transformed from ~0 on the reactant side to ~P on the product side (shown in red). The gamma components on the receptors are omitted since they do not explicitly affect this process. pLb is a parameter that specifies the first order phosphorylation rate constant.

Because patterns used in rules can get large, it helps to sort the specified structures into **reaction center** and **reaction context** to aid their comprehension and discussion. The reaction center is the set of structures that are modified by the rule and thereby defines the action of the rule. The reaction center of rule R1 specified above is the set of binding sites fc and alpha on the reactant side, and the fc-alpha bond on the product side. The reaction center of rule R4 is the internal state of the beta component that was modified from ~0 to ~P. The reaction context includes the remaining structures that are specified in the rule but are not modified by the rule. This establishes the set of local conditions under which the action of the rule is allowed to happen. For rule R1, the reaction context is the presence of a second unbound fc site. For rule R4, the reaction context is the unbound status of the beta site that was phosphorylated and the set of three bonds that constitute the Lyn-recruited-to-dimer configuration. Given a rule, the reaction center is identified by the differences between the reactants and products of the rule and the reaction context is identified by structures preserved on both reactants and products.

Rules interact with each other when the reaction center of one rule overlaps with the reaction context of another. For example, the fc-alpha bond that is formed in rule R1 is necessary for the Lyn-recruited-to-dimer configuration that is context for rule R4, implying that R1 enables R4. These interactions constitute the flow of signal through the system and reaction rules enable reconstituting a signaling pathway from the fundamental kinetic processes. The FceRI model used in this chapter has 19 reaction rules: 1 for ligand-binding, 1 for receptor crosslinking by ligand, 2 for Lyn binding to receptor, 2 for Syk binding to receptor, 6 for transphosphorylation by Lyn on receptor and Syk sites, 2 for transphosphorylation by Syk on Syk, and

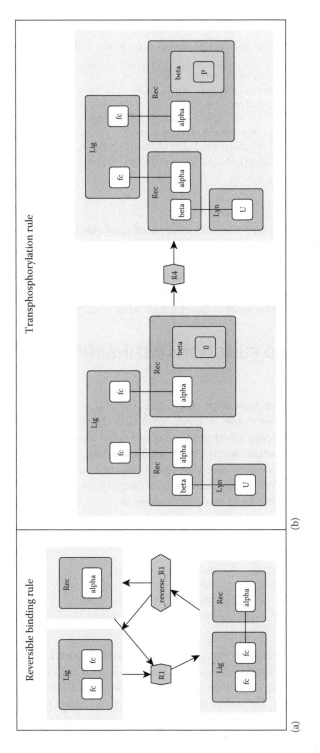

Figure 5.4 Reaction Rules. In a reaction rule, only the parts necessary for a kinetic process need to be specified. **(a)** Reversible Binding. Reaction rule R1 models reversible binding of free ligand and receptor. On the receptor pattern, only alpha subunit is specified because of the assumed independence between ligand-binding and other binding processes. **(b)** Transphosphorylation Rule. Reaction rule R4 models phosphorylation of beta domain by Lyn recruited to the adjacent (trans) receptor in a dimer. The pattern used indicates the minimum conditions for this process: a cross-linked dimer, an unphosphorylated beta domain substrate on side of the dimer, and Lyn bound to beta domain on the other side.

6 for background dephosphorylation processes, respectively. In the BioNetGen model file, rules are listed in the `reaction rules` block:

```
begin reaction rules
# Ligand-receptor binding
R1: Rec(alpha) + Lig(fc,fc) <-> Rec(alpha!1).Lig(fc!1,fc)  kp1, km1
# Receptor-aggregation
R2: Rec(alpha) + Lig(fc,fc!0).Rec(alpha!0) <-> \
Rec(alpha!1).Lig(fc!1,fc!0).Rec(alpha!0)  kp2, km2
# Constitutive Lyn-receptor binding
R3: Rec(beta~0) + Lyn(U,SH2) <-> Rec(beta~0!1).Lyn(U!1,SH2)  kpL, kmL
# Transphosphorylation of beta by constitutive Lyn
R4: Lyn(U!1).Rec(beta!1,alpha!2).Lig(fc!2,fc!3).Rec(alpha!3,beta~0)->\
Lyn(U!1).Rec(beta!1,alpha!2).Lig(fc!2,fc!3).Rec(alpha!3,beta~P) pLb
...
...
end reaction rules
```

Text beginning with # and ending on a line break can be used to provide useful comments and annotations anywhere in the model, and they are ignored by the BioNetGen processor. The character \ can be used to split rules across lines when the rules get really large. Within patterns, the order of components between brackets does not matter. Similarly, the specific bond index used for bonds does not matter, as long as the intended pair of components has the same unique bond index. BioNetGen also allows more complex specifications for the rate law that are out of the scope of this chapter (Chylek et al., 2015).

5.6 OBSERVABLES AND FUNCTIONS DEFINE THE OUTPUTS OF THE MODEL

There are two types of outputs in the BioNetGen model: measurements of species concentrations called observables and functions of those observables. In a rule-based model, pattern matching can be exploited to generate sums of species automatically. Observables are of two types: counting unique complexes only, or counting individual matches of patterns within complexes. These are specified using the `Species` and `Molecule` keywords respectively within the observables block. For the FcεRI model, we are interested in the partitioning of individual receptor and Syk molecules into various configurations, so we will only use `Molecule` observables. The observables block used for this model is:

```
begin observables
      Molecules     Dimer       Rec(alpha!1).Lig(fc!1,fc!2).Rec(alpha!2)
      Molecules     TotalRec    Rec()
      Molecules     ActiveSyk   Syk(aloop~P)
      Molecules     TotalSyk    Syk()
      Molecules     BetaP       Rec(beta~P!?)
      Molecules     GammaP      Rec(gamma~P!?)
end observables
```

Here, the pattern Rec(alpha!1).Lig(fc!1,fc!2).Rec(alpha!2) counts all ligand-crosslinked dimer species, of which there are 300 types in the model. Since it is a `Molecule` observable and the pattern will match twice into each dimer, each dimer will be counted twice and the resultant sum will be the total number of receptors in dimers. The pattern Syk(aloop~P) counts number of Syk molecules with phosphorylated activation loop, and the patterns Rec(beta~P!?) and Rec(gamma~P!?) count receptor molecules that are respectively phosphorylated on beta and gamma. Here !? was used to ensure that the observable counted both unbound and bound forms of beta and gamma components. This was not necessary for aloop since there are no binding rules specified for aloop. Also, the two observables for β and γ

phosphorylation will have some species that are counted for both observables since receptors can be phosphorylated on both `beta` and `gamma` sites. Finally, observables `Rec()` and `Syk()` simply count all receptor molecules and Syk molecules in the system respectively, as no component-matching terms are specified.

Functions of observables can be defined in the `functions` block. For the FcεRI model, we will consider three outputs: fraction of receptor in dimers, fraction of Syk that is active (i.e., phosphorylated on the activation loop), and ratio of phosphorylated gamma and beta sites on receptors.

```
begin functions
        DimerFraction                     Dimer/TotalRec
        AutoPhosphorylatedSykFraction     ActiveSyk/TotalSyk
        GammaBetaPhosphorylationRatio     GammaP/BetaP
end functions
```

5.7 PARAMETERIZING A MODEL REQUIRES GEOMETRIC TERMS, RATE CONSTANTS, AND SPECIES CONCENTRATIONS

Parameterizing a BioNetGen model requires a self-consistent set of units for concentrations and rate constants. For this particular model, we have only used unimolecular and bimolecular reactions and we would like to measure protein fluxes in molecules per second. We will limit ourselves to considering a single cell surrounded by a milieu of freely diffusing ligand. We will also specify units as comments using # symbol in order to be clear to the modeler. These comments will be ignored by BioNetGen.

First, we will need to specify fundamental constants such as π and Avogadro's number N_A to be used in our calculations.

```
NA          6.023e23        # units: molecules/mol
pi          3.14159         # no unit
```

Next, we will need to specify concentrations of proteins and ligands that reflect the experimental setup. Ligand concentration for this system is typically provided in nanomolar values and has to be converted to molecule numbers. One molar concentration is one mol/liter, so the conversion is achieved by multiplying molar concentration with the Avogadro constant and volume of the external milieu, which in turn is estimated from a cell density of million cells per milliliter. A conversion factor of 1e3 is required to convert milliliter volumes to liters.

```
celldensity     1e6*1e3             # units: cells/L
vol_ext         1/celldensity       # units: L/cell*(1 cell) = L
Lig_conc        1e-9                # units: molar
Lig_tot         Lig_conc*vol_ext*NA # units: molecules
```

Receptor numbers are usually provided as molecule numbers per cell, so they are used directly. Lyn and Syk numbers are estimated relative to receptor numbers, so they are specified using proportional factors.

```
Rec_tot     4e5                 # units: molecules
fLyn        0.07
fSyk        1
Lyn_tot     fLyn*Rec_tot
Syk_tot     fSyk*Rec_tot
```

Unimolecular rate constants such as those for phosphorylation, dephosphorylation, and bond dissociation are usually known or estimated in per second units, so they can be used directly. Here, we show one example of each: ligand dissociation constant (km1), rate of β -phosphorylation by Lyn (pLb), and rate of background dephosphorylation at the membrane (dm).

```
km1             0.01    # units: /s
pLb             30      # units: /s
dm              20      # units: /s
```

Bimolecular association rate constants are usually provided in units of "per molar per second". Converting to per molecule per second requires dividing by Avogadro constant and the respective volume in which the bimolecular association occurs. We show three examples below: association rate constant for free ligand that needs to be scaled by external volume (kp1), association rate constant for ligand crosslinking that occurs in the membrane (kp2), and association rate constant for Lyn binding to unphosphorylated β site that occurs in the cytoplasm (kpL). For a simple BioNetGen model, scaling of association rate constants can be performed manually, but for more complicated systems it is recommended to use the compartmental extension to the BioNetGen framework (Harris et al., 2009a) where such scaling is performed automatically.

```
kp1     1e7/(NA*vol_ext)      # units: /molecule/s
kp2     1e6/(NA*vol_mem)      # units: /molecule/s
kpL     4.2e7/(NA*vol_cell)   # units: /molecule/s
```

External volume was calculated previously from cell density. Volume of the membrane is specified by multiplying surface area of the cell with an effective width of 10 nanometers (Harris et al., 2009a). Volume and surface area of the cell are both estimated by assuming a spherical cell with 7 micron radius. Cubic meter volume is converted to liter units by multiplying by 1e3.

```
rad_cell    7e-6                      # units: meter
vol_cell    1e3*(4/3)*pi*rad_cell^3   # units: L
surf_area   4*pi*rad_cell^2           # units: squared meter
eff_width   10e-9                     # units: meter
vol_mem     1e3*surf_area*eff_width   # units: L
```

Here, the association constant for membrane reactions (kp2) was specified as a three-dimensional association rate constant (units: per molar per second, i.e., per "mol per liter" per second), which necessitates a conversion of the two-dimensional surface area of the membrane to a three-dimensional volume using an effective width term. An alternate parameterization would be to use a two-dimensional association rate constant (units: per "mol per squared meter" per second), in which case it is sufficient to multiply by surface area only and not the effective width.

The parameters and parameter expressions are specified in the parameters block in the model file.

```
begin parameters
    NA              6.023e23                  # units: molecules/mol
    pi              3.14159
    rad_cell        7e-6                      # units: meter
    vol_cell        1e3*(4/3)*pi*rad_cell^3   # units: L
    celldensity     1e6*1e3                   # units: cells/L
    vol_ext         1/celldensity             # units: L/cell*(1 cell)= L
    Lig_conc        1e-9                      # units: molar
    Lig_tot         Lig_conc*vol_ext*NA       # units: molecules
    ...
    ...
end parameters
```

Initial concentrations for chemical species are specified in the seed species block. The concentrations can be specified in terms of parameter expressions defined in the parameters block.

```
begin seed species
     Lig(fc,fc)                            Lig_tot
     Lyn(U,SH2)                            Lyn_tot
     Syk(tSH2,linker~0,aloop~0)            Syk_tot
     Rec(alpha,beta~0,gamma~0)            Rec_tot
end seed species
```

In the seed species block, only fully defined molecules and complexes must be specified. In other words, every molecule should have every component present, and every component should have internal and binding states clearly specified. For this model, the unbound and unphosphorylated forms of all molecules are considered to be the seed species. Depending on how the system is simulated the remaining species that can occur in the system will either be generated by iterative application of the rules to the seed species by a process called network generation, or they will be discovered "on-the-fly" as the system is simulated and rules modify the state of the initial species (Faeder et al., 2009).

5.8 MODEL ACTIONS ARE USED TO SIMULATE AND ANALYZE A MODEL

The complete model specification has blocks for parameters, molecule types, reaction rules, observables, and seed species, and is stored in a text file with the extension ".bngl". Model actions are appended to the end of the model file in order to call tools that use the model specification. This enables the specified model to be converted into a reaction network, simulated using multiple available methods, exported to other frameworks, visualized at different resolutions, and also scanned over parameter ranges to reveal parameter sensitivity and bifurcation properties. A comprehensive actions and arguments guide is available at http://bionetgen .org. Here, we will discuss the use of three model actions: generate _ network(), simulate(), and parameter _ scan().

5.8.1 REACTION NETWORK CAN BE GENERATED FROM A RULE-BASED MODEL

The following action is used to generate a reaction network whose kinetics are equivalent to the specified rule-based model:

```
generate_network({overwrite=>1})
```

This command iteratively applies the reaction rules to the seed species in order to generate new configurations of molecules and complexes and new reactions (Faeder et al., 2009). The full state space of molecules, complexes, and reactions is written to a file with the extension ".net". The overwrite command is to ensure that when network generation is performed a second time, any past generated networks of the same model are overwritten. For the full model with four seed species and 19 rules, the generate _ network() action results in 354 total number of species and 3680 reactions (Faeder et al., 2003).

One of the features of network generation is that the calculation of statistical factors for reactions is handled automatically. For this reason, it is advantageous to build rule-based models even for small reaction networks. We will show using simple examples how BioNetGen handles symmetry and multiplicity.

Multiplicity factors are needed when the same rule can be applied to multiple identical parts of the same reactant species, which increases the effective rate by a factor. For example, consider the molecule types A(b) and B(a,a) and the reaction rule:

```
R_AB:   A(b) + B(a) <-> A(b!1).B(a!1) kf,kr
```

Now consider how to parameterize two pairs of reversible binding reactions generated from the rule: binding in which both sites on B are free, and binding in which one of the sites is already occupied.

```
A(b)  + B(a,a)          <->     A(b!1).B(a!1,a)
A(b)  + B(a,a!1).A(a!1) <->     A(b!2).B(a!2,a!1).A(b!1)
```

The pattern B(a) matches to species B(a,a) in two different ways, i.e., using one or the other free binding site. This means that the effective rate of the reaction is double what one would expect if there was only one free site on B. BioNetGen would detect this and calculate a multiplicity factor of 2 for the forward reaction, i.e.:

```
A(b)  + B(a,a)          <->     A(b!1).B(a!1,a)                    2*kf,kr
```

For the second pair of reactions, the product pattern A(b!1).B(a!1) would match twice into the species A(b!2).B(a!2,a!1).A(b!1)since there are two identical bonds that could be matched. In this case, it is the reverse reaction that needs to be multiplied by two, since the presence of two identical bonds would double the effective rate of bond breaking, i.e.:

```
A(b)  + B(a,a!1).A(a!1) <-> A(b!2).B(a!2,a!1).A(b!1)   kf,2*kr
```

Symmetry factors are needed when the action of a rule modifies at least two instances of a species simultaneously and identically. For example, consider the molecule type A(b~0~1) and the reaction rule:

```
R_AA:   A(b)  + A(b)  -> A(b!1).A(b!1)   kf
```

The reaction rule would generate three reactions:

```
A(b~0)  + A(b~1)  -> A(b~0!1).A(b~1!1)
A(b~0)  + A(b~0)  -> A(b~0!1).A(b~0!1)
A(b~1)  + A(b~1)  -> A(b~1!1).A(b~1!1)
```

The first reaction involves two different reactant species: A(b~0) and A(b~1). If N_0 and N_1 are the concentrations of A(b~0) and A(b~1) respectively, then the first reaction would have a rate of $k_f N_0 N_1$.

The second reaction operates on two instances of the same species A(b~0), and the rate is determined to be $kf \frac{N_0(N_0-1)}{2}$, where $\frac{N_0(N_0-1)}{2}$ is the number of ways to select two molecules out of N_0 molecules. For high N_0, $k_f \frac{N_0(N_0-1)}{2} \approx k \frac{N_0^2}{2}$, but a rate calculation similar to the first reaction would only yield $k_f N_0^2$. Therefore, a factor of ½ needs to be applied for the second reaction and not the first. Similarly, the third reaction would also have an effective rate of $k_f \frac{N_1^2}{2}$ since it operates on two instances of the same species A(b~1). Using graph isomorphism calculations (Hogg et al., 2014), BioNetGen estimates the correct symmetric factor adjustment for the rate constants of all generated reactions, i.e.:

```
A(b~0)  + A(b~1)  -> A(b~0!1).A(b~1!1)   kf
A(b~0)  + A(b~0)  -> A(b~0!1).A(b~0!1)   0.5*kf
A(b~1)  + A(b~1)  -> A(b~1!1).A(b~1!1)   0.5*kf
```

5.8.2 MODEL SIMULATION AND PARAMETER SCANS REVEAL INSIGHT ABOUT MODEL BEHAVIOR

The specified model is simulated using the simulate() action.

```
simulate({method=>"ode",t_end=>600,n_steps=>10,print_functions=>1})
```

There are three simulation methods that can be used: ODE integration (method=>"ode"), Gillespie's stochastic simulation algorithm (method=>"ssa") (Gillespie, 1977) and network-free stochastic simulation (method=>"nf"). The ODE and SSA methods require the reaction network to be generated prior to simulation. Network-free simulation uses the NFsim algorithm (Sneddon et al., 2011), which was designed to exactly simulate kinetics without having to generate the full reaction network in advance of the simulation. It generates results indistinguishable from SSA and is useful for models that generate disproportionately large or infinite reaction networks, e.g., models with oligomerization rules. In these networks, the number of unique species may be much larger than the actual number of molecules and complexes present during simulation and only a fraction of the state space may be populated at any given time. In practical terms, the network-free simulation method typically leads to faster simulations than the corresponding SSA when the number of possible species is more than several hundred to a thousand (Sneddon et al., 2011).

The outputs of the simulate() action are trajectory files with extensions ".cdat" and ".gdat". The ".cdat" file is generated by ODE and SSA methods and contains concentrations of all molecules and complexes over time. The ".gdat" file is generated by all three methods and contains the measured values over time for the observables defined in the observables block. If the print_functions=>1 flag is used, then the ".gdat" files include columns for each of the specified functions in the functions block also. The trajectory files can be imported into any data-processing software such as Microsoft Excel, OpenOffice Calc, or MatLab.

BioNetGen provides additional actions in order to run multiple simulations of the same model at different parameter settings, such as setParameter(), setConcentrations(), resetConcentrations(), etc. It also provides a command to run batch simulations called parameter_scan(), which enables scanning over a particular parameter given a range of values while keeping other parameters constant. parameter_scan() takes the same arguments as simulate() shown above, and additionally takes arguments that specify the range of values to be scanned over and the reset behavior between simulations. The results of parameter_scan() are stored in a similar form to ".gdat" and ".cdat" files, but with the extension ".scan". Here, we show how parameter scans can be used to elucidate aspects of model behavior.

Shown in Figure 5.5 are results from three parameter scans for each of the three outputs defined in the functions block, i.e., receptor fraction in dimers, ratio of γ / β phosphorylation, and active Syk fraction. The parameter scan over ligand concentration was performed using the command:

```
parameter_scan({method=>"ode",parameter=>"Lig_conc",par_min=>1e-12, \
par_max=>1e-,n_scan_pts=>50, log_scale=>1,reset_conc=>1, \
print_functions=>1,t_end=>600,n_steps=>5})
```

Note that method, print_functions, t_end and n_steps arguments are used the same as in the simulate() command. Additionally, parameter specifies the parameter to scan over, par_min and par_max establish the minimum and maximum of the range of values to be used, n_scan_pts determines how many points to sample within the range. log_scale=>1 sets the spacing between points to be logarithmic, which enables scanning over many orders of magnitude. For smaller ranges, the default setting of log_scale=>0 is used, which ensures that the sampled points are spaced equally. reset_conc=>1 ensures that when a new simulation is run, all parameter values and species concentrations are reset instead of being carried over from the previous simulation. In the parameter_scan() command shown above, we enable scanning over ligand concentration from 1e-12 M to 1e-3 M. The other two parameter_scan() methods shown below scan over Lyn/receptor ratio and Syk/receptor ratio between the range of 0.01 to 10 and use the same remaining arguments as the first one. Action statements can also be split across multiple lines using the \ character.

```
parameter_scan({parameter=>"fLyn",par_min=>0.01,par_max=>10,\
n_scan_pts=>50,log_scale=>1,...})
parameter_scan({parameter=>"fSyk",par_min=>0.01,par_max=>10,\
n_scan_pts=>50,log_scale=>1,...})
```

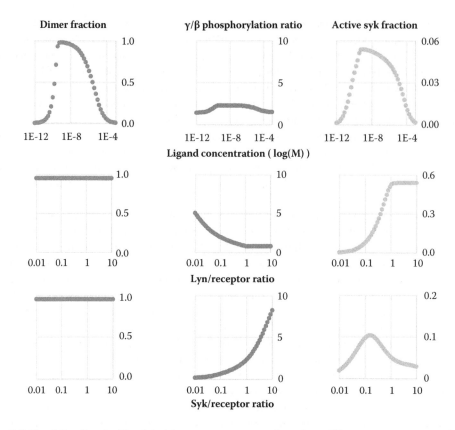

Figure 5.5 Simulation Results. Simulated dose-response curves from three different parameter scans (rows) of the model. For each scan, the outputs measured were fraction of receptors in dimers, ratio of phosphorylation between γ and β sites, and fraction of Syk that is active (columns). Varying ligand concentration showed that dimerization and Syk activation are inhibited at high ligand doses. Varying Lyn/receptor ratio showed that high concentrations of Lyn protect β sites from dephosphorylation. Varying Syk/receptor ratio showed that high concentrations of Syk protect γ sites from dephosphorylation.

In systems such as the FcεRI model where crosslinking by a ligand or scaffold is necessary for signaling, one can observe a phenomenon called high dose inhibition. As seen in Figure 5.5, at high concentrations of ligand, the fraction of receptors in dimers actually decreases to negligible values, and there is a corresponding decrease in the active Syk fraction. This phenomenon occurs because binding of free ligand competes with the crosslinking mechanism for free monomeric receptors, and free ligand binding dominates at high ligand concentrations, leading to decreased crosslinking and fewer dimers (Nag et al., 2010). Another mechanistic insight that can be derived for this system is the modulation of γ / β phosphorylation by Lyn and Syk numbers. In the model, β sites are phosphorylated by Lyn, as well as protected by Lyn-binding. On the other hand, γ sites are phosphorylated by Lyn, but protected by Syk-binding. As Lyn numbers increase, the ratio of γ / β phosphorylation decreases, since more β sites are being protected by Lyn-binding (Faeder et al., 2003). Similarly, as Syk numbers increase, the ratio of γ / β phosphorylation increases, since more γ sites are being protected by Syk-binding (Faeder et al., 2003).

5.9 ADVANCED METHODS

In the previous section, we covered elementary actions that can be applied to BioNetGen models, such as network generation and simulation by ODE, SSA (Gillespie, 1977), or NFsim (Sneddon et al., 2011). In addition to the basic specification demonstrated in this chapter, extensions to the BioNetGen language include specification of compartments and transport rules (Harris et al., 2009a), use of observables and local functions in rate laws (Sneddon et al., 2011), and preservation of detailed balance (Hogg, 2013). In addition to these, a number of improvements to simulation algorithms have been developed that are centered on the BioNetGen specification. For models where network-free simulation can occupy too much memory due to large numbers of certain molecules and complexes, a hybrid approach between network-based and network-free methods can be used (Hogg et al., 2014). The efficiency of each SSA simulation can be improved by enabling tau-leaping procedures (Harris et al., 2009b), and the sampling of rare stochastic events can be improved by weighted ensemble simulation (Donovan et al., 2013). A comprehensive BioNetGen actions and arguments guide is available at http://bionetgen.org.

A number of external software have interfaces to BioNetGen or utilize BioNetGen as a back end. These include modeling environments that facilitate model construction using programmatic, tabular, or graphical interfaces, such as VCell (Moraru et al., 2008), pySB (Lopez et al., 2013), rxncon (Tiger et al., 2012), and BioUML (Kolpakov et al., 2006). Parameter sensitivity analysis and fitting to experimental data can be performed for BioNetGen models using the ptempest toolbox for MatLab (Hogg, 2013) and the BioNetFit software (Thomas et al., 2015). Recently, we have developed advanced visualization tools for showcasing individual rules and interactions between rules (Sekar et al., 2017), ported BioNetGen model specification for the MCell simulator that explicitly simulates spatial diffusion and reactions (Stefan et al., 2014), and enabled conversion of reaction networks to rule-based specifications (Tapia and Faeder, 2013). Kappa (http://kappalanguage.org/) and Simmune (http://simmune.org) are other rule-based modeling frameworks with similar rule-based specifications to BioNetGen, and they have their own constellations of related tools and software. A common interchange format SBML-Multi is being developed to enable models to be translated and analyzed across rule-based frameworks (http://sbml.org).

5.10 RESOURCES

The BioNetWiki (http://bionetgen.org) is the main resource for all BioNetGen related tools. On the Downloads page, links are provided for the standalone BioNetGen distribution as well as the distribution bundled with RuleBender, a graphical user interface. Currently, precompiled packages are distributed for Windows, OSX, and Linux platforms. On the Tutorials page, one can find models that have been presented or published as parts of tutorials, including the model used in this chapter. For a comprehensive reference of BioNetGen syntax and usage, see Faeder, Blinov, and Hlavacek (2009). An updated online version is maintained on the wiki, with additional documentation on model visualization, bifurcation analysis, tau leaping, SBML import, and other advanced tools. Also on the wiki is a comprehensive reference for model actions and arguments used in BioNetGen. Sekar and Faeder (2012) provide a more detailed tutorial on BioNetGen that includes compartmental specification and the reconstruction of a large signaling pathway. Chylek et al. (2013) provide a current review of rule-based methods and Chylek et al. (2015) give examples that illustrate a number of advanced modeling features. The formalisms used in BioNetGen are explained in Blinov et al. (2006) and Hogg et al. (2014). For more detailed examples of rule-based models of immunoreceptor signaling, see the libraries of rules for FcεRI (Chylek et al., 2014b) and the large scale model of T cell receptor signaling (Chylek et al., 2014a), as well as Chapter 13 in this volume.

REFERENCES

Aldridge, B.B., Burke, J.M., Lauffenburger, D.A., and Sorger, P.K. (2006). Physicochemical modelling of cell signalling pathways. *Nat Cell Biol 8*, 1195-1203.

Blinov, M.L., Yang, J., Faeder, J.R., and Hlavacek, W.S. (2006). Graph theory for rule-based modeling of biochemical networks. In C. Priami, A. Ingolfsdottir, B. Mishra, H.R. Nielson (Eds.), *Transactions on Computational Systems Biology VII* (89-106). Berlin Heidelberg: Springer-Verlag Berlin Heidelberg.

Borisov, N.M., Markevich, N.I., Hoek, J.B., and Kholodenko, B.N. (2005). Signaling through receptors and scaffolds: Independent interactions reduce combinatorial complexity. *Biophys J 89*, 951-966.

Chylek, L.A., Akimov, V., Dengjel, J., Rigbolt, K.T.G., Hu, B., Hlavacek, W.S., and Blagoev, B. (2014a). Phosphorylation Site Dynamics of Early T–cell Receptor Signaling. *PLoS One 9*, e104240.

Chylek, L.A., Harris, L.A., Faeder, J.R., and Hlavacek, W.S. (2015). Modeling for (physical) biologists: An introduction to the rule-based approach. *Phys Biol 12*, 045007.

Chylek, L.A., Harris, L.A., Tung, C.-S., Faeder, J.R., Lopez, C.F., and Hlavacek, W.S. (2013). Rule-based modeling: A computational approach for studying biomolecular site dynamics in cell signaling systems. *Wiley Interdiscip Rev Syst Biol Med 6*, 13-36.

Chylek, L.A., Holowka, D.A., Baird, B.A., and Hlavacek, W.S. (2014b). An Interaction Library for the FcεRI Signaling Network. *Front Immunol 5*, 172.

Danos, V., Feret, J., Fontana, W., Harmer, R., and Krivine, J. (2007a). Rule-based Modelling of Cellular Signaling. In L. Caires, and V.T. Vasconcelos (Eds.), *CONCUR 2007 - Concurrency Theory, Lecture Notes in Computer Science* (17-41). Berlin Heidelberg: Springer-Verlag Berlin Heidelberg.

Danos, V., Feret, J., Fontana, W., and Krivine, J. (2007b). Scalable Simulation of Cellular Signaling Networks. In Z. Shao (Ed.), *Lect Notes Comput Sci 4807* (139-157). Berlin Heidelberg: Springer-Verlag Berlin Heidelberg.

Donovan, R.M., Sedgewick, A.J., Faeder, J.R., and Zuckerman, D.M. (2013). Efficient stochastic simulation of chemical kinetics networks using a weighted ensemble of trajectories. *J Chem Phys 139*, 115105.

Faeder, J.R., Blinov, M.L., and Hlavacek, W.S. (2009). Rule-based modeling of biochemical systems with BioNetGen. *Methods Mol Biol 500*, 113-167.

Faeder, J.R., Hlavacek, W.S., Reischl, I., Blinov, M.L., Metzger, H., Redondo, A., Wofsy, C., and Goldstein, B. (2003). Investigation of early events in Fc epsilon RI-mediated signaling using a detailed mathematical model. *J Immunol 170*, 3769-3781.

Gillespie, D.T. (1977). Exact stochastic simulation of coupled chemical reactions. *J Phys Chem 81*, 2340-2361.

Harris, L.A., Hogg, J.S., and Faeder, J.R. (2009a). Compartmental rule-based modeling of biochemical systems. In *Proceedings of the 2009 Winter Simulation Conference (WSC)* (908-919). IEEE.

Harris, L.A., Piccirilli, A.M., Majusiak, E.R., and Clancy, P. (2009b). Quantifying stochastic effects in biochemical reaction networks using partitioned leaping. *Phys Rev E - Stat Nonlinear, Soft Matter Phys 79*.

Hlavacek, W.S., Faeder, J.R., Blinov, M.L., Perelson, A.S., and Goldstein, B. (2003). The Complexity of Complexes in Signal Transduction. *Biotechnol Bioeng 84*, 783-794.

Hlavacek, W.S., Faeder, J.R., Blinov, M.L., Posner, R.G., Hucka, M., and Fontana, W. (2006). Rules for modeling signal-transduction systems. *Sci STKE signal Transduct Knowl Environ 2006*, re6.

Hogg, J.S. (2013). *Advances in Rule-Based Modeling: Compartments, Energy, and Hybrid Simulation, with Application to Sepsis and Cell Signaling*. (Unpublished Doctoral Dissertation). University of Pittsburgh, Pittsburgh, PA.

Hogg, J.S., Harris, L.A., Stover, L.J., Nair, N.S., and Faeder, J.R. (2014). Exact hybrid particle/population simulation of rule-based models of biochemical systems. *PLoS Comput Biol 10*, e1003544.

Kitano, H. (2002). Systems biology: A brief overview. *Science 295*, 1662-1664.

Kolpakov, F., Puzanov, M., and Koshukov, A. (2006). BioUML: Visual modeling, automated code generation and simulation of biological systems. In, *Proceedings of The Fifth International Conference on Bioinformatics of Genome Regulation and Structure* (281-284).

Lodish, H.F., Berk, A., Zipursky, S.L., Matsudaira, P., Baltimore, D., and James, D. (2008). *Molecular Cell Biology* (6th ed.). New York, NY: W.H. Freeman.

Lopez, C.F., Muhlich, J.L., Bachman, J.A., and Sorger, P.K. (2013). Programming biological models in Python using PySB. *Mol Syst Biol 9*, 646.

Meier-Schellersheim, M., Xu, X., Angermann, B., Kunkel, E.J., Jin, T., and Germain, R.N. (2006). Key role of local regulation in chemosensing revealed by a new molecular interaction-based modeling method. *PLoS Comput Biol 2*, 0710-0724.

Moraru, I.I., Schaff, J.C., Slepchenko, B.M., Blinov, M.L., Morgan, F., Lakshminarayana, A., Gao, F., Li, Y., and Loew, L.M. (2008). Virtual cell modelling and simulation software environment. *IET Syst Biol 2*, 352-362.

Nag, A., Faeder, J.R., and Goldstein, B. (2010). Shaping the response: The role of FcεRI and Syk expression levels in mast cell signalling. *IET Syst Biol 4*, 334-347.

Nelson, D.L., and Cox, M.M. (2013). *Lehninger Principles of Biochemistry* (6th ed.). John Wiley & Sons, W. H. Freeman: New York, NY.

Owen, J.A., Punt, J., Stranford, S.A., Jones, P.P., and Kuby, J. (2013). *Kuby Immunology* (7th ed.). W.H. Freeman.

Sekar, J.A.P., and Faeder, J.R. (2012). Rule-Based Modeling of Signal Transduction: A Primer. *Methods Mol Biol 880*, 139-218.

Sekar, J.A.P., Tapia J.J., and Faeder, J.R. (2017). Automated visualization of rule-based models. *PLoS Computational Biology 13*(11), e1005857.

Siraganian, R.P., de Castro, R.O., Barbu, E.A., and Zhang, J. (2010). Mast cell signaling: The role of protein tyrosine kinase Syk, its activation and screening methods for new pathway participants. *FEBS Lett 584*, 4933-4940.

Smith, A.M., Xu, W., Sun, Y., Faeder, J.R., and Marai, G.E. (2012). RuleBender: Integrated modeling, simulation and visualization for rule-based intracellular biochemistry. *BMC Bioinformatics 13*, S3.

Sneddon, M.W., Faeder, J.R., Emonet, T. (2011). Efficient modeling, simulation and coarse-graining of biological complexity with NFsim. *Nat Methods 8*, 177-183.

Stefan, M.I., Bartol, T.M., Sejnowski, T.J., and Kennedy, M.B. (2014). Multi-state Modeling of Biomolecules. *PLoS Comput Biol 10*.

Tapiam, J.-J., and Faeder J.R. (2013). The Atomizer: Extracting Implicit Molecular Structure from Reaction Network Models. In *Proceedings of the International Conference on Bioinformatics, Computational Biology and Biomedical Informatics (BCB'13)* (726-727). New York, NY: ACM.

Thomas, B.R., Chylek, L.A., Colvin, J., Sirimulla, S., Clayton, A.H.A, Hlavacek, W.S., and Posner, R.G. (2015). BioNetFit: A fitting tool compatible with BioNetGen, NFsim, and distributed computing environments. *Bioinformatics*, btv655.

Tiger, C.-F., Krause, F., Cedersund, G., Palmér, R., Klipp, E., Hohmann, S., Kitano, H., and Krantz, M. (2012). A framework for mapping, visualisation and automatic model creation of signal-transduction networks. *Mol Syst Biol 8*, 1-20.

Zhang, F., Angermann, B.R., Meier-Schellersheim, M. (2013). The Simmune Modeler visual interface for creating signaling networks based on bi-molecular interactions. *Bioinformatics 29*, 1229-1230.

Boolean models in immunology

REINHARD LAUBENBACHER AND ELENA DIMITROVA

6.1 INTRODUCTION

The use of mathematical models in immunology goes back to the 1970s, mostly focused on capturing the dynamics of different cell populations in a host, generally with the aid of ordinary differential equations (see, e.g., [1]). Since then, modeling has become an important technology in this field. Systems of ordinary differential equations still represent a key modeling framework, but they have been joined by models of other types, in particular Boolean models and their generalizations as well as agent-based models. Modeling with differential equations as well as agent-based modeling is discussed elsewhere in this volume. In this chapter, we focus on the use of Boolean models and their generalizations in immunology.

The immune system has emerged as a tremendously complex "complex system" that is still very poorly understood. It has been recognized early on that mathematical models of various kinds are indispensable for a quantitative understanding of the myriad interconnected dynamic processes comprising the immune system. Broadly speaking, the majority of published models can be divided into two types. One type focuses on intracellular molecular networks involved in gene regulation, signaling, and other molecular processes. The other type focuses on systemic aspects of immune system dynamics, primarily capturing cell populations.

The choice of mathematical modeling framework, as always, depends primarily on the kind of problem to be solved and the types of data and information that is available for the task. Boolean network models are best suited to capture the regulatory logic that connects different molecular species or different cell populations. Such models consist of a collection of nodes, representing, e.g., genes or cell types. Each node can take on a finite number of different states, such as "high/low," "active/inactive," or "low/normal/high." Classical Boolean network models allow two possible states per node, but the framework can accommodate any finite number of states. Different types of directed arrows between these nodes represent relationships through which one node can influence the state of another node, e.g., activation or inhibition. The result is a graphical representation of a network, which can be viewed as a type of wiring diagram commonly used in the immunology literature. Furthermore, each node is equipped with a logical rule that integrates the different causal relationships and serves as a mechanism to drive the temporal evolution of the network in discrete time. That is, if node A is in state a at time t, $A(t) = a$, it is regulated by nodes B and C, and its logical rule is denoted by f, then the state of A at time $t + 1$ can be described by the functional relationship

$$A(t+1) = f\big(B(t), C(t), a\big).$$

Iterating this process, we obtain the temporal evolution of node A. We illustrate this framework with a simple abstract example for an entire network.

Let A, B, C, D represent four transcription factors, each of which can be either *expressed* (1) or *not expressed* (0). We presuppose the following regulatory relationships between these: A upregulates B, B and C synergistically downregulate D, that is, both B and C need to be present to exert this action, B inhibits expression of C, C activates A, and A inhibits C (see Figure 6.1 for a wiring diagram of this network).

The logical rules for the four nodes are as follows

$$A(t+1) = C(t),$$
$$B(t+1) = A(t),$$
$$C(t+1) = \big[\text{NOT } A(t)\big] \text{ OR } \big[\text{NOT } B(t)\big],$$
$$D(t+1) = B(t) \text{ AND } C(t).$$

Table 6.1 shows the transition table for node A. These rules can be interpreted via the following "transition tables." The table for node A is given in Figure 6.1, and is similar to that for node B. Table 6.2 describes the rules for node C, with node D regulated as in Table 6.3.

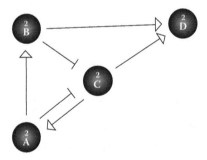

Figure 6.1 Wiring diagram for example network. The diagram was built using the software tool PlantSimLab (plantsimlab.org). The numeral 2 above the node names indicates that the node takes on two possible values.

Table 6.1 Transition table for node A

A(t)	C(t)	A(t + 1)
0	0	0
0	1	1
1	0	1
1	1	1

Note: If A is not expressed at time t, and C is expressed, then it will upregulate expression of A at time $t + 1$. On the other hand, if A is expressed already, then, in the framework of binary states, C does not have any effect on A. That is, each row of the table can be interpreted as a biological statement about regulation of A by C, and the four rows cover all possible combinations of the states of A and C at time t.

Table 6.2 Transition table for C

A(t)	B(t)	C(t)	C(t + 1)
0	0	0	0
1	0	0	0
0	1	0	0
0	0	1	1
1	1	0	0
1	0	1	0
0	1	1	0
1	1	1	0

Note: The only scenarios in which A and B exert an action on C is when C is expressed and A or B (or both) are expressed (rows 6–8).

Table 6.3 Transition table for D

B(t)	C(t)	D(t)	D(t + 1)
0	0	0	0
1	0	0	0
0	1	0	0
0	0	1	1
1	1	0	1
1	0	1	1
0	1	1	1
1	1	1	1

Note: The only effect of B and C on D takes place when B and C are expressed and D is not expressed (row 5).

We can now successively apply all these rules and generate the global dynamics of the network. This can be done by drawing another graph that has all possible network states as nodes, in this case all binary 4-tuples, representing all possible combinations of states of A-D. In this case, there will be $2^4 = 16$ such states. An arrow from state x to state y indicates that the system transitions from x to y when the transition rules are applied to each of the four coordinates of x. This graph can be seen in Figure 6.2. Notice that the system has two steady states: when all nodes are ON and when all nodes are OFF. All other states eventually transition to one of these two states.

The different processes governing the nodes of the network do not typically happen at the same time scale, and some of them may be stochastic, due to, e.g., low copy number. In those cases, the procedure above of

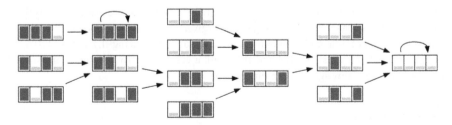

Figure 6.2 State space graph of example network. There are 16 possible states, each represented by a rectangle comprising four bars, which correspond to the network nodes in the order (A, B, C, D). A solid bar indicates that the corresponding node is ON, a empty bar that it is OFF. An arrow from one state to another indicates that upon application of the logical rules, the state at the source of the arrow transitions to the state at the tip. The diagram was built using the software tool PlantSimLab (plantsimlab.org).

updating all the nodes at the same time is biologically not realistic. There are several possible alternatives, all of which, in one form or another, update variables sequentially instead. One approach to this problem is taken in the paper in the first case study below, where, at each time step, a sequential update order is chosen at random. Another approach is taken in [2], where each node is updated at a given time step with a given probability. For slow processes, this probability is lower than for fast processes. It is worth noting that applying sequential rather than parallel update does not change the steady states of the network, but it may well change periodic behavior, and it may change the trajectories from a given network state to a steady state.

Before we give a partial survey of published Boolean models of immunological processes, we describe in detail two published models, one at the intracellular and one at the population level, in order to give the reader an opportunity to become familiar with the framework described above in an immunological context.

6.2 TWO CASE STUDIES

6.2.1 CASE STUDY 1. BOOLEAN MODELS OF IMMUNE RESPONSES AGAINST SINGLE AND CO-INFECTIONS WITH *BORDETELLA BRONCHISEPTICA* AND *TRICHOSTRONGYLUS RETORTAEFORMIS* [3]

Co-infections with more than one infecting agent can alter the immune response against each individual pathogen and can also alter the relative severity and persistence of the infections within the host. The main reason is that the immune system is not compartmentalized within the host but acts as a whole to allow the host to maintain control of the infections as well as repair damaged tissues and avoid immuno-pathology. Thakar et al. [3] investigated the network of immune responses against single and co-infections with the respiratory bacterium *Bordetella bronchiseptica* and the gastrointestinal helminth *Trichostrongylus retortaeformis*. The goal was to identify representative mediators and functions that could capture the essence of the host immune response as a whole, and to assess how their relative contribution dynamically changes over time and between single and co-infected individuals.

To this end, the authors built three Boolean network models: (1) A single *B. bronchiseptica* infection model; (2) A single *T. retortaeformis* infection model; and (3) A *B. bronchiseptica*-*T. retortaeformis* co-infection model.

The network of interactions against *B. bronchiseptica* was based on infection in the lungs, the crucial organ for bacterial clearance, and constructed following knowledge of the dynamics of *B. bronchiseptica* infection in mice. The immune network mounting a response against *T. retortaeformis* was built on the knowledge of helminth infections in mice and focused on the duodenum, where the majority of *T. retortaeformis* colonization and immune activity has been observed.

The networks were then developed into Boolean models in which each node was categorized by two qualitative states, ON and OFF, which are determined from the regulation of the focal node by upstream nodes given in the network. The nodes in the ON state are assumed to be above an implicit threshold that can be defined as the concentration necessary to activate downstream immune processes; below this threshold the node is considered to be in an OFF state. The regulation is given by a Boolean transfer function. For example, dendritic cells (DC) induce differentiation of naïve T cells (T0) by producing IL4 and IL12. IL4 is also produced by differentiated Th2 cells, and IL4 and IL12 inhibit each other. These interactions are reflected in Figure 6.3 [4] and modeled through Boolean functions as:

$$T0(t+1) = \text{DCII}(t),$$
$$\text{IL12II}(t+1) = \text{DCII}(t) \text{ AND } T0(t) \text{ AND } \big(\text{NOT IL4II}(t)\big),$$
$$\text{IL4II}(t+1) = ((\text{DCII}(t) \text{ AND } T0(t)) \text{ OR Th2II}(t)) \text{ AND (NOT IL12II}(t)) \text{ AND (NOT IFNgII}(t)).$$

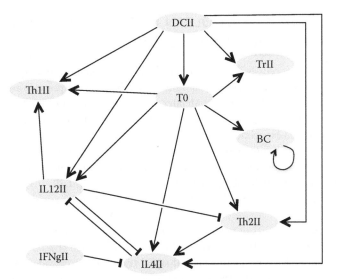

Figure 6.3 A portion of the network of immune components considered in single *B. bronchiseptica* infection. IL4lI: Interleukin 4 in the systemic compartment; IL12I: Interleukin 12 in lungs; BC: B cells; DCII: Dendritic cells in the systemic compartment; Th1lI: T helper cell subtype I in the systemic compartment; T0: Naïve T cells; TrlI: T regulatory cells in the systemic compartment; Th2lI: Th2 cells in the systemic compartment; IFNgI: Interferon gamma in the lungs. Figure drawn in *CellDesigner*. (From Kitano, H. et al, *Nat Biotechnol, 23* (8), 961–966, 2005.)

The status of the system across time was simulated by repeatedly applying the Boolean rules for each node until a steady state was found. Since the kinetics and timescales of the individual processes represented as edges are not known, a random order asynchronous update was selected in which the timescales of each regulatory process were randomly chosen in such a way that the node states were updated in a randomly selected order during each time-step. The time-step of the model approximately corresponds to nine days. The randomized asynchronicity of the model does not alter the steady states of the dynamical system but causes stochasticity in the trajectory between the initial conditions and the steady states, and thus it can sample more diverse behaviors than synchronous models.

To explicitly quantify the interactions between *B. bronchiseptica* and *T. retortaeformis* the two single immune networks were connected and the co-infection network simulated as a single entity without changing the Boolean rules built for the single networks, except for the adjustments necessary for assembly. The link between networks was established through cytokines, which maintain the communication between the systemic and local immune processes as well as the cross-interactions between infections. For example, IL4 or IL12 can be produced by *B. bronchiseptica*- or *T. retortaeformis*-specific T subtypes or dendritic cells.

The co-infection model was verified by empirical findings. Simulations based on the model revealed, among other things, that a T helper cell mediated antibody and neutrophil response led to phagocytosis and clearance of *B. bronchiseptica* from the lungs. The model also revealed a few unexpected results: first, the faster clearance of *T. retortaeformis* in co-infected compared to single infected individuals, which was observed in the model simulations and confirmed in the empirical data. Another surprising finding based on the model was that *B. bronchiseptica* infection in the lungs was not significantly altered by the concurrent helminth infection, despite the increase in local IL4 expression observed in both the simulations and the experiment. Furthermore, perturbation analysis of the models through the knockout of individual nodes identified the cells critical to parasite persistence and clearance both in single and co-infections. The model, combined with experimental data, captured the within-host immuno-dynamics of bacteria-helminth infection and identified key components that can be crucial for explaining individual variability between single and co-infections in natural populations.

6.2.2 CASE STUDY 2. A BOOLEAN MODEL OF THE TERMINAL DIFFERENTIATION OF B CELLS [5]

Terminal differentiation of B cells is an essential process for the humoral immune response in vertebrates and is achieved by the concerted action of several transcription factors in response to antigen recognition and extracellular signals provided by Thelper cells. Méndez and Mendoza [5] built a Boolean model of the regulatory network controlling terminal B cell differentiation and analyzed its dynamic behavior under normal and mutant conditions. They used experimental data from the literature referring to the key molecules involved in the control of terminal B cell differentiation from the precursor B cell (Naive) to GC, Mem, or PC cell types (Figure 6.4) [4]. The network contains 22 nodes representing functional molecules or molecular complexes, namely AID, Ag, Bach2, Bcl6, BCR, Blimp1, CD40, CD40L, ERK, IL2, IL2R, IL4, IL4R, IL21, IL21R, Irf4, NFκB, Pax5, STAT3, STAT5, STAT6, and XBP1. These nodes have 39 positive and negative regulatory interactions among them.

The regulatory network consists of two sets of nodes, i.e., those pertaining to a core module integrated by the master transcriptional regulators of terminal B cell differentiation (Bach2, Bcl6, Blimp1, Irf4, Pax5, and XBP1) and a set of nodes representing several signal transduction cascades (Ag/BCR/ERK, CD40L/CD40NFκB, IL2/IL2R/STAT5, IL4/IL4R/STAT6, and IL21/IL21R/STAT3) transmitting key external signals required for the control of the differentiation process. The nodes corresponding to these signaling pathways are active (ON) if an external stimulus is present. If an extracellular molecule is available, it is recognized by a specific receptor that transduces the signal via a messenger molecule, which, in turn, regulates the expression of the transcription factors in the core regulatory network. For example, BCR is activated by the input node Ag, simulating the presence of extracellular antigen and so resulting in the Boolean function

$$BCR(t+1) = Ag(t),$$

which determines the next state of BCR. Furthermore, BCR cross-linking promotes ERK activation after Ag simulation, which is expressed as a Boolean function as

$$ERK(t+1) = BCR(t).$$

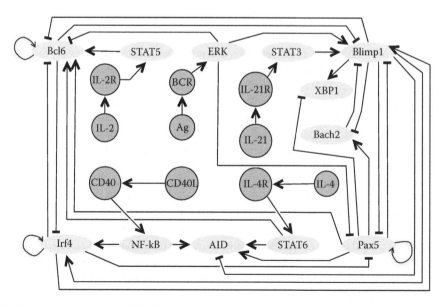

Figure 6.4 The regulatory network of B cells. Figure drawn in *CellDesigner*. (From Kitano, H. et al, *Nat Biotechnol*, 23 (8), 961–966, 2005.)

The Boolean function of AID is an example of a more complicated regulatory relationship. AID is positively regulated by the presence of Pax5 in response to CD40 and IL-4 signals, transduced by NFκB and STAT6, respectively. AID is active only if its inhibitor Blimp1 is absent. This is expressed as a Boolean function as

$$\text{AID}(t+1) = (\text{STAT6}(t) \text{ OR } (\text{NF-}\kappa\text{B}(t) \text{ AND } \text{Pax5}(t))) \text{ AND } (\text{NOT } \text{Blimp1}(t)).$$

To study the dynamic behavior of the system, the steady states of the Boolean models were obtained by exhaustively testing the behavior of the network from all possible initial conditions. The system reaches four steady states: The first steady state (Naive), where the nodes Pax5 and Bach2 are active, can be interpreted as the activation pattern of naive cells. The second steady state (GC), with high levels of Bcl6, Pax5, and Bach2, corresponds to the GC cell type. The third steady state (Mem), with high levels of Irf4, Pax5, and Bach2 and the absence of Bcl6 can be interpreted as the Mem cell fate. Finally, the fourth steady state (PC), with high Blimp1, Irf4, and XBP1, corresponds to the pattern of the cell type PC. The basins of attraction of these steady states, i.e., the collection of states that all transition eventually to a given steady state, do not partition the state space evenly. The percentages of initial states leading to each of the steady states are as follows: Naive = 56.25%, GC = 6.25%, Mem = 6.25%, and PC = 31.25%. The authors suggest that the size of the basins reflects how a steady state can be attained from different initial configurations and may indicate the relative stability of each steady state.

To gain further insight into the dynamical behavior of the B cell regulatory network the authors simulated all possible single loss and gain-of-function mutants and evaluated the severity of each mutation by comparing the resulting steady states with those of the wild type model. Loss-of-function mutations were simulated by fixing at OFF the value of a node, whereas gain-of-function mutations were simulated by fixing at ON the same activation state of a node. For each mutant, its attractors were found through an exhaustive simulation. The mutants were grouped according to whether a mutant effect results in the loss of one or more steady states with respect to the wild type model or if it results in the appearance of atypical attractors not found in the wild type model. The model was able to describe most of the reported mutants for the six master regulators that form the core of the network. For instance, the simulated loss-of-function of the Blimp1 node results in the disappearance of the PC attractor, which is in accordance with the experimentally acknowledged role of Blimp1 as an essential regulator for PC differentiation. As another example, for the Blimp1 null mutant a distinct steady state was found showing low Pax5 and high Irf4 levels. It has been reported that Pax5 inactivation along with Irf4 induction precedes Blimp1 expression and, while Irf4 activation is not sufficient to rescue PC differentiation in the absence of Blimp1, the coordinate expression of both factors is necessary for complete terminal B cell differentiation. Therefore, this attractor may represent a cellular state prior to the PC state.

Despite the lack of quantitative information, a Boolean modeling framework made it possible to reconstruct the regulatory network of B cells and propose a basic regulatory architecture. This Boolean model proposes the existence of some missing regulatory interactions and activation states not documented in the literature that might play an important role in the context of terminal B cell differentiation. These interactions constitute specific predictions that can be tested experimentally. Furthermore, the results suggest that the dynamic behavior of the B cell regulatory network is to a large extent determined by the structure of the network rather than the details of the kinetic parameters.

6.3 BOOLEAN MODELS IN THE RECENT LITERATURE

The (generalized) Boolean modeling framework is being used increasingly in efforts to understand a wide range of processes, in particular those related to the immune system. Reviews of general techniques and existing Boolean models can be found in, e.g., [6,7]. It is worth noting that one of the earliest applications of the generalized Boolean network framework, so-called logical models, was toward the understanding of the immune response based on the interaction between different T cell types [8]. Here, we focus on a representative collection of recently published models related to immunology. As described earlier in the context of [3], Boolean models have been used successfully to capture the dynamics of cell populations. At the molecular level, an important focus of recent modeling efforts is on signal transduction and gene regulatory networks, which we discuss now. We have chosen models that illustrate the capabilities of Boolean models beyond the basic setup described in the introduction.

One of the most exciting recent developments in the fight against cancer is a new approach to enhance the capability of the patient's immune system to attack cancer cells. Several immune therapy drugs have been approved and have shown great initial promise. These drugs target receptors on T cells that regulate T cell activity through downstream signaling. On the other hand, the treatment of autoimmune diseases, for instance, requires the suppression of T cell activity. In either case, it is important to understand the signaling pathways downstream of different receptors and their cross talk. In [9], this was done for the signal transduction pathways for two receptors, the T cell receptor for antigen (TCR) and the interleukin-2 (IL-2) receptor. The role of TCR is to recognize peptides bound to proteins of the major histocompatibility complex (MHC), encoded by the human leukocyte antigen genes (HLA) and to regulate the activation of T cells. In activated T cells, the production of both IL-2 and its receptor IL-2R is upregulated. The authors constructed a Boolean model of an IL-2R signaling pathway from information available in the literature (Figure 5 in [9]), and validated it with cell culture experiments, using peripheral human T cells derived from healthy volunteers. This network is then integrated with a TCR signaling pathway, also derived from literature information. The combined network includes 150 molecules and 167 regulatory relationships. Even though the two individual pathways are well known, a detailed study of the merged network illuminated several important effects of what the authors call "off-target" interactions across pathways. Since these two pathways are also heavily involved in T cell differentiation, this model may also shed light on the processes involved, possibly by combining this model with a Boolean T cell differentiation model [10], as the authors suggest. One might also consider combining it with the T cell differentiation model discussed below.

An interesting technical feature of the model is the use of two different time scales, representing interactions that happen only early in the signaling process and others that happen later. The resulting two networks (early and late) are considered separately.

In recent years, T cell differentiation has received much attention, as new T cell types are discovered. The plasticity of T cells, their ability to dynamically differentiate into types with different properties, e.g., inflammatory or anti-inflammatory, depending on the environment makes them a versatile component of the immune system. A recent Boolean model of CD4+ T cell differentiation [11] models the regulatory network that directs the cell to one of eight phenotypes: Th0, Th1, Th2, Th17, Tfh, Th9, iTreg, and Foxp3-independent T regulatory cells. It is a combination of transcriptional regulation and signaling events, with the environment represented by different cytokines, obtained from the literature. Each of the different phenotypes corresponds to the steady state of the model for a particular choice of external parameters (cytokine presence/absence), triggered by transient activation/inhibition of transcriptional regulation. The model was analyzed using model reduction techniques to reduce computational complexity, an important step without which large Boolean models are difficult or impossible to analyze, since the size of the state space of a model is exponential in the number of nodes. The authors also validated the model by building a continuous model that exhibited the same basic dynamic features.

Cytokine signaling is one of the central mechanisms of the immune response and takes place via complex signaling cascades. In [12], the authors construct comprehensive large-scale Boolean network models for the signaling networks of the two pro-inflammatory cytokines interleukin 1 (IL-1) and 6 (IL-6), based on a synthesis of the available literature. These are known to be involved in a multitude of processes, from the immune response to pathogens to cancer-related processes and the regulation of inflammatory processes linked to insulin resistance. The models were optimized using available proteomics data from human hepatocytes. Analysis of the network suggests several model modifications in order to better fit available knowledge and data, which can be regarded as experimental hypotheses to be pursued.

The networks discussed so far capture signaling and regulatory cascades involved in a wide range of processes that are part of the immune response. We conclude this section with a brief discussion of a model that connects the immune response to a viral, pathogen, HIV, to demonstrate how Boolean modeling can be used for the purpose of modeling host-pathogen interactions.

In its aim to replicate within its human host, human immunodeficiency virus type 1 (HIV-1) manipulates host cellular processes by interacting with proteins that are involved in signaling processes. The dynamics of this process are not well understood. The focus of [13] is an effort to model the interaction of HIV-1 with the signaling network involved in the activation of CD4+ T lymphocytes. Using the HIV-1 Human Interaction Database, the authors constructed a Boolean network model that included 137 proteins (16 HIV-1, the remainder human proteins) and 336 protein-protein interactions. The model was validated with publicly available experimental data, and its analysis revealed a number of key host cell factors relevant to T cell activation that can be manipulated by the virus to hijack the host's molecular machinery.

The selection of models we have described here is only a small part of the extant literature of the recent past. Other articles we could have focused on, instead or in addition, include but are not limited to [10,14–23].

6.4 THE RELATIONSHIP BETWEEN BOOLEAN AND CONTINUOUS MODELS

While this chapter is focused on the use of Boolean models in immunology, there are of course many continuous models in this field, described elsewhere in this volume. It is natural to ask what the relationship is between Boolean models and models of the same biological system described by a collection of ordinary differential equations (ODEs). This question is quite difficult to answer in general. Concepts that are fundamental for ODEs, such as stability, multistationarity, etc., do not always translate in a straightforward way, in part because Boolean models do not typically have parameters that can be varied. Nonetheless, some results are available, which we review briefly. The process of constructing a Boolean model for a molecular network from available information typically proceeds by first constructing a wiring diagram of the network, which captures the dependency relationships between the molecular species in the network. Then, for each node, a choice must be made of a Boolean function that integrates the variables corresponding to each incoming edge. This function captures the regulatory logic of the node. The result is a Boolean network. To construct an ODE model of the same network, one needs to determine a continuous function for each node that represents its regulatory mechanisms, by which its concentration is affected by the concentrations of the input nodes. Common choices include Hill functions, viewing the network as a biochemical reaction network (which it might not be, if regulatory interactions are phenomenological and don't correspond directly to chemical reactions). The next step typically is to estimate the numerical parameters in the model from experimental data and/or the literature. Thus, a significant part of the construction process for an ODE model and the information used is the same as that for a Boolean model, and so it is not surprising that there should be a relationship between the resulting dynamics. An obvious question to focus on, which has received some attention, is a comparison of the steady states of the two model types.

The most general results about this question can be found in [24]. The main theorem, Theorem 3.4, gives conditions under which there is a one-to-one correspondence between a system of ODEs and a properly defined discrete dynamical system. One possible application of this result is the possibility to study some properties of an ODE model by studying instead properties of a derived discrete system. This result generalizes work done on this question in [25–28]. In [25], on the other hand, the motivation for studying this question was to begin with a Boolean network model and construct from it an ODE model that could be used for more quantitative studies of networks. Much less extensively studied are periodic attractors. One of the very few studies of this type is [29], in which the authors study the relationship between general attractors of a Boolean and a corresponding continuous system, using a case study. While the results obtained so far by these and other authors show that there is likely a rich relationship between these model types, much of it remains to be understood through a general theoretical study.

6.5 MODEL STANDARDS AND SOFTWARE

Tools for the construction, analysis, and sharing of (generalized) Boolean models are of the utmost importance in moving the field forward. Unfortunately, in comparison to the situation for continuous models, tool availability is still sparse. For model sharing, standards are essential, and the development of the Systems Biology Markup Language (SBML) was a major advance. Unfortunately, SBML was intended initially to only cover models that consisted of systems of ordinary differential equations. A recent effort by the discrete modeling community has resulted in an extension of SBML to discrete models [30].

Several software packages for the construction of Boolean models are available. Each has different features, strengths, and weaknesses. Examples include GINsim [31], BoolNet [32], and the Cell Collective [33], to name a few. Some are stand-alone web tools, such as GINsim, others are implemented in, e.g., R or Matlab. The individual needs of the user will dictate the appropriate package to use.

6.6 DISCUSSION

As the survey in this chapter shows, Boolean models have been used successfully to model key aspects of the immune system and its role in a variety of diseases. They can be viewed as a "coarse-grained" representation of biological mechanisms, that is qualitative, rather than quantitative, in the sense that they provide qualitative output. This drawback is balanced by the advantage that they only require qualitative input, in the form of relational statements between the entities to be modeled, capturing the logic of their relationships. It is also worth observing that, in the process of building a differential equations model of a signaling pathway, for example, one is forced to collect together essentially all the information needed to build a Boolean model. Therefore, such models can serve as a first step in a process that ultimately results in a quantitative model. In the end, as always with modeling, the model type to be used needs to be commensurate with the questions to be answered and the information and data available.

The sampling of models we discussed shows the versatility of modeling the immune system using Boolean networks and the richness of insights one can gain. At the intracellular level, models capture a variety of signaling events, most importantly signal transduction networks emanating from receptors, engaging downstream in crosstalk. We have included network models of the regulation of T cell differentiation and activation and cytokine signaling. Finally, we have seen a model that captures the interactions between a human host and a pathogen. At the systemic level, we have seen a model that depicts the immune response to co-infection.

The picture that emerges is one of a patchwork of models, many of which are related, especially in the context of T cell signaling. It is tempting to work toward larger systematic integrated models of signaling networks that include some of the complexity that is neglected when we look at individual pathways. This is to be balanced by the substantial computational cost that comes with large Boolean networks and their analysis. As mentioned earlier, an analysis of the dynamics of a Boolean network requires that we explore a space whose size is exponential in the number of variables of the network. There are some systematic approaches to deal with this combinatorial explosion; see, e.g., [34]. However, even if model analysis is feasible, it is not always straightforward to interpret the output of large models with many hundreds or even thousands of nodes. Ultimately, both approaches will be required, together with modeling tools with matching complexity. As the immune system is playing an ever-larger role in human health, mathematical models will become an indispensable technology, with Boolean models as a valuable resource.

REFERENCES

1. Perelson, A.S., Mirmirani, M., and Oster, G.F. (1976). Optimal strategies in immunology. I. B-cell differentiation and proliferation. *J Math Biol* 3(3–4), 325–367.
2. Murrugarra, D. et al. (2012). Modeling stochasticity and variability in gene regulatory networks. *EURASIP J Bioinform Syst Biol* 2012(1), 5.

3. Thakar, J. et al. (2012). Network model of immune responses reveals key effectors to single and co-infection dynamics by a respiratory bacterium and a gastrointestinal helminth. *PLoS Comput Biol* 8(1), e1002345.

4. Kitano, H. et al. (2005). Using process diagrams for the graphical representation of biological networks. *Nat Biotechnol* 23(8), 961–966.

5. Mendez, A., and Mendoza, L. (2016). A network model to describe the terminal differentiation of B cells. *PLoS Comput Biol* 12(1), e1004696.

6. Abou-Jaoude, W. et al. (2016). Logical modeling and dynamical analysis of cellular networks. *Front Genet* 7, 94.

7. Samaga, R., and Klamt, S. (2013). Modeling approaches for qualitative and semi-quantitative analysis of cellular signaling networks. *Cell Commun Signal* 11(1), 43.

8. Kaufman, M., Urbain, J., and Thomas, R. (1985). Towards a logical analysis of the immune response. *J Theor Biol* 114(4), 527–561.

9. Beyer, T. et al. (2011). Integrating signals from the T-cell receptor and the interleukin-2 receptor. *PLoS Comput Biol* 7(8), e1002121.

10. Naldi, A. et al. (2010). Diversity and plasticity of Th cell types predicted from regulatory network modelling. *PLoS Comput Biol* 6(9), e1000912.

11. Martinez-Sanchez, M.E. et al. (2015). A minimal regulatory network of extrinsic and intrinsic factors recovers observed patterns of CD4+ T cell differentiation and plasticity. *PLoS Comput Biol* 11(6), e1004324.

12. Ryll, A. et al. (2011). Large-scale network models of IL-1 and IL-6 signalling and their hepatocellular specification. *Mol Biosyst* 7(12), 3253–3270.

13. Oyeyemi, O.J. et al. (2015). A logical model of HIV-1 interactions with the T-cell activation signalling pathway. *Bioinformatics* 31(7),1075–1083.

14. Aslam, B. et al. (2014). On the modelling and analysis of the regulatory network of dengue virus pathogenesis and clearance. *Comput Biol Chem* 53PB, 277–291.

15. Clarke, D.C., and Lauffenburger, D.A. (2012). Multi-pathway network analysis of mammalian epithelial cell responses in inflammatory environments. *Biochem Soc Trans* 40(1), 133–138.

16. Farooqi, Z.U. et al. (2016). Logical analysis of regulation of Interleukin-12 expression pathway regulation during HCV infection. *Protein Pept Lett*.

17. Ganguli, P. et al. (2015a). Temporal protein expression pattern in intracellular signalling cascade during T-cell activation: A computational study. *J Biosci* 40(4), 769–789.

18. Ganguli, P. et al. (2015b). Identification of Th1/Th2 regulatory switch to promote healing response during leishmaniasis: A computational approach. *EURASIP J Bioinform Syst Biol* 2015, 13.

19. Hegde, S.R. et al. (2012). Understanding communication signals during mycobacterial latency through predicted genome-wide protein interactions and boolean modeling. *PLoS One* 7(3), e33893.

20. Kang, C.C. et al. (2011). A genetic algorithm-based Boolean delay model of intracellular signal transduction in inflammation. *BMC Bioinformatics* 12 Suppl 1, S17.

21. Niarakis, A. et al. (2014). Computational modeling of the main signaling pathways involved in mast cell activation. *Curr Top Microbiol Immunol* 382, 69–93.

22. Raman, K., Bhat, A.G., and Chandra, N. (2010). A systems perspective of host-pathogen interactions: Predicting disease outcome in tuberculosis. *Mol Biosyst* 6(3), 516–530.

23. Saez-Rodriguez, J. et al. (2007). A logical model provides insights into T cell receptor signaling. *PLoS Comput Biol* 3(8), e163.

24. Veliz-Cuba, A. et al. (2012). On the relationship of steady states of continuous and discrete models arising from biology. *Bull Math Biol* 74(12), 2779–2792.

25. Wittmann, D.M. et al. (2009). Transforming Boolean models to continuous models: Methodology and application to T-cell receptor signaling. *BMC Syst Biol* 3, 98.

26. Kauffman, S., and Glass, L. (1973). The logical analysis of continuous, nonlinear biochemical control networks. *J Theor Biol* 39, 103–129.

27. Mendoza, L., and Xenarios, I. (2006). A method for the generation of standardized qualitative dynamical systems of regulatory networks. *Theor Biol Med Model* 3(13), 1–18.

28. Snoussi, E. (1989). Qualitative dynamics of piecewise linear differential equations: A discrete mapping approach. *Dyn Stab Syst 4*(3), 189–207.

29. Sun, M., Cheng, X., and Socolar, J.E. (2013). Causal structure of oscillations in gene regulatory networks: Boolean analysis of ordinary differential equation attractors. *Chaos 23*(2), 025104.

30. Chaouiya, C. et al. (2015). The systems biology markup language (SBML) level 3 package: Qualitative models, version 1, release 1. *J Integr Bioinform 12*(2), 270.

31. Chaouiya, C., Naldi, A., and Thieffry, D. (2012). Logical modelling of gene regulatory networks with GINsim. *Methods Mol Biol 804*, 463–479.

32. Mussel, C., Hopfensitz, M., and Kestler, H.A. (2010). BoolNet--an R package for generation, reconstruction and analysis of Boolean networks. *Bioinformatics 26*(10), 1378–1380.

33. Helikar, T. et al. (2012). The Cell Collective: Toward an open and collaborative approach to systems biology. *BMC Syst Biol 6*, 96.

34. Veliz-Cuba, A. et al. (2014). Steady state analysis of Boolean molecular network models via model reduction and computational algebra. *BMC Bioinformatics 15*, 221.

From evolutionary computation to phenotypic spandrels
Inverse problem for immune ligand recognition

PAUL FRANÇOIS AND MATHIEU HEMERY

7.1 INTRODUCTION

Discrimination between self and not-self is an example of complex multiscale cellular computation. Immune T cells have to perform sensitive and specific detection of foreign ligands (Feinerman et al., 2008a), taking "decision on the fly" (Siggia and Vergassola, 2013) without triggering devastating auto-immune response in the presence of vast amounts of self ligands (Lalanne and François, 2015). Biochemical nature of foreign ligands is highly diverse, and specific recognition strategies must be implemented to ensure good immune coverage (Mayer et al., 2015). At the population scale, immune cells must coordinate with each other to ensure proper organismal response (Tkach et al., 2014; Voisinne et al., 2015).

The structure of the underlying biochemical networks performing so many complex decisions appeared through Darwinian evolution, and we expect organization features of those networks to reflect the daunting complexity of their task. It is then quite natural to ask an "inverse problem" question: given such biological function or other phenotypic constraints, can we predict anything on the underlying network structure? A priori, answering such question appears hopeless for many reasons: for instance, the phenotype to genotype mapping is known to be highly complex and degenerate. One could also imagine that networks performing such functions are so complex that only billions of years of evolution will be able to explore the "actual and the possible" (to paraphrase François Jacob (Jacob, 1981)) or that the specific network performing a biological function is just a random unremarkable element within a vast ensemble of possible working solutions.

A useful starting point is to consider Gene Regulatory Networks (GRN) formalism to describe dynamics within a cell. This approach consists in approximating gene activities by continuous or discrete variables, with interaction terms corresponding to regulations. Dynamics of those networks can then be simulated in the computer or even sometimes studied analytically, and mapping of phenotypes (i.e., dynamics of variables) to genotypes (i.e., parametrized interactions between variables) studied in simple coarse-grained models. With sufficient computational power, one can then explore all possible (small) networks corresponding to a well-defined biological function, as done in the examples of biochemical adaptation (Ma et al., 2009) and stripe formation in development (Cotterell and Sharpe, 2010). Such enumeration techniques are nevertheless limited because they can not deal with combinatorial explosion of interactions when considering bigger networks.

An alternative approach is to get inspiration from biology and search for networks using a genetic algorithm (or *in silico* evolution) approach. Genetic algorithms use Darwinian evolution as a general optimization method for complex problems with many degrees of freedoms or parameters. In recent years, genetic algorithms have been applied to optimization problems posed by biology itself, using GRNs inspired formalism. The overall idea is to automatically generate and select GRNs to build networks performing a pre-defined biological function, with the hope of understanding better both structure and function of actual biological networks. In that sense *in silico* evolution is an instance of two increasingly popular trends: machine learning (Duvenaud et al., 2013) and "automatized science" (Schmidt and Lipson, 2009; Lobo and Levin, 2015; Daniels and Nemenman, 2015).

Examples of *in silico* evolution are numerous and include but are not limited to selection for oscillators or multistable systems (François and Hakim, 2004), developmental networks (François et al., 2007; Fujimoto et al., 2008; ten Tusscher and Hogeweg, 2011), selection of modularity (Kashtan and Alon, 2005), or allostery in varying environments (Hemery and Rivoire, 2015). In this review, we use the example of immune recognition as a case-study to introduce the general method of evolutionary computation. We first define the biological function of interest, then introduce the general evolutionary algorithm used for this specific problem, discussing in particular the important problem of the choice of the objective function. Then we review the results of such evolution before finally linking to actual biology and reviewing lessons and possible extensions.

7.2 FRAMING THE QUESTION

One of the first steps of immune response is the recognition of foreign ligands by immune T cells. The primary level of recognition is the interaction of T cell receptors (TCR) with peptides presented by Antigen Presenting Cells (APC). Then, depending on the nature of the ligand, T cells are activated (or not) and more complex immune response is triggered. The first important quantitative question is the definition (biochemically speaking) of the nature of the ligand. Years of experimental (Kersh et al., 1998; Gascoigne et al., 2001) as well as theoretical explorations (McKeithan, 1995) have suggested that one of the main determinant of the nature of ligand is the binding time τ of ligands to TCRs. Schematically, higher binding times define agonists (considered as foreign ligands) while lower binding times are non agonists, defining the so-called "lifetime dogma" (Feinerman et al., 2008a). It should be pointed out immediately that this is a simplification of a complex reality, see e.g., (Lever et al., 2014; Govern et al., 2010) for exceptions to this rule; however, recent chimeric receptors built with DNA indeed confirm the existence of a very sharp discrimination based on binding times (Taylor et al., 2017). Importantly, the decision is characterized by a "golden triangle" of properties:

- sensitivity: only few ligands can trigger response,
- specificity: a three-fold change of binding time τ separates agonist from non-agonist, suggesting discrimination is based on relative values of τ compared to a critical binding time τ_c,
- speed: decision is reached within a couple of minutes at most.

The combination of these properties raises an interesting problem: how can we have "absolute discrimination" (François and Altan-Bonnet, 2016) purely based on τ and (almost) *independent* from ligand concentration? We would naively expect that more ligands (irrespective of their binding times) would create more "signal", so why do the tens of thousands of ligands just below binding time threshold not trigger response while only a few ligands above threshold do? Furthermore, this picture is complexified by the existence of antagonism: not only do ligands with binding times just below τ_c not trigger a response, but it is also known that they antagonize the response of agonists (Altan-Bonnet and Germain, 2005). These different properties are summarized in Figure 7.1.

Before our work, a complex quantitative model recapitulating all these properties was proposed in 2005 by Altan-Bonnet and Germain (Altan-Bonnet and Germain, 2005). It relies on the exhaustive description of the many biochemical components of the system and of their interactions. The three main components of this model are:

- a kinetic proofreading backbone, as first proposed in this context by McKeithan (McKeithan, 1995), allowing for amplification of differences based on τ,
- a negative feedback loop mediated by the tyrosine-protein phosphatase SHP-1, putting a "brake" on cascade progression,
- a positive feedback loop mediated by an extracellular signal-regulated kinase (ERK) that relieves the SHP-1 brake allowing for full decision.

Importantly, this model accounts for the golden triangle, experimental antagonism, and was later used in a predictive way to study the digital/analog components of this signaling cascade (Feinerman et al., 2008b). However, despite later theoretical attempts (Lipniacki et al., 2008), the origin of the different quantitative properties remains obfuscated. For instance, is there any simple way to understand what defines the critical binding time for response τ_c? Are we doomed to "hairball" biology (Lander, 2010), where multiple biochemical interactions emerge in an intractable way into phenotypes, or can we envision methods to unknot those interactions to get more intuitive understanding?

This is a typical case where the relative simplicity of the observed phenotypes (discrimination based on τ value irrespective of concentration) allows for an inverse problem approach, starting with a genetic algorithm.

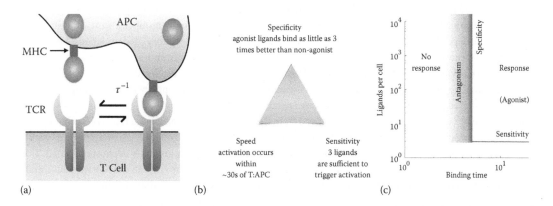

Figure 7.1 Setting the problem. **(a)** For our model, the quality of the ligands is mostly determined by his binding time τ. **(b)** A sketch of the "Golden triangle" for immunology. **(c)** Qualitative phase diagram of the ligands response in the (L, τ) space. (b. Reproduced from François, P., and Altan-Bonnet, G., *Journal of Statistical Physics*, 162(5), 1130–1152, 2016.)

7.3 GENETIC ALGORITHM

Our algorithm mimics the three essential pillars of evolution: selection, reproduction, and mutation. The algorithm presented here has been successfully applied to study a wide range of problems in signaling and development, reviewed in (François, 2014). In the Appendix, we give a very simple illustration of this algorithm on a basic biological function.

In summary, starting from an initial population of networks, we begin by ranking them according to a score function, traditionally called fitness, that measures the performance of each network at a predefined goal. Then in order to mimic the action of Darwinian selection, we cut the population to only keep the best half and duplicate it, randomly inserting mutations during the duplication step. This last step gives the next generation that serves as initial population for the next iteration of the process as depicted in Figure 7.2a.

This type of algorithm is of very general usage and may be applied in nearly every optimization problems, albeit its usefulness may vary from field to field. Three main components should retain our attention: namely, the description of the network, the mutation operator, and the fitness function. We now describe each of these parts in detail in our chosen example of early immune response.

7.3.1 NETWORK DEFINITION AND BIOCHEMICAL GRAMMAR

Many choices are possible to simulate a given biochemical network. Including all possible proteins in a given pathway (similar to what has been done in (Altan-Bonnet and Germain, 2005)) would be in principle possible, but would be too computationally expensive for network exploration with *in silico* evolution. Rather we evolve so-called "phenotypic models" (François et al., 2013; Lever et al., 2014), by considering some minimal set of coarse-grained interactions necessary for the complex functions of interest. This implements a compromise between the necessary freedom to generate many classes of possible models while being small and tractable enough to be functionally understandable yet predictive of biology.

The immune problem we consider here consists in the single cell detection of ligands by immune T cells. The networks considered simulate biochemical interactions in response to ligand exposure within a single T cell. We consider only phosphorylation/catalytic networks: the assumption is that the time-scale considered is small enough so that the total number of proteins does not change much during a recognition event by a T cell. However, these proteins can be interconverted into different forms, based on catalytic interactions with other proteins.

Possible interactions are:

- in the cell, we assume there is an ensemble of kinases or phosphatases that can be themselves phosphorylated multiple times or dephosphorylated. We make a "well-mixed" assumption, meaning that the concentration/activity of each of these proteins is described by one single number for the whole cell.
- at the surface of the cell, the ligand-receptor complex can be itself phosphorylated or dephosphorylated multiple times, to mimic the multiple phosphorylation states of the Immunoreceptor Tyrosine-based Activation Motifs (ITAMs)—the functional intracellular part of the receptor. We will call C_k the ligand receptor complex phosphorylated k times. Phosphorylations and dephosphorylations are implemented by the shared pool of kinases or phosphatases inside the cell.
- we include a dissociation rate τ^{-1} of the ligand from the receptor. This dissociation rate will be characteristic of the ligand's nature and the basis for discrimination between ligand quality. We make the important assumption that upon ligand dissociation, the receptor gets immediately and fully dephosphorylated. This phenomenologically implements a kinetic segregation mechanism (Davis and van der Merwe, 2006), and is known to be the basis for ligand proofreading (as first proposed by (McKeithan, 1995)).

Within our computational formalism, a network is represented by a graph of biochemical species (typically proteins) and interactions (e.g., ligand receptor interactions). This graph is bipartite: proteins can only be linked to interaction and interaction to proteins. Possible interactions are randomly combined by the algorithm yielding families of complex networks, an example shown in Figure 7.2b.

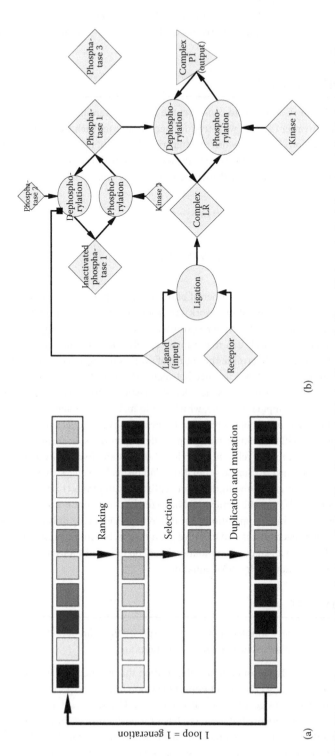

Figure 7.2 **(a)** Schematic representation of our genetic algorithm. Black and white levels encode fitness (darker = better); the expectation is that as evolution goes, average performance increases. **(b)** An example of a network as represented by our program. It illustrates some of the possible interactions (ellipses) between biochemical species (polygons).

Given this network, we are able to derive the dynamical equations governing the concentration of each species and integrate them numerically to determine the response of the system for a given set of input. In our biological example, the inputs are both the concentration and the type of the ligand τ (allowing us to explore the phase diagram of Figure 7.1c). One species in the network is taken as the output, and the fitness function is computed on it (see below).

7.3.2 NETWORK DYNAMICS

The representation of the network allows us to construct the set of differential equations that corresponds to the dynamic of the system. In order to do so, we introduce one variable for each free species in the system and then look at the different reactions in the network to determine the rate of interconversion of this species. As an explicit example, assume kinase K phosphorylates species S into S_p with rate $\alpha(K) = \alpha K$, while phosphatase P dephosphorylates S_p into S with rate $\beta(P) = \beta P$, then we write the dynamical equations:

$$\dot{S} = \beta P S_p - \alpha K S \tag{7.1}$$

$$\dot{S}_p = \alpha K S - \beta P S_p \tag{7.2}$$

Note that $\dot{S} + \dot{S}_p = 0$ meaning that total number of phosphorylated plus unphosporylated species is conserved. We also assume that phosphorylations work far from saturation, explaining why the respective interconversion rates are linear in S and S_p. We write similar equations for every single biochemical species accounting for all their interactions, and turn to a numerical solver to compute the whole dynamic of the system. This dynamic will be used to determine the course of evolution through the fitness function.

Again, our choice of formalism strikes a balance between a detailed description of the system and the need to keep a tractable computation time. More detailed stochastic or molecular dynamics like-simulation would induce a great expense in computation time, which would make evolutionary exploration impossible. Furthermore, there is no real reasons to opt for such a refinement given the fact that the large number of receptors at the surface of a cell will result in an averaging of all the quantities we are looking at, implying that our equations might already capture the relevant behavior of the system. Eventually, once a working structure has been obtained, more refined stochastic simulations can be made to check that the evolved structure works within a more detailed framework and under more realistic assumptions (Lalanne and François, 2013; François et al., 2013). A completely opposite limit would be to read our network not as chemical reactions but as a Boolean network performing binary operations, the different species being only present or not. This has effectively been done for other mechanisms and can give good results, but in the present problem, we expect discrimination to be first based on an analog computation based on the continuous biochemical parameter τ, so it is natural to consider continuous differential equations.

7.3.3 MUTATION LIST

At the beginning of the evolutionary simulation, we have to specify the kind of mutations that can act on a network during simulated Darwinian evolution. Those mutations are:

- **Modification of parameters.** The most obvious modification that our network does is to change the value of an existing parameter, e.g., the rate of phosphorylation of a given species.
- **Adding/Deleting a species.** The algorithm may also add a new kinase/phosphatase to the network, at first it may play no role in the network but it offers a basis for new future evolutionary innovations.
- **Adding/Deleting an interaction.** New interactions are added to the network by linking existing species, defining a new interaction. Here, there are only two kinds of interactions: phosphorylations and dephosphorylations of kinases/phosphatase in the system or of receptors. Note that appending a phosphorylation step to the complex receptor-ligand corresponds here to the addition of a proofreading step.

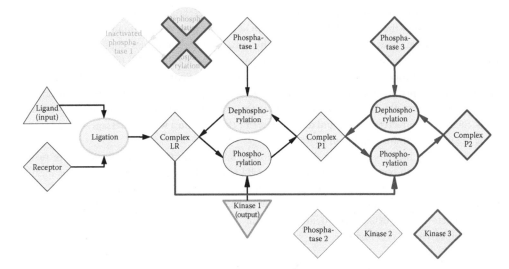

Figure 7.3 The different kinds of mutation of our algorithm, acting on the network of Figure 7.2, are depicted here. Ligation and dephosphorylation, for example, have modified parameters. The algorithm has also changed the topology of the network: the cross indicates deletion of an interaction and its child species, a kinase has been added as well as a new phosphorylation step of the main complex. Moreover, the output of the system has changed.

- **Choose a new output.** The nature of the output considered for fitness computation itself is under mutation, and can be changed during the course of evolution. For instance, it could potentially be any complex in the receptor phosphorylation cascades, or a free kinase/phosphatase. Not constraining the output is another way to unleash evolutionary forces as much as we can.

Possible mutations are illustrated on Figure 7.3. Relative mutation rates (i.e., the probability of mutations) are predefined by the user for a given simulation, and the algorithm is generally run in a regime where modifications of parameters are much more probable than changes of network topologies, and where removal of interactions are much more probable than addition of new biochemical species or interactions. We also rescale mutation rates at each generation so that on average there is one mutation per network per generation: this prevents an uncontrolled combinatorial explosion of the network (due to the fact number of interactions increases quadratically with number of biochemical species present) and implements the phenomenological Drake rule that mutation rates (inversely) scale with genome size (Lynch, 2007).

7.3.4 MUTUAL INFORMATION AS FITNESS FUNCTION

The success of evolutionary computation crucially resides in the choice of the fitness function, namely the function that allows us to rank the different networks with respect to their performance in the task of ligand discrimination. Apart from the obvious fact that this function should describe a form of discrimination, it should also be loose enough in order to start sorting the network even at the very first step of our numerical evolution, a point at which the networks are still very simple and—truly speaking—perform very badly. Moreover, the fitness function must be as abstract as possible in order not to guide evolution in a predefined implementation of the function. In short, we want to let evolution express its creativity!

A natural formalism to formulate the discrimination problem here is the information theory developed by Shannon (Shannon, 1948), which offers quantitative ways to assess questions such as "How well does the output of our network correlate with the nature of the input ligand"? Or more precisely, how much information about the ligand do I have by looking at the steady state concentration of some output?

For the sake of clarity, let us take a first simple example (unrelated to biology). I roll a die twice and announce that the sum is 6. What can you say about the value of the first roll? What if the sum is not 6 but 12? It is clear that even if there is an unknown variable (here the result of the second roll) you can extract some piece of information from the sum of the two rolls. For instance, if we know the sum is 6, we are sure that the first result cannot be itself 6, so we have (slightly) reduced the uncertainty (or increased the information) on the first die. If we know the sum is 12, both dice should be 6 so we have maximum information (and 0 uncertainty) on the first die. Now, imagine we can add a hypothesis: if we know the second die is strongly loaded and only results in 1 or 6, we then are almost certain that the first die rolled a 5 if the sum is 6.

In information theory, the key concept of *entropy*, defined by Shannon (Shannon, 1948), is a measure for the unpredictability of a random event. The higher the entropy of this event, the less predictable it is. In communication theory, this is also a convenient measure for information because the more unpredictable an event is, the more "characters" you would need to describe this event in a written message. Roughly speaking, entropy is a measure of this number of characters.

To have a usable measure, Shannon designed it to be additive, meaning that the entropy of two events should be the sum of the entropy of each one. As is well known, adding two independent events means multiplying the possibilities: the logarithm thus seems to be a good function to express this. For example, the entropy of a fair six sided die may be log(6), two dice would have an entropy of $\log(6^2) = 2\log(6)$, as it should be.

The complete formula extends this definition to non-uniformly distributed events. The entropy of a discrete random variable X is defined as:

$$\varepsilon(X) = -\sum_{x \in X} p(X = x)\log_2(p(X = x)),$$
(7.3)

where $p(X = x)$ is the probability of the output x. We take the $\log_2$ because it is the more widespread in information theory due to the very binary nature of the used tools. But using any other logarithm would not change the picture. The unit of entropy (with $\log_2$) is the Shannon or Bit. Entropy quantifies the uncertainty about a random event. An entropy near 0 means that there is practically no uncertainty: the event is highly predictable. Conversely, an event that is uniformly distributed between 2^N states has an entropy of $-\sum_N 1/2^N \log_2 2^N = N$ bits.

When dealing with several variables, the correct concept to use for such problems is the *mutual information*. The mutual information of two discrete random variables X and Y, is defined as

$$I(X,Y) = \sum_{x \in X} \sum_{y \in Y} p(x,y)\log_2\left(\frac{p(x)p(y)}{p(x,y)}\right),$$
(7.4)

It measures the amount of information, expressed in bits, that you can acquire about one of the two variables by reading the other one. Mathematically we can express mutual information as the difference of two entropies:

$$I(X,Y) = \varepsilon(X) - \varepsilon(X|Y)$$
(7.5)

where we have introduced $\varepsilon(X|Y)$, the entropy of X conditional to the knowledge of variable Y.* So we see that mutual information has an intuitive meaning: it is the difference between the uncertainty that we have on X with the uncertainty that we have on X *if we know another variable Y*. To come back to our previous example, X would be for instance the value of the first die, while Y would be the value of the sum of the dice. If X and Y are totally independent unrelated events, the uncertainty we have on X does not change if we know Y, i.e., $\varepsilon(X|Y) = \varepsilon(X)$, which means that the mutual information is 0 as expected. If conversely, Y completely determines X, then $\varepsilon(X|Y) = 0$ (no uncertainty on X) and we see that the mutual information $I(X|Y) = \varepsilon(X)$ and is maximum, as entropy is a positive quantity.

---

* Defined as $\varepsilon(X|Y) = -\sum_{y \in Y} p(Y = y)\left[\sum_{x \in X} p(X = x|Y)\log_2\left(p(X = x|Y)\right)\right]$

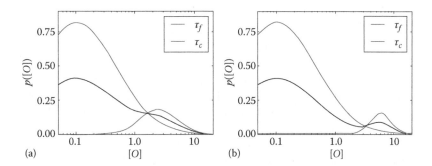

Figure 7.4 Example of mutual information computation for two different output responses. On each panel, the left curve describes the typical response to a non-agonist ligand and the right one to an agonist ligand. The intermediate curve represents the output of the system when both types can be seen with equal probability. The left panel shows a mutual information between the output and the ligand type of IM = 0.32, while the right one has IM = 0.60, highlighting the fact that the intermediate curve on the right panel is more bimodal and hence more informative about the type of ligand encountered.

Coming back to the immune discrimination problem, the first die (X) corresponds to the nature of the ligand (agonist or non agonist, called T), the unknown information the concentration of the ligand, and the announcement of the sum (Y) to the concentration of some output of the biochemical recognition network (that we call o). That gives

$$I(T,O) = \sum_{\tau \in T} \sum_{o \in O} p(\tau,o) \log_2 \left(\frac{p(\tau)p(o)}{p(\tau,o)} \right) \tag{7.6}$$

$$= \varepsilon(T) - \varepsilon(T \mid O) \tag{7.7}$$

Assuming we fix $\varepsilon(T)$, then having maximum mutual information between type and output concentrations means that $\varepsilon(T|O)$ (uncertainty of the type given the Output value) should be minimum, i.e., the knowledge of the Output concentration completely determines the type of ligands. This is what we expect from a biochemical decision process where for instance some internal switch unambiguously distinguishes between two situations.

We ran our evolutionary computation with $I(T,O)$ as objective function to maximize (once O has reached steady state). Now the value of the mutual information clearly depends on the distribution of ligands presented to the cells (i.e., not only the probability $P(T)$ but also the possible ligand concentrations presented to the cells). Unfortunately, we do not know precisely what these distributions are, so (conservative) assumptions should be made. For computational evolution, we chose a uniform distribution of log-ligand concentrations (to account for the fact that discrimination should be possible over large range of ligand concentrations), and probability 1/2 to have agonist (defined by binding time $\tau = 10s$) or non agonist (defined by binding time $\tau = 3s$). Figure 7.4 illustrates possible distribution of ligands and binding times with different mutual information: panel B is more "bimodal" than panel A, and the corresponding mutual information is higher, meaning there is more information on the nature of ligands encountered.

7.4 RESULTS OF EVOLUTIONARY COMPUTATION

At the very beginning of the evolutionary simulation, the network is initialized with a simple ligand-receptor interaction, which gives a first ligand-receptor complex that we call C_0. Then the algorithm randomly implements different network modifications based on a biochemical grammar defining all possible interactions within a network as described previously and selects them based on the mutual information fitness described in previous section.

7.4.1 ADAPTIVE SORTING

Apart from the junk networks* that unavoidably appear through the course of evolution, the core mechanism that performs the function of interest is always the same for all of our runs. This surprising fact is a good advocate for the use of inverse problems to unravel the mystery of biological system. For a given function, the number of typical implementations that can be found through evolution may actually be quite low. This not only means that we may hope to recover the correct architecture through our *in silico* evolution, but also that the same kind of solution may appear in various context—an intuition that will be reinforced later—making the detailed analysis of a particular problem even more fruitful.

The benchmark to analyze our results will be the golden triangle of selectivity, sensitivity, and speed. The network should correctly separate the correct and the false ligand irrespectively of their concentrations and in a time that is comparable with the one found in real system. For example, the *kinetic proof reading* (KPR) mechanism that was first proposed in (McKeithan, 1995), despite displaying interesting properties with respect to the selectivity does not account for the sensitivity in the range of concentration found *in vivo* and would need much longer times than effectively observed as discussed in (Altan-Bonnet and Germain, 2005). We ran the genetic algorithm using mutual information between type of ligands T and number of Outputs O as an objective function to optimize for our networks. Simulations very systematically converge towards a simple category of networks, which is depicted in Figure 7.5 (Lalanne and Francois, 2013). The core network is built upon a one-step KPR mechanism: the antigen starts binding with the receptor to form the complex C_0 which then produces the complex C_1 corresponding to our output. Building upon this KPR mechanism, the unphospho-rylated complex C_0 controls the activity of the kinase K responsible for its own phosphorylation. This is done through the regulation of the phosphorylation of K. The feedforward loop thus created effectively controls the output so that it depends mainly on r irrespectively of the ligand concentration (see curves for different τ on Figure 7.6a'). To understand why, we need to write down the equations for the three main species:

$$
\begin{aligned}
\dot{C}_0 &= \kappa RL - \left(\alpha K + \tau^{-1}\right)C_0, \\
\dot{C}_1 &= \alpha K C_0 - \tau^{-1}C_1, \\
\dot{K} &= -\delta C_0 K + \epsilon K^*
\end{aligned}
\tag{7.8}
$$

Introducing $K_T = K + K^*$, the total concentration of K, the last line gives $K = \dfrac{\epsilon K_T}{\delta C_0 + \epsilon}$ at a steady state, which would be clearer if we introduce $C_* = \dfrac{\epsilon}{\delta}$ so that $K = \dfrac{K_T C_*}{C_0 + C_*}$. Then, the second line gives the final output

$$
C_1 = \alpha K_T \tau \frac{C_0 C_*}{C_0 + C_*},
\tag{7.9}
$$

which, while still being a function of C_0, is already very informative about the behavior of the feedback loop. Indeed, it appears a function of the form $f(x) = \dfrac{\alpha x}{\alpha + x}$ which has two obvious asymptotes with $f \simeq x$ for $x \ll a$ and $f \simeq x$ for $x \gg a$. This means that our network introduces a threshold concentration C_* above which the network saturates, effectively buffering the high concentrations to a predefined level. Most importantly, the saturation level is

$$
C_1^{sat} = \alpha K_T C_* \tau
\tag{7.10}
$$

---

* This term is of course reminiscent of the well-known junk DNA. It is similar in his causes as it is produce by the very structure of the evolutionary algorithm as a part which is under no real selective pressure and so just remain here apparently without purpose. Now, this junk DNA may actually be quite useful, providing raw material for the evolution to build upon. The same is probably true for our own networks but have not been quantified.

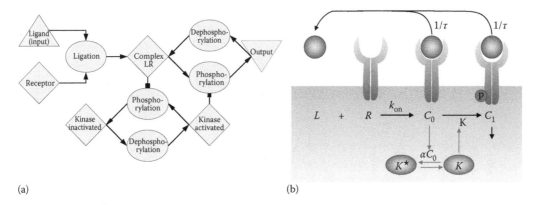

Figure 7.5 (a) The adaptive sorting mechanism as represented by our algorithm and **(b)** a corresponding more intuitive biological reaction scheme. The kinetic proofreading part of the network is depicted in bold, the incoherent feedforward loop that transform it into an adaptive sorting mechanism is depicted in grey. (Adapted from François, P., and Altan-Bonnet, G., *Journal of Statistical Physics*, 162(5), 1130–1152, 2016.)

i.e., is proportional to τ. Thus, C_1 realizes a direct measure of τ almost independently from ligand concentration! One can then imagine that a downstream sensor can measure the level of C_1 and triggers a response when it is higher than a predefined threshold, i.e., $C_1 \geq \Theta$. Thus, the threshold of detection for the binding time r is directly defined by:

$$\tau_c = \frac{\Theta}{\alpha K_T C_*} \tag{7.11}$$

The key mechanism to explain this is the incoherent feedforward loop (Mangan and Alon, 2003) between the complex and the kinase that perform its phosphorylation. The term incoherent here means that the complex C_0 effectively restrains its own phosphorylation in order to buffer the effect of high ligand concentration on the final output. This renders the concentration of C_1 almost insensitive to the ligand concentration L presented: this is indeed a well-known mechanism in classical biochemical adaptation, see e.g., (François and Siggia, 2008; Ma et al., 2009), thus the name of "adaptive sorting" for this absolute discrimination process. Lastly, it should be pointed out that in this model, different receptors are independent with respect to ligand binding, but coupled via the kinase K that is assumed to be shared between all receptors.

By construction, adaptive sorting satisfies specificity and sensitivity. Speed is related to an implicit issue: the low number of molecules implicated. If we want to detect a small number of ligands L, in a more realistic setting, we should observe huge stochastic fluctuations in the number of biochemical species of the detection network, and this can only be filtered out by more or less sophisticated test (e.g., (Siggia and Vergassola, 2013)). We chose a conservative approach where we assumed that some variable is present to average fluctuations: then indeed decision can be taken in at most a couple of minutes even with very low ligand concentration (Lalanne and François, 2013). So in the end adaptive sorting is a simple elegant solution naturally realizing the golden triangle of Figure 7.1.

7.4.2 ANTAGONISM

But an interesting phenotypic surprise lies at the heart of the adaptive sorting solution. Despite the fact that this was not explicitly selected for* in the adaptive sorting model, ligands below threshold of detection τ_c are antagonists, very similarly to what is observed in reality (François et al., 2013; François and Altan-Bonnet, 2016). This is illustrated on Figure 7.6a": when cells are exposed to ligands below thresholds τ_c, one needs many more agonist ligands to trigger response.

---

* And as it is a detrimental feature, we would never think of selecting our networks for that!

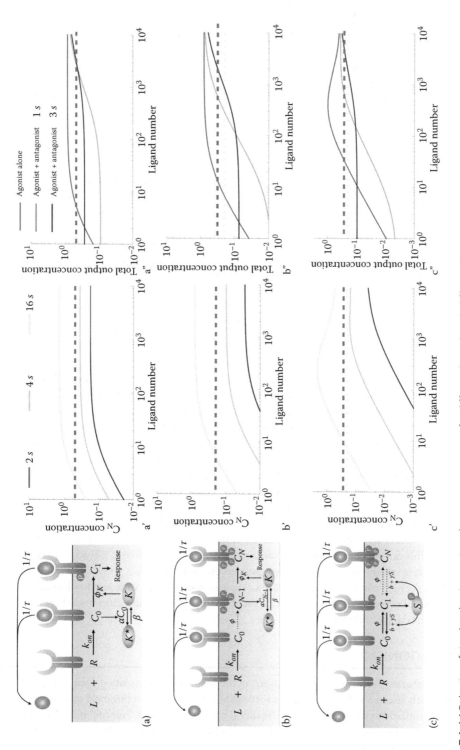

Figure 7.6 (a) Behavior of simple adaptive sorting: dose response curves for different ligands with different binding times τ in a', and dose response curves of agonists in presence of 10^4 antagonists in a". Dashed line indicates threshold for detection, so that only ligands with $\tau = 16s$ will trigger response in a'. **(b)** Behaviour of adaptive sorting with more upstream proofreading steps. Antagonism is mitigated but does not completely disappear (compare b" and a"). **(c)** Behaviour of immune system model from (François et al., 2013). (Adapted from François, P., and Altan-Bonnet, G., *Journal of Statistical Physics*, 162(5), 1130–1152, 2016.)

Antagonism has a very simple and intuitive explanation: it originates from the existence of the shared pool of kinase K. When one type of ligands is present, deactivation of kinase K exactly balances direct induction of signal, to give rise to a response that is concentration independent but sensitive to binding time τ. When several types of ligands are presented, they still all deactivate kinase K. But then ligands below threshold yield less signal than ligands above threshold, so that the overall response is lower. Thus ligands below threshold "antagonize" ligands above threshold.

Mathematically, calling C and D the complex corresponding to ligands above (L_f, τ_f) and below (L_s, τ_s) threshold simultaneously presented to the same cell, we have now

$$
\begin{aligned}
&\dot{C}_0 \kappa R L_f - \left(\alpha K + \tau^{-1}\right) C_0, \\
&\dot{C}_1 = \alpha K C_0 - \tau_f^{-1} C_1, \\
&\dot{D}_0 = \kappa R L_s - \left(\alpha K + \tau^{-1}\right) D_0, \\
&\dot{D}_1 = \alpha K D_0 - \tau_s^{-1} D_1, \\
&\dot{K} = -\delta (C_0 + D_0) K + \epsilon K^*.
\end{aligned}
\tag{7.12}
$$

At steady state, we thus have $K = \dfrac{K_T C_*}{C_0 + D_0 + C_*}$ so that in the limit where $C_0 + D_0 \gg C_*$, the total phosphorylated receptor is

$$
C_1^{sat} + D_1^{sat} = \alpha K_T C_* \frac{\tau_f C_0 + \tau_s D_0}{C_0 + D_0}
\tag{7.13}
$$

Now imagine that τ_s is very small, then

$$
C_1^{sat} + D_1^{sat} = \alpha K_T C_* \frac{\tau_f C_0}{C_0 + D_0} < \alpha K_T C_* \tau_f
\tag{7.14}
$$

which means that if decision is based on thresholding of this variable, we are farther below threshold and thus might lose response. This effect is clearly coming from the presence of D_0 in the denominator of the left hand side of Equation 7.14, accounting for the fact that ligands below threshold decrease K but do not contribute to final signaling because of low τ_s.

Putting realistic numbers together, an extra difficulty appears: with realistic biological parameters, even self ligands (with $\tau \simeq 0.1$s) would be strong antagonists with the simple adaptive sorting scheme, and thus immune detection in presence of self ligands would be impossible! To solve this last conundrum, we turned to computational evolution again, by re-running all our simulations so that our networks should perform detection in the presence of self ligands. A natural solution appearing in evolution is simply to add a couple of proofreading steps, upstream of the control of kinase K (Figure 7.6b). For instance, if there are N total proofreading steps and m steps upstream of K, we now get for the output variable:

$$
C_N^{sat} + D_N^{sat} \simeq \frac{\tau_f^N C_0 + \tau_f^N D_0}{\tau_f^m C_0 + \tau_s^m D_0}
\tag{7.15}
$$

In that case, if $\tau_s \ll \tau_f$, contributions of D_0 on *both* the numerator and the denominator are negligible compared to C_0, which means that detection in presence of subthresholds ligands is possible because antagonism is strongly mitigated (compare Figure 7.6a" and b"). So while proofreading appears crucial as first proposed by McKeithan (McKeithan, 1995) it is in an unexpected way: proofreading helps detection primarily by preventing antagonism by self. An analogy can be made using decision theory: in McKeithan's original model, proofreading ensures that self ligands do not trigger response, i.e., "decreases" the possibility of false positives due to self. In adaptive sorting, proofreading ensures that decision can be taken despite presence of potentially antagonizing self, i.e., "decreases" the possibility of false negatives due to self.

Connections to decision theory for those models have been more formally studied in (Lalanne and François, 2015). Finally, when performing evolution in presence of self, new solutions appear where the buffering role of K is played by phosphatases instead of a kinase.

7.5 LINKING BACK TO BIOLOGY AND EXTENSIONS

Once principles have been identified by computational evolution, one can check if candidates for the different processes at the heart of adaptive sorting exist in actual TCR recognition network.

7.5.1 A NEGATIVE FEEDBACK MODEL FOR RECOGNITION BY T CELL

The kinetic proofreading backbone is generally assumed to correspond to successive phosphorylations of ITAMs on receptor intracellular domains (Kersh et al., 1998). Fast dephosphorylations are due to kinetic segregation mechanisms (Davis and van der Merwe, 2006). This connection was actually implicit in our biochemical grammar.

Adaptive sorting presented in previous section predicts an internal loop, where an early complex in the cascade prevents further phosphorylations via titration of a kinase (i.e., repression of an effector). In the real system, it seems a phenomenological similar effect is the activation of the SHP-1 phoshpatase (i.e., consisting in the activation of a repressor). SHP-1 has been clearly established as a negative component of the system in seminal papers by Dittel et al. (Dittel et al., 1999), and Stefanová et al. (Stefanová et al., 2003). Most of this negative effect has been shown via antagonistic experiments, where recruitment of SHP-1 by receptors bound to antagonist ligands leads to dephosphorylation of ITAMs. Furthermore, this effect is infectious within the same cell: once SHP-1 is active, it can act even on receptors unbound to antagonist. Later quantitative experiments have refined this view, and in particular have shown how level of SHP-1 modulates response (Altan-Bonnet and Germain, 2005). In particular, increase of SHP-1 activity has been associated to a "digital" loss of response (Feinerman et al., 2008b) when negative effects overwhelm any possible activation.

This led us to propose a simplified phenotypic model including only kinetic proofreading and negative influence by SHP-1 (François et al., 2013) (Figure 7.6c). Behavior of this model is very similar to adaptive sorting, with a "flattening" of dose response curve over several orders of magnitude of ligand concentration at the threshold for binding time τ_c (Figure 7.6c'). A difference with adaptive sorting models is that SHP-1 acts on all proofreading steps, while we need kinase K to be specific to one proofreading step in models of Figure 7.6a and b. Thus, in some sense, the more realistic immune model represents a parsimonious solution implementing adaptive sorting with non-specific enzymes.

This model is semi-analytic and reproduces all aspects of absolute discrimination by T cells described in this chapter: sensitivity, specificity, speed, and antagonism (Figure 7.6c" and (François et al., 2013) for an experimental study). It is also able to recover the digital loss of response seen in (Feinerman et al., 2008b) when SHP-1 is over-expressed. Interestingly, a new prediction of this model is that for intermediate activity of SHP-1, response might be lost first at high concentration of ligands, yielding a non-monotonic response curve, which has been indeed checked experimentally (François et al., 2013).

7.5.2 THE ACTUAL AND THE POSSIBLE: PHENOTYPIC SPANDREL AND GENERALIZATION TO OTHER SYSTEMS

It thus appears in retrospect that the principle of adaptive sorting derived by our computational approach is at the core of early immune recognition. We also saw how some internal negative variables can act as a "brake" on the system and are responsible for antagonism. Antagonism appears to be detrimental to the system because it can prevent agonists from triggering response. Furthermore, even when we select against antagonism in our evolutionary simulations while new proofreading steps appear, there is still some antagonism for subthreshold ligands (Lalanne and François, 2013). Can we get perfect discrimination without antagonism?

The answer to this question is no, under broad generic assumptions. One can simply show mathematically (François et al., 2016) that a biochemical system with the ability to sort chemical compounds with respect to a kinetic parameter τ_{eff}, *independently* from their concentration, presents two properties:

- independence of concentration for detection implies that they are biochemically adaptive right at the threshold τ_c for detection of chemical parameter τ_{eff},
- because of this biochemical adaptation, antagonism necessary ensues.

The reason why antagonism derives from biochemical adaptation is rather intuitive: if the response of a system is biochemically adaptive, i.e., does not depend on stimulus concentration, then some variable in the system buffers for ligand concentration to ensure a completely flat dose response curve (see e.g., (François and Siggia, 2008; Ma et al., 2009)). This internal variable then plays the exact same role as the kinase described in the above section on adaptive sorting: when it is activated by subthreshold ligands, antagonism ensues. This is completely independent of the specific biochemistry of the system. Interestingly, it turns out that we can find other systems potentially performing absolute discrimination, with completely different biochemistry, that indeed display antagonism as expected. For instance, in another immune context, FCReRI signalling pathways display a so-called "dog in the manger effect" (Torigoe et al., 1998), where ligands sub threshold have been shown to indeed titrate the kinase responsible for the activation of the response, which is exactly the effect predicted by adaptive sorting.

Thus, the theory developed in (François et al., 2016) ends up fully solving the inverse problem of absolute discrimination under fairly general assumptions: adaptive sorting, defined as an adaptive process combined to a τ sensitive mechanism, is the generic solution to the absolute discrimination problem close to threshold τ_c. It can nevertheless be implemented biochemically in many different ways (some examples are given in (François et al., 2016)). However, adaptive sorting appears as a local property in a specific region of parameter space at $\tau = \tau_c$. It does not preclude more complex non-linear effects for different τ: for instance, for the simplest linear model, antagonism grows when τ gets further below threshold (François et al., 2016), while for proofreading-based models, antagonism reaches a maximum slightly below threshold, then entirely disappears for ligands with very small τ. Finally, for more realistic biochemical models, absolute discrimination might not be perfect and work only for relatively high L ligand concentrations, but interestingly antagonism can still be observed, indicating that the associated mathematical constraints persist even for imperfect discrimination (François et al., 2013).

Finally, turning back to evolution, the fact that antagonism always works hand in hand with absolute discrimination is reminiscent of the classical "spandrel" debate in evolutionary biology. Gould and Lewontin (Gould and Lewontin, 1979) proposed in the late 1970s that not all functional biological traits result from evolutionary adaptation. Their idea was that some phenotypes could simply come as a byproduct of the "true" selected phenotypes, just as the elaborated spandrels of the Basilica San Marco in Venice were primarily the architectural consequences of the positioning of domes on pillars. They argued that many complex phenotypes might simply be consequences of deeper evolutionary constraints. In turn, these spandrel phenotypes might be later tinkered by evolution, leading to the notion of exaptation (Gould and Vrba, 1982). So it could potentially be that many complex biological features are first born as spandrels, and studying the origin of spandrels might be crucial to understand macroevolution in general. Our mathematical study (François et al., 2016) thus clearly establishes that antagonism in our evolutionary simulations indeed is a spandrel of absolute discrimination, showing that evolutionary computation can indeed lead to interesting insights on evolution itself (François and Siggia, 2012).

7.6 WHAT WE HAVE LEARNED

Based on the example of immune recognition at the level of the gene regulatory network, we have shown in this chapter how the joint use of phenotypic models and genetic algorithm can help us to derive simplified principles—here the "adaptive sorting" model for immune recognition. With a broader view, it appears that once we succeed to identify the abstract goal of evolution-discriminating ligand irrespectively of their concentration for our example, such procedure may give us much simpler pictures and deeper insights than what was first expected. This success comes from the use of evolutionary computation approach as a method for performing the inverse problem of biological systems, an approach that is finally close to the original thought of the father of genetic algorithm (Holland, 1992). It is likely that other problems can be formulated in a similar way, and by such a combination of numerical simulations and pen and paper reasoning we might be able to highlight the meaningful flow of information hiding beneath the hairball of biological interactions.

This method not only helps us to understand the very basis of system such as adaptive sorting, but, by comparing our result to the known biochemistry of the system and refining our hypotheses to account of those facts, it also reveals the role of the different parts of the real system in a modular fashion. In our example, the upstream proofreading step appears to be a response to the presence of self as can be seen as it evolves to avoid the detrimental effects of antagonism, only when this feature of the environment is explicitly introduced in our model. Similarly, we can go back to our pens and build a model where some hypothesis are relaxed, on specificity of phosphorylations. This allowed us to reformulate a simplified realistic model of what happens in real immune detection.

On a more fundamental level, we might expect that the existence of "phenotypic spandrels," that is the appearance of complex features as by-products of the physical and chemical constraints from another evolved trait may be a general principle of evolution. The antagonism is so tightly linked with the absolute discrimination that each case of evolved absolute discrimination exhibits its own form of antagonism. This allows us, at a more abstract level, to connect several systems with completely different biochemistry, and thus we might have discovered a unifying principle of absolute discrimination. At an even higher scale, this suggests that spandrels might be give important constraints on evolution, as first intuited by Gould and Lewontin (Gould and Lewontin, 1979; Gould and Vrba, 1982). We have been able at least in this situation to formalize and confirm this intuition.

APPENDIX

As a textbook example for evolutionary computation of a gene network, let us look a simple example: a biological "chronometer," estimating the duration of a given signal. How can a purely transcriptional network measure duration? Our algorithm is tailored to answer such questions. To frame the problem, we assume there is an input signal. We take the simplest possible form: a gate function. The input thus has a value I between time 0 and τ and is 0 otherwise. We would like our system to have an output where we could read τ independently of the level of I.

To evaluate the performance of a given network, we launch several integrations (tries) for different value of the parameters τ, I and collect the final value of one predefined output O_f. Then we fit the function $O_f = A\tau$ and take the squared error as a measure of how well the network allow us to read the time up to a multiplicative constant (the lower, the better):

$$\phi = \sum_{tries} \left(\frac{O_f}{A\tau} - 1 \right)^2 \tag{7.16}$$

where A has been fit over all the tries.

After several generations, some of our runs are found to have a very good performance (see Figure 7.7). The networks that constitute the population of working networks are quite complex. We can then (manually or automatically) modify several parameters while preserving their performance and prune the networks. After removing every unnecessary part, we end up with the simplest working network, where an output with a very low degradation rate is simply activated by the input. A simple equation for this network is:

$$\frac{dO}{dt} = r \frac{I^n}{I^n + h^n} - \delta O \tag{7.17}$$

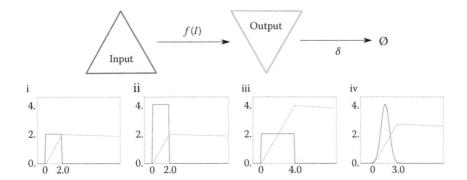

Figure 7.7 A simple evolved biological chronometer, where an Input activates an Output. i to iv represents the behavior of the network for different signal shape and durations, the level of the Output is clearly proportional to the duration of the signal—as indicated by its behavior linear in time—illustrating robustness of the solution.

Indeed, if the output starts from 0 and $\delta \simeq 0$, the level of the output will simply time-integrate when the signal is present $O(t) \simeq r \int_0^t \frac{I(t')^n}{I(t')^n + h^n} dt'$. To get rid of the I-dependency, the activation is saturated even for low value of I, i.e., $h \simeq 0$ so that $O \simeq r\tau$. During an evolutionary run, activation of O by I is first selected, then parameters are optimized so that both δ and h go to 0. This situation exemplifies many of our evolutionary simulations: while solutions found can be very simple, they are quite robust and furthermore there might be some hidden constraints (here saturation of activation with respect to I) that are biologically predictive and might not be obvious a priori for more complex problems.

REFERENCES

Altan-Bonnet, G., and Germain, R.N. (2005). Modeling T cell antigen discrimination based on feedback control of digital ERK responses. *PLoS Biology 3*(11), e356.

Cotterell, J., and Sharpe, J. (2010). An atlas of gene regulatory networks reveals multiple three-gene mechanisms for interpreting morphogen gradients. *Molecular Systems Biology 6*, 425.

Daniels, B.C., and Nemenman. I. (2015). Automated adaptive inference of phenomenological dynamical models. *Nature Communications 6*, 8133.

Davis, S.J., and van der Merwe, P.A. (2006). The kinetic-segregation model: TCR triggering and beyond. *Nature Immunology 7*(8), 803-809.

Dittel, B.N., Stefanova, I., Germain, R.N., and Janeway, C.A. (1999). Cross-antagonism of a T cell clone expressing two distinct T cell receptors. *Immunity 11*(3), 289-298.

Duvenaud, D., Lloyd, J.R., Grosse, R., Tenenbaum, J.B., and Ghahramani, Z. (2013). Structure Discovery in Nonparametric Regression through Compositional Kernel Search.

Feinerman, O., Germain, R.N., and Altan-Bonnet, G. (2008a). Quantitative challenges in understanding ligand discrimination by $\alpha\beta$ T cells. *Molecular Immunology 45*(3), 619-631.

Feinerman, O., Veiga, J., Dorfman, J.R., Germain, R.N., and Altan-Bonnet, G. (2008b). Variability and Robustness in T Cell Activation from Regulated Heterogeneity in Protein Levels. *Science 321*(5892), 1081-1084.

François, P. (2014). Evolving phenotypic networks in silico. *Seminars in cell & developmental biology 35*, 90-97.

François, P., and Altan-Bonnet, G. (2016). The Case for Absolute Ligand Discrimination: Modeling Information Processing and Decision by Immune T Cells. *Journal of Statistical Physics 162*(5), 1130-1152.

François, P. and Hakim, V. (2004). Design of genetic networks with specified functions by evolution in silico. *Proc Natl Acad Sci U S A 101*(2), 580-585.

François, P. and Siggia, E.D. (2008). A case study of evolutionary computation of biochemical adaptation. *Physical Biology 5*(2), 26009.

François, P. and Siggia, E.D. (2012). Phenotypic models of evolution and development: Geometry as destiny. *Current Opinion in Genetics & Development 22*(6), 627-633.

François, P., Hakim, V., and Siggia, E.D. (2007). Deriving structure from evolution: Metazoan segmentation. *Molecular Systems Biology 3*, 9.

François, P., Voisinne, G., Siggia, E.D., Altan-Bonnet, G., and Vergassola, M. (2013). Phenotypic model for early T-cell activation displaying sensitivity, specificity, and antagonism. *Proc Natl Acad Sci U S A 110*(10), E888-997.

François, P., Hemery, M., Johnson, K.A., and Saunders, L.N. (2016). Phenotypic spandrel: Absolute discrimination and ligand antagonism. *Physical Biology 13*(6), 066011.

Fujimoto, K., Ishihara, S., and Kaneko, K. (2008). Network Evolution of Body Plans. *PLoS ONE 3*(7), e2772.

Gascoigne, N.R., Zal, T., and Alam, S.M. (2001). T-cell receptor binding kinetics in T-cell development and activation. *Expert Reviews in Molecular Medicine 2001*(06), 1-17.

Gould, S.J., and Lewontin, R.C. (1979). The spandrels of San Marco and the Panglossian paradigm: A critique of the adaptationist programme. *Proceedings of the Royal Society of London. Series B, Containing Papers of a Biological Character 205*(1161), 581-598.

Gould, S.J., and Vrba, E.S. (1982). Exaptation-a missing term in the science of form. *Paleobiology.*

Govern, C.C., Paczosa, M.K., Chakraborty, A.K., and Huseby, E.S. (2010). Fast on-rates allow short dwell time ligands to activate T cells. *Proc Natl Acad Sci U S A 107*(19), 8724-8729.

Hemery, M., and Rivoire, O. (2015). Evolution of sparsity and modularity in a model of protein allostery. *Physical review E, Statistical, Nonlinear, and Soft Matter Physics 91*(4).

Holland, J.H. (1992). *Adaptation in Natural and Artificial Systems: An Introductory Analysis with Applications to Biology, Control, and Artificial Intelligence.* Cambridge, MA: Bradford Book.

Jacob, F. (1981). *Le Jeu des possibles: Essai sur la diversité du vivant.* Fayard.

Kashtan, N., and Alon, U. (2005). Spontaneous evolution of modularity and network motifs. *Proc Natl Acad Sci U S A 102*(39), 13773-13778.

Kersh, E.N., Shaw, A.S., and Allen, P.M. (1998). Fidelity of T cell activation through multistep T cell receptor zeta phosphorylation. *Science 281*(5376), 572-575.

Lalanne, J-B., and François, P. (2013). Principles of adaptive sorting revealed by in silico evolution. *Physical Review Letters 110*(21), 218102.

Lalanne, J-B., and François, P. (2015). Chemodetection in fluctuating environments: Receptor coupling, buffering, and antagonism. *Proc Natl Acad Sci U S A 112*(6), 1898-1903, Jan. 2015.

Lander, A.D. (2010). The edges of understanding. *BMC Biology 8*, 40.

Lever, M., Maini, P.K., van der Merwe, P.A., and Dushek, O. (2014). Phenotypic models of T cell activation. *Nature Reviews Immunology 14*(9), 619-629.

Lipniacki, T., Hat, B., Faeder, J.R., and Hlavacek, W.S. (2008). Stochastic effects and bistability in T cell receptor signaling. *Journal of Theoretical Biology 254*(1), 110-122.

Lobo, D., and Levin, M. (2015). Inferring Regulatory Networks from Experimental Morphological Phenotypes: A Computational Method Reverse-Engineers Planarian Regeneration. *PLoS Comput Biol 11*(6), e1004295.

Lynch, M. (2007). *The origins of genome architecture.* Sinauer Associates Inc.

Ma, W., Trusina, A., El-Samad, H., Lim, W.A., and Tang, C. (2009). Defining network topologies that can achieve biochemical adaptation. *Cell 138*(4), 760-773.

Mangan, S., and Alon, U. (2003). Structure and function of the feed-forward loop network motif. *Proc Natl Acad Sci U S A 100*(21), 11980-11985.

Mayer, A., Balasubramanian, V., Mora, T., and Walczak, A.M. (2015). How a well-adapted immune system is organized. *Proc Natl Acad Sci U S A 112*(19), 5950-5955.

McKeithan, T.W. (1995). Kinetic proofreading in T-cell receptor signal transduction. *Proc Natl Acad Sci U S A 92*(11), 5042-5046.

Schmidt, M., and Lipson, H. (2009). Distilling Free-Form Natural Laws from Experimental Data. *Science 324*(5923), 81-85.

Shannon, C.E. A Mathematical Theory of Communication. (1948). *Bell System Technical Journal 27*(3), 379-423.

Siggia, E.D., and Vergassola, M. (2013). Decisions on the fly in cellular sensory systems. *Proc Natl Acad Sci U S A 110*(39), E3704-12, Sept. 2013.

Stefanová, I., Hemmer, B., Vergelli, M., Martin, R, Biddison, W.E., and Germain, R.N. (2003). TCR ligand discrimination is enforced by competing ERK positive and SHP-1 negative feedback pathways. *Nature Immunology 4*(3), 248-254.

Taylor, M.J., Husain, K., Gartner, Z.J., Mayor, S., and Vale, R.D. (2017). A DNA-Based T Cell Receptor Reveals a Role for Receptor Clustering in Ligand Discrimination. *Cell 169*(1), 108-119

ten Tusscher, K.H., and Hogeweg, P. (2011). Evolution of Networks for Body Plan Patterning; Interplay of Modularity, Robustness and Evolvability. *PLoS Comput Biol 7*(10), e1002208.

Tkach, K.E., Barik, D., Voisinne, G., Malandro, N., Hathorn, M.M., Cotari, J.W., Vogel, R., Merghoub, T., Wolchok, J., Krichevsky, O., and Altan-Bonnet, G. (2014). T cells translate individual, quantal activation into collective, analog cytokine responses via time-integrated feedbacks. *eLife 3*, e01944.

Torigoe, C., Inman, J.K., and Metzger, H. (1998). An unusual mechanism for ligand antagonism. *Science 281*(5376), 568-572.

Voisinne, G., Nixon, G.B., Melbinger, A., Gasteiger, G., Vergassola, M., and Altan-Bonnet, G. (2015). T Cells Integrate Local and Global Cues to Discriminate between Structurally Similar Antigens. *Cell Reports 11*(5), 1-12.

Zen and the art of parameter estimation in systems biology

CHRISTOPHER R. MYERS

8.1 INTRODUCTION

A mathematical model describes a space of possibilities. As this volume illustrates, models come in many shapes and sizes, and discerning an appropriate form of a model for a given problem is in many ways as much art as science, suggested by an intuitive feel for a problem and a drive to distill the important degrees-of-freedom needed to capture some phenomenon of interest. Alongside the poetry of identifying an ideal model form lies the more prosaic work of estimating the values of parameters that provide reality to that form.

Broadly speaking, mechanistic mathematical models typically consist of state variables, interaction rules among those variables, and parameters that quantify aspects of those state variables and interaction rules. Parameters dictate the space of possible model outputs, given a specified model structure. Thus, parameters represent a class of model inputs that impact what possible predictions a model can make. Parameter estimation is the process by which a modeler, having identified a plausible model structure, endeavors to determine the numerical values of parameters within that model in order to be able to assess model outcomes. As such, parameter estimation is an aspect of inference, and typically refers to a process of fitting parameters to data through their collective effects in a model; if one were able to measure parameters directly and with sufficient certainty, one would simply use those measured values as parameter inputs. But for many biological systems of interest, carrying out such measurements is not easy or may not be possible, and one is left instead with the process of reverse engineering plausible parameter values from measurements of state variables (or functions thereof) rather than forward simulation based on experimentally determined parametric inputs.

Many models of interest in the field of systems biology contain many unknown parameters, resulting in high-dimensional parameter spaces that must be characterized, with complex structure that is not well understood. Understanding such structure, and how it impacts the predictivity of models and the potential for the construction of alternative models, is an active area of research. I will begin by providing an overview of some of the mechanics of parameter estimation, although "mechanics" more perhaps in the style of *Zen and the Art of Motorcycle Maintenance* [1] than in that of the Chilton manuals for auto repair. Just as importantly, however, I will also endeavor to consider parameter estimation within the broader context of modeling, to describe how it relates to model construction, inference, selection, reduction, and analysis. I will close with some thoughts about the somewhat fractured and multifaceted field of systems biology, highlighting how issues of parameterization and parameter estimation lie at the crossroads of different schools of thought.

Even though I will mostly address mechanistic models of cellular processes, many of the concepts and techniques introduced here are broadly applicable to a wide range of models relevant not just to immunology and systems biology, but to other fields as well [2]. In the field of immunology, this might include statistical models, or descriptions at other levels of biological resolution, such as models of the population dynamics of pathogens replicating within hosts, or spreading among hosts [3]. Where possible, I will endeavor to point out generalities and abstractions that are useful across different classes of models, while also noting some of the particular aspects that arise in analyzing complex cellular networks.

8.2 THE MECHANICS OF PARAMETER ESTIMATION

8.2.1 ESTIMATING PARAMETERS FROM DATA

Let us assume that we have a set of M state variables $\mathbf{x}(t) = x_1(t),\ldots, x_M(t)$. Since we are focused here primarily on dynamical models, we assume there are a set of initial conditions $\mathbf{x}^0(t = 0)$, and a prescription for solving for the dynamics of the system at later times. If our model is deterministic, this prescription might involve formulating and integrating a set of coupled ordinary differential equations (ODEs) describing the time rate of change of chemical concentrations; if the model is stochastic, we might instead use a stochastic simulation algorithm such as Gillespie's method [4] to step the system forward in time. The particular trajectory that the system traces out in its state space will also depend on the choice of model parameters. We will denote this set of N parameters $\theta = \theta_1,\ldots, \theta_N$ and denote the trajectory's dependence on parameters as $\mathbf{x}(t;\theta)$. The goal of parameter estimation is to infer the numerical values of the parameters θ based on available data. For the case of deterministic dynamics described by ODEs, the state variables will unfold in time according to the dynamical equation $d\mathbf{x}/dt = \mathbf{f}(\mathbf{x},t;\theta)$, where $\mathbf{f}$ reflects the sum of all the reaction fluxes in and out of the states.

Experimental data might reflect individual state variables at specific time points $x_i(t_j;\theta)$, or they might reflect functions of multiple state variables. Often, one is able to measure the abundance of some chemical entity, but is unable to distinguish its participation in different molecular compounds or states; in such a case, the relevant observed quantity would reflect some weighted sum of individual state variables. In other cases, data might be available on reaction fluxes, which are (potentially nonlinear) functions of state variables. We might have measurements of the system under different experimental conditions, such as with different initial amounts of chemical species, or in a mutant where we have knocked out or overexpressed some particular component. Let $y^*_{o,c}(t_j)$ represent the value of observable o in condition c at time t_j; denote the uncertainty of that measurement as $\sigma_{o,c}(t_j)$; and let $y_{o,c}(t;\theta)$ represent the corresponding predictions of the model for a given set of parameters θ. We are interested in finding a choice of parameters θ for which the model trajectories

$\mathbf{y}(t;\theta)$ best approximate the measured values $y^*_{o,c}(tj)$. We can define a cost function $C(\theta)$ that represents the squared deviation of a given set of model predictions from the data:

$$C(\theta) = \frac{1}{2} \sum_{o,c,t_j} \left(\frac{y_{o,c}\,(t_j;\,\theta) - y^*_{o,c}\,(t_j)}{\sigma_{o,c}\,(t_j)} \right)^2,$$

where t_j refers to the timepoints at which the data are measured. The best fitting parameter set θ^* is that which minimizes the cost: $\theta^* = argmin[C(\theta)]$.

In statistics, one is often interested in computing the *likelihood* of a particular model, that is, the probability of observing the particular data measured given a set of parameters θ. If the model residuals are independent and normally distributed, then the cost function $C(\theta)$ corresponds to the negative logarithm of the likelihood $P(Data|\theta)$, where "Data" refers here to the full set of measured observables [5]:

$$P(Data|\theta) = \prod_{o,c,t_j} \frac{1}{\sqrt{2\pi}\sigma_{o,c,t_j}} \exp\left(-\frac{1}{2} \frac{y_{o,c}\,(t_j;\,\theta) - y^*_{o,c}\,(t_j)}{\sigma_{o,c}\,(t)}\right)^2$$

Minimizing the cost $C(\theta)$ corresponds to maximizing the likelihood function. Different statistical frameworks emphasize different aspects of this data-fitting problem: frequentist statistics typically focuses on estimating the parameters that maximize the likelihood, while Bayesian statistics uses the likelihood to estimate the posterior distribution, reflecting the probability of estimating different sets of parameters given the data. A nice discussion that emphasizes distinctions between frequentist and Bayesian statistical treatments of parameter estimation for models in systems biology can be found in [6].

Our goal is not just to fit the data, however, since the whole point of building a model is to be able to make predictions about situations for which we do not have data. One common pitfall in parameter estimation is overfitting, typically from having an overly complicated model with many parameters that can fit the existing data very well but which has poor predictive performance on unseen data. In such a case, the data are often "overfit" in the sense that the power of the model is used to fit random fluctuations in the data rather than the underlying trend of the data. Having laid this groundwork, we will now consider parameter estimation in the context of some specific models of biological networks.

8.2.2 Examples: JAK-STAT signaling and Epo receptor trafficking

Information processing lies at the core of many important biological functions, implemented by molecular networks supporting signal perception and integration. A central function of the immune system is to process signals in the environment and to decide whether those signals are associated with self or non-self. An important class of perception and signaling networks, relevant both to immune system function and other biological processes, is the JAK-STAT pathways [7,8]. JAK-STAT signaling involves the perception of extracellular ligands (cytokines, growth factors, etc.) by membrane-bound receptors (so-called Janus kinases, or JAKs) that trigger the activation of an intracellular molecular complex that subsequently translocates to the nucleus and affects gene transcription (so-called signal transducers and activators of transcription, or STATS). A schematic figure of this pathway is shown in Figure 8.1(a). This basic structural theme is played out again and again throughout systems biology, although this relatively simple signaling architecture is more reminiscent of bacterial two-component signaling systems [9] than the more deep and elaborate signaling cascades that have evolved in animals. In mammals, there are seven different JAK proteins and four different STATS. Therefore, this basic architecture can in principle be instantiated in various forms by combining different JAKs and STATs, although this molecular flexibility can also introduce the possibility of crosstalk among different components [10]. Whereas engineered communication systems can be constructed to support efficient

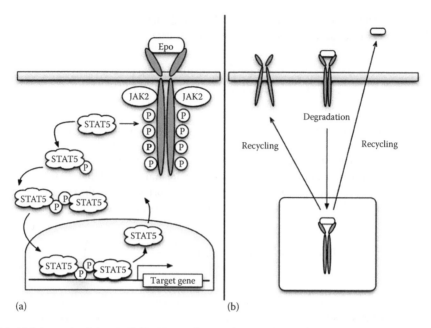

Figure 8.1 **(a)** Schematic of the JAK2-STAT5 signaling pathway (Adapted from Swameye, I et al., *Proceedings of the National Academy of Sciences of the United States of America*, 100(3), 1028–1033, 2003.), in which binding to extracellular Epo induces recruitment and phosphorylation of intracellular STAT5 via JAK2. Phosphorylated STAT5 dimerizes and translocates to the nucleus, where it regulates expression of target genes, followed by recycling of monomeric STAT5 back to the cytoplasm. **(b)** Schematic of receptor trafficking, involving the degradation and recycling of receptor proteins and ligands; an example is EpoR trafficking (Adapted from Becker, V. et al., *Science*, 328(5984),1404–1408, 2010.), in which bound Epo-EpoR complexes are internalized, and either degraded or recycled back to the membrane as free EpoR.

and nonambiguous codes [11], living systems that communicate through the interaction of many paralogous components evolving through duplication and divergence face the nontrivial challenge of communicating reliably in the face of constraints posed by crosstalk [12,13].

The development and analysis of mathematical models of JAK-STAT signaling has a rich history in the field of systems biology, with particular relevance to the problem of parameter estimation. Owing largely to the work of Timmer and colleagues, various models of JAK-STAT pathways have been constructed, fit to experimental data, and used to assess new theoretical and computational tools for parameter estimation and sensitivity analysis. Much of this work has centered on the JAK2-STAT5 pathway, which is involved in detecting the growth factor erythropoietin to stimulate the production of red blood cells.[1] The original JAK-STAT signaling model developed by Timmer and collegues [14,15] emphasized the importance of inference through "databased modeling," and worked through a series of related models to demonstrate the importance of STAT recycling from the nucleus back to the cytoplasm and time delays associated with that process. That model has been used as an application example on parameter estimation in various software packages, such as the SBML-PET Parameter Estimation Toolkit [16], SloppyCell [17,18], and Data2Dynamics [19]. Raue et al. examined this same model in their use of the profile likelihood to analyze structural and practical parameter identifiability [20]. Vanlier et al. used the model and underlying data to probe the relationship between parameter estimation and experimental design [21]. And Toni and Stumpf revisited JAK-STAT signaling as an application example to highlight their use of Approximate Bayesian Computation [6]. Readers interested in both the details of JAK-STAT signaling and the intricacies of parameter estimation are encouraged to dig through that rich history of research.

I will consider briefly a related model, involving not the downstream signaling through the JAK-STAT pathway, but the regulation and trafficking of membrane-bound receptors involved in Epo recognition at the gateway of JAK-STAT. Signaling networks are not static scaffolds along which information is communicated (as is often the case with our hard-wired engineered systems), but are instead dynamic entities themselves subject to regulation and control, as indicated schematically in Figure 8.1(b). The regulation and organization of membrane-bound receptors is important in a number of problems in systems biology [22,23,24] and their misregulation is sometimes implicated in diseases such as cancer, where an excess of growth factor receptors can lead to enhanced rates of cell growth. The model in question here was developed by Becker et al. as part of a larger study considering Epo receptor (EpoR) trafficking [23]. I will address here only the "core" model presented in [23]. The dynamical equations for the core model described the concentrations of various molecular states and complexes:

$$\frac{d}{dt}\Big[EpoR\Big] = k_t B_{max} - k_t\Big[EpoR\Big] - k_{on}\Big[Epo\Big]\Big[EpoR\Big] + k_{off}\Big[Epo-EpoR\Big] + k_{ex}\Big[Epo-EpoR_i\Big]$$

$$\frac{d}{dt}\Big[Epo\Big] = -k_{on}\Big[Epo\Big]\Big[EpoR\Big] + k_{off}\Big[Epo-EpoR\Big] + k_{ex}\Big[Epo-EpoR_i\Big]$$

$$\frac{d}{dt}\Big[Epo-EpoR\Big] = k_{on}\Big[Epo\Big]\Big[EpoR\Big] - k_{off}\Big[Epo-EpoR\Big] - k_e\Big[Epo-EpoR\Big]$$

$$\frac{d}{dt}\Big[Epo-EpoR_i\Big] = k_e\Big[Epo-EpoR\Big] - k_{ex}\Big[Epo-EpoR_i\Big] - k_{di}\Big[Epo-EpoR_i\Big] - k_{de}\Big[Epo-EpoR_i\Big]$$

$$\frac{d}{dt}\Big[dEpo_i\Big] = k_{di}\Big[Epo-EpoR_i\Big]$$

$$\frac{d}{dt}\Big[dEpo_e\Big] = k_{de}\Big[Epo-EpoR_i\Big]$$

While the model contains these six state variables, experimentally the authors were only able to measure pools of Epo in various compartments: Epo in the extracellular medium (Epo_medium = [Epo] + [dEpoe]), Epo at the cellular membrane (Epo_membrane = [Epo-EpoR]), and Epo in the interior of the cell (Epo_cells = [Epo-EpoR_i] + [dEpo_i]).

8.2.3 DATA FITTING

The actual process used by the authors for parameter estimation for this Epo receptor trafficking model is much more complicated than the simplified analysis that I will present here [23]. A variety of different assays were carried out to characterize and estimate subprocesses within the model, such as the binding of Epo to EpoR. In addition, multiple model variants were developed (the "core" model, the "core model + k_{mob}," and the "auxiliary" model), and parameter estimation was performed simultaneously for both the core and auxiliary model. I will not delve into all the complexity of the estimation process presented in [23], but will simply use the model and some of the data to illustrate some basic points.

As noted, experimental data are available characterizing the levels of Epo in various pools in three different locations: extracellular, on the membrane, and internal to the cell [25]. Experiments provide these levels at six time points (ranging from approximately 1 to 300 minutes after introduction of Epo) for three replicated versions of the experiment. From the replicated data, we can estimate the average levels of Epo in each location and at each time point: if we have no intrinsic information about the uncertainties inherent in the experimental data, we can estimate uncertainties in these mean quantities by computing the standard error of the triplicate points. From these 18 data points and their uncertainties, we can estimate the best-fitting set of model parameters. In [23], the parameter B_{max} was fixed based upon estimation from other data, as was the ratio of $K_D = k_{off}/k_{on}$; in this example, I will leave k_{off} and k_{on} as separate parameters and fit them to the time-course data. Thus the set of parameters to fit includes: k_t, k_{on}, k_{off}, k_e, k_{ex}, k_{di}, k_{de}. Using SloppyCell, a Python package we have developed to support the simulation and analysis of reaction networks, I can import the SBML version of the core model deposited by the authors at BioModels.net (BIOMD0000000271.xml, which encodes the reaction network and associated kinetic laws in the dynamical equations above), define a model which links together the experimental data and the model, add some priors to keep the parameters within broad ranges identified by the authors, and optimize the parameters to fit the data. Details on these sorts of operations can be found in the SloppyCell user's guide (http://sloppycell.sourceforge.net/user.pdf). The best-fit time-courses for the three observables are shown in Figure 8.2(a).

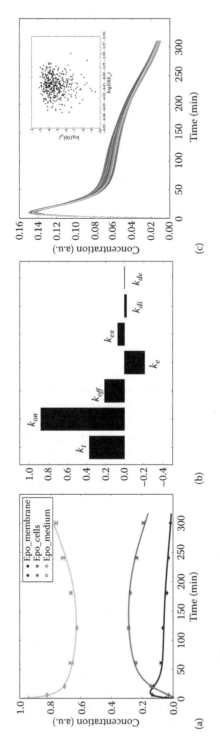

Figure 8.2 (a) Best-fit time courses in the Epo-EpoR model for the observed data. **(b)** Stiffest eigenvector of the approximate Hessian J^TJ at the best-fit set of parameters. **(c)** Main panel: Ensemble of trajectories for [Epo_membrane] over a sampled parameter ensemble. Inset: projection of parameter ensemble in the (k_{on}, k_{off}) plane.

Much of the power that one gains in dissecting complex biological systems arises from the ability to perturb such systems in a sufficiently diverse set of conditions so as to tease apart the contributions of different components and subsystems. If every such condition required estimation of an entirely new and disjoint set of parameters, nothing would be gained by combining different experiments. For example, suppose one could alter the pH within a cell, and conduct a series of experiments at different pH levels, but without having a model that incorporates the effects of pH directly, and with no idea how model parameters should vary as a function of pH. Every experiment would effectively be independent of all others, involving a different and unrelated parameter for each pH, even if all models shared the same underlying mathematical structure.[2] Fortunately, many experimental perturbations are often local in nature, affecting a node or an edge in a biochemical reaction network. In such a situation, one can fit data to different variants of a reaction network, differing only in these local perturbations. Unless there is reason to think otherwise, one can fit these multiple variants of a network—each of which makes different predictions about the specific experimental conditions relevant to that variant—to multiple datasets. More concretely, if we knock out some component of a network, we expect to be able to estimate the same numerical values for parameters elsewhere in the network that are not involved in that knockout. Different model variants that share parameters can typically have those parameters fit to system-specific data across all relevant experimental conditions.

In order to fit model parameters across sets of different conditions, one needs to coordinate the integration of experimental data with the appropriate model variants, running each model variant separately to fit the relevant data. One advantage to using existing tools targeted specifically for parameter estimation in reaction networks is that there is often support for that sort of data integration. The SloppyCell system, for example, stitches together objects representing collections of Experiments with objects representing collections of Calculations in order to carry out the combined inference. The Data2Dynamics system provides additional intelligence in this regard, automatically creating model variants for different experimental conditions and organizing output data accordingly [25,27]. These sorts of multi-experiment parameter estimation problems can be complicated in their structure, however: witness the different sets of experiments and estimation processes involved in Epo receptor trafficking discussed in [23]. The field of systems biology has been accelerated through the development of a standard format for the specification of reaction network models (the Systems Biology Markup Language, or SBML (sbml.org)), and there have been related efforts to develop additional ontologies and formats to standardize other aspects of the modeling process (e.g., characterization of simulation time courses, http://sed-ml.org). Given the importance of parameter estimation to the modeling process and the potential complexities inherent in carrying it out in practice, it might be worthwhile for the community to focus on the development of standard formats and data structures to organize parameter estimation activities, to enable the reuse and exchange of data, metadata and models for parameter estimation in the same way that SBML facilitates the reuse of the underlying model specifications themselves.

8.2.4 OPTIMIZATION

Abstracted appropriately, the specific form of a mathematical model is irrelevant insofar as the numerical optimization of the cost function is concerned, as long as it can evaluate the least-squares deviation of a model from data for a given set of parameters θ. Optimizing an arbitrary nonlinear function of a set of variables is a widespread problem throughout all of science, and accordingly, much algorithmic and development work has been devoted to producing numerical tools capable of carrying out this essential computational task. Numerical optimization is something of an art: there is a vast set of different algorithms that one might possibly make use of, and determining which is most appropriate for a given problem can require a bit of experimentation. Perhaps the most relevant distinguishing feature among different algorithms are those that are capable of identifying global optima and those that make do with finding local optima. In some cases, there can be multiple distinct local minima of the cost function $C(\theta)$ separated by barriers of higher cost. This can complicate the process of finding the global minimum, especially since most numerical minimization routines move locally downhill. Some optimization algorithms are in fact designed to avoid getting stuck in local minima, and one can often use local methods in conjunction with multiple independent restarts in order to converge to different minima. Several of those methods are addressed specifically in the context of biological parameter estimation in [28] and [27]. A more subtle complication in finding a global minimum, even in cases where there may be no other competing local minima, arises from a near degeneracy in the cost function near the minimum. This degeneracy is often associated with long, thin canyons in parameter space, resulting in multiple different combinations of parameters that are able to fit the data within the underlying uncertainty, along which the numerical values of individual parameters might vary wildly. I will return to this issue in more detail below in describing parametric sloppiness, but note here that in some cases a detailed understanding of the structure of cost surfaces under evaluation can lead to the development of novel optimization algorithms that exploit that structure, such as those involving geodesic flow along model manifolds [29].

8.2.5 SENSITIVITY ANALYSIS

Parameter sensitivity analysis quantifies how model trajectories depend upon variations in parameters. Formally, one can differentiate the dynamical equation for a system of interest with respect to parameters, and then reorder derivatives to arrive at a set of sensitivity equations for the parametric derivatives that can be solved alongside the underlying dynamical equations:

$$\frac{\partial}{\partial t} \frac{\partial x}{\partial \theta} = \frac{\partial f}{\partial x} \frac{\partial x}{\partial \theta} + \frac{\partial f}{\partial \theta}$$

Carrying out this sensitivity integration with analytically calculated derivatives is generally preferable to numerically estimating such sensitivities using finite-difference approximations to derivatives by imposing small variations on parameter values. Finite-difference approaches to sensitivity analysis generally do a poorer job of characterizing complicated cost surfaces, especially those plagued with long, thin, shallow canyons. Tools such as SloppyCell and Data2Dynamics calculate these analytic derivatives from the underlying kinetic laws and reaction network topology, supporting sensitivity integration.

One is not limited to characterizing sensitivities with respect to single parameters, and deeper insights come from considering the collective effects of interactions among parameters. This can be done by examining the structure of the Hessian matrix of parametric second derivatives $Hij = \partial^2 C / \partial \theta_i \partial \theta_j$ or its approximation $J^T J$, where J represents the Jacobian matrix of first derivatives. Local sensitivities to combined parameter variation can be assessed by computing the eigenvalues and eigenvectors of H, as described in detail elsewhere [5,30]. For the Epo-EpoR trafficking model, sensitivity integration can be used to compute $J^T J$, and subsequently its eigenvalues and eigenvectors. Figure 8.2(b) shows the "stiffest" parameter combination associated with the fit of the Epo-EpoR model to the experimental data, that is, the eigenvector associated with the largest eigenvalue of $J^T J$. Nonlocal exploration of parameter space can be undertaken using parameter sampling approaches, as described below.

8.2.6 PARAMETER SAMPLING, POSTERIOR DISTRIBUTIONS, AND IDENTIFIABILITY

Identifying a single set of parameters which best fits the available data does not acknowledge that other parameter sets might be almost as effective in describing observations. Within the framework of Bayesian statistics, one aims to ascertain posterior distributions on parameters, that is, the probability of parameters (and hence a model) given the available data. Bayes' theorem, along with the ability to compute the likelihood of the probability of the data given the parameters, allows us to compute the posterior distribution $P(\theta|Data)$:

$$P(\theta \,|\, Data) \propto P(Data) P(Data \,|\, \theta)$$

Markov Chain Monte Carlo (MCMC) sampling can be used to explore parameter space, sampling from the posterior distribution to identify an ensemble of parameter sets that fit the data within the experimental uncertainty [30,5]. For the Epo-EpoR model, Figure 8.2(b, inset) shows a projection of such an ensemble in the k_{on}, k_{off} plane. While the distribution of k_{on} values is well-localized about a central value, the values of k_{off}

vary by several orders of magnitude. In the original Epo-EpoR paper, however, additional binding kinetics data were incorporated into the estimation process that enabled the authors to estimate and fix a value for the dissociation constant $K_D = k_{off}/k_{on}$.

The goal of parameter estimation is to identify the values of model parameters, but this is often confounded for a variety of reasons. The subject of "parameter identifiability" (or, of greater concern, nonidentifiability) addresses such issues [31,32]. Typically a distinction is made between *structural nonidentifiability* and *practical nonidentifiability*. Structural identifiability refers to the way that two or more parameters enter into the mathematical structure of a model; for example, if two parameters only ever enter a model in terms of their ratio or their product, then the separate values of those parameters cannot be determined. Mathematically, relationships associated with structural nonidentifiabilities correspond to zero modes of the Hessian, that is, eigenvectors of the Hessian matrix of second derivatives of the cost function $H_{ij} = \partial^2 C/\partial\theta_i \partial\theta_j$ with zero eigenvalue. In such cases, it is best to first mathematically reformulate the problem in order to replace nonidentifiable parameters.

Practical nonidentifiability is a more subtle problem, involving parameters that are not strictly degenerate but which are difficult to disentangle in practice. A canonical example of this arises in problems with a separation of time scales, such as in the case of binding-unbinding kinetics that is fast compared to other reactions. I will return to the issue of practical nonidentifiability below in the context of sloppy parameter sensitivities.

8.2.7 QUANTIFYING PREDICTION UNCERTAINTIES

One constructs a model in order to make predictions, and thus for those predictions to be testable through further experimentation, it is necessary to indicate what it means for the model to be wrong. (Of course, "all models are wrong" [33], so it may seem odd that I would need to delineate under what conditions any particular model is wrong.) But to test predictions, we need to quantify the uncertainty of those predictions, given the information they are built upon. Just in the same way that uncertainties and errors can be propagated through simple arithmetic calculations, we can propagate parameter uncertainties (derived from the sorts of sampling procedures described above) through the action of mathematical models, in order to specify model prediction uncertainties.

Either the local analysis of sensitivities, or the nonlocal sampling of parameter space, can be used to estimate prediction uncertainties. Figure 8.2(c), for example, shows a set of trajectories for [Epo_membrane] for the parameter sets contained in the sampled ensemble. Even though some parameters in the ensemble vary considerably, the ensemble of trajectories shows much less variation.

It should be noted that much of the machinery described above assumes that there are experimental data available to fit to. Often there are, and clearly one will be on uneasy ground making predictions from models that are not built on a foundation of experimental verifiability. Nonetheless, the reality is that many mathematical models are published with parameters that are not systematically fit to data, but which are instead estimated based on values in the literature or assumed to be of the right order of magnitude based on data. One is often nonetheless interested in understanding the sensitivity of model predictions to parameters (e.g., to suggest possible perturbations of interest) and can use many of the same methods described above. In this case, we are interested not in fitting to experimental data, but rather to synthetic data generated by the model itself.

8.2.8 RESOURCES FOR PARAMETER ESTIMATION IN SYSTEMS BIOLOGY

Several excellent treatments and reviews of many of the issues touched upon here are available in the literature, with specific application to mechanistic systems biology models [5,6,28,34]. A summary of lessons learned in computational approaches to parameter estimation—with specific application to the JAK-STAT and EpoR models discussed above—can be found in [27]. In addition, while parameter estimation is a generic problem in many different areas of mathematical modeling, software tools specifically engineered to support parameter estimation and related analyses in the area of systems biology are available in several packages, including Copasi, Data2Dynamics, ABC-SysBio, the MATLAB SimBiology toolbox, and SloppyCell. Many such systems make use of the SBML standard for encoding models of reaction networks, which facilitates not only model interchange but also model meta-analyses such as those contained in [35] and [36]. The Data2Dynamics website contains numerous examples that weave together computational models and associated experimental data for fitting, and the ABC-SysBio system is described in considerable detail in a protocol article describing its use [37].

8.2.9 STOCHASTIC MODELS

Most of the discussion here has focused on deterministic descriptions of biological processes, whereby a given choice of parameters and initial conditions always leads to the same set of model predictions. Models of this sort, typically in the form of coupled ODEs describing the dynamics of molecular concentrations, are most appropriate when fluctuations are insignificant, although they are sometimes used even if that is not the case due to the relative ease with which they can be analyzed. Investigation of a stochastic model is complicated by the fact that (a) system trajectories will vary from realization to realization [4], and (b) solving the master equation for the joint probability distribution characterizing those variable trajectories becomes prohibitively expensive as the system size grows due to the combinatorial explosion of the configuration space [38]. The process of parameter estimation for stochastic models is further complicated by the fact that estimating the likelihood is not as tractable as for the case of deterministic models with normally distributed noise. A discussion of inference methods for stochastic models is beyond the scope of this article, but several useful theoretical descriptions and computational tools supporting these types of analyses are available [37,39,40,41,42,43].

8.3 PARAMETER ESTIMATION AND THE PROCESS OF MODELING

Having laid out some of the basic procedures involved in parameter estimation (and pointed to references where much more detailed and expert descriptions are available), I will now step back to examine how the process of parameter estimation relates to other aspects of modeling. As noted above, parameter estimation is not an end in itself, but a means to an end of making predictions about new behaviors or analyzing the structure of existing behaviors. As such, parameter estimation functions as an inner loop in service of these other goals.

8.3.1 SLOPPINESS AND THE GEOMETRY OF PARAMETER SENSITIVITIES

I alluded above to long, thin canyons in high-dimensional parameter spaces, and collective interactions among parameters in the sensitivity of model predictions to parameter variation. These features are related to a phenomenon that my colleagues and I have termed "sloppiness," whereby system dynamics are very insensitive to some particular combinations of parameter changes while being very sensitive to others; see Figure 8.3(a). This wide range of sensitivities, involving a few stiff modes that determine system dynamics and a large space of sloppy modes that do not impact system behavior, is seen in a number of complex, multiparameter, nonlinear models [2,30,35]. This anisotropy in parameter sensitivities can be quantitatively characterized by the eigenvalue spectrum of the Hessian matrix as described above, which has a characteristic form where the eigenvalues decay by a roughly constant factor, implying that only a few stiff modes contribute significantly [44]. Parameter ensembles generated by MCMC sampling can exhibit large variation in individual parameters, some fluctuating by many orders of magnitude over an ensemble [45]. These parameters are practically nonidentifiable, but it is possible for a model with a set of widely divergent parameter estimates to nonetheless show well-constrained model predictions. This is counterintuitive, since one usually expects that if one puts junk into a model (in the form of un-characterized parameter values) one would expect junk out (in the form of useless predictions). But sloppiness reveals that due to internal redundancies and correlations in parameter sensitivities, constrained and therefore testable predictions can often be made from sloppy models. More recent work by Transtrum, Machta, and Sethna has extended this theory by combining insights from sloppy models with techniques from differential geometry and information geometry to characterize the underlying manifolds associated with how models map from parameter space to data space [29,46].

There are a variety of implications arising from this characteristic geometric structure of sensitivities. Unless all model parameters can be well-constrained through other measurements, model predictions can vary substantially if even one parameter is not so constrained [35]. Efficient sampling of parameter space in

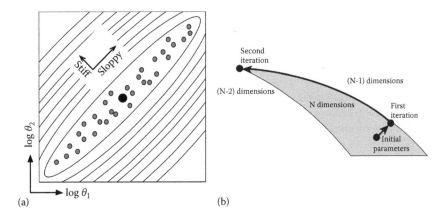

Figure 8.3 (a) Schematic of the cost surface of a sloppy model (Adapted from Gutenkunst, R.N. et al., *PLoS Computational Biology* 3(10), e189 EP, 2007.), projected on a two-dimensional parameter subspace (θ_1, θ_2). Curved lines/ellipses represent contours in the cost surface $C(\theta)$ in the vicinity of the best-fit set (large black dot). Stiff directions are directions in parameter space where system behavior changes rapidly with parameters; in sloppy directions, behavior is largely insensitive to parameter variations. The anistropy of the cost contours is proportional to the square root of the eigenvalues of the Hessian matrix. Gray dots represent other parameter sets near the cost minimum, generated by MCMC sampling. **(b)** Schematic depicting model reduction via the manifold boundary approximation method (Reprinted with permission from Transtrum, M.K., and Qiu, P., *Physical Review Letters*, 113(9), 098701, 2014. Copyright by the American Physical Society). The manifold associated with N-dimensional parameterization of the full model is bounded by lower-dimensional facets, edges, and corners. Model reduction proceeds by repeatedly flowing to boundaries and lumping parameters together in accordance with the zero mode that emerges at the boundary, resulting at each step in a new model with one less parameter.

MCMC requires taking step sizes in different directions consistent with the underlying anisotropy [47]. As described in some more detail below, simplified models with better-identified parameters can be constructed using model reduction procedures that leverage the hierarchical structure of model manifolds. And we have hypothesized that sloppiness in complex biological networks might provide a mechanism for evolution to explore extended parametric neutral spaces, allowing for robustness to some types of parameter variation while enabling evolvability of new phenotypes [26].

8.3.2 MODEL INFERENCE, REFINEMENT, SELECTION, AND REDUCTION

Traditionally, parameter estimation has served as a separate inner loop within the broader processes of model construction, inference, refinement, selection, and reduction. One posits a model structure, attempts to fit parameters in that model, and refines the model structure if it is unable to describe the data. A model successfully fit to data can be used to make predictions about unseen scenarios, although whether those predictions are falsifiable depends on how constrained they are by the available data. (New scenarios might involve, for example, different initial conditions, or the knockout, inhibition, or overexpression of particular model components.) Upon making a falsifiable prediction about a new condition and testing it experimentally, one will find either that the prediction is validated, or that it is not. Those experiments might suggest possible changes to the model structure, as well as contribute additional data to feed into the parameter estimation pipeline.

A key aspect of model inference, as a first step, and model refinement subsequently is experimental design [48,49]. In some cases, separate experiments can be carried out in order to estimate particular parameter values and then fix those values in subsequent efforts to estimate other parameters from different types of data; the multistage estimation efforts carried out in [23] and [50] are representative of this approach. A significant part of the experimental design literature aims to address issues of parameter non-identifiability. Within the context of the sorts of sloppy parameter sensitivities described above, papers by Tonsing et al. [51], Apgar et al. [52], and Hagen et al. [53] have demonstrated that appropriate design of experiments can reduce most of the uncertainty in parameter estimates observed in sloppy models, albeit by introducing more complex sorts of experiments [5]. That is, despite the ubiquity of sloppiness arising in parameter estimation for many different models, it is not intrinsic, as both model reparameterizations and targeted experiments can result in identifiable parameters. Motivated by the sense that constraining prediction uncertainties is a more fruitful endeavor than constraining parameter uncertainties per se, Casey et al. used experimental design techniques to propose and test new measurements needed to optimally reduce prediction uncertainties for a molecular complex identified as relevant to the regulation of EGF receptor trafficking [24].

Model selection refers broadly to the process of deciding from among a set of competing models based on their ability to describe available data and to make testable predictions about unseen data. Likelihood ratio tests are one common method for formally characterizing the goodness of fit of different competing models; the early papers on modeling the JAK-STAT pathway, for example, show this practice in great detail [14]. In situations where a large amounts of training data are available, cross-validation is a common approach to model comparison: some portion of the available data are included in a training set for parameter estimation, while the remaining data are left out for validation. Unfortunately, while technological advances have placed some facets of biology squarely in the land of Big Data, parameterization of many complex dynamical models of biological networks is still usually on more barren terrain, often with barely more data points than parameters to be estimated.

The term "model selection" also refers somewhat more specifically to methods for deciding among different structural models that contain different numbers of parameters. Within this latter context, one acknowledges that structurally different models are inherently unequal, in that one might expect a more complex model to be more able to fit existing data simply because it contains more fitting degrees-of-freedom. (Although the caveats of having complicated models that overfit the data must be heeded.) In this sense, model selection echoes Occam's razor, a principle encouraging the development of parsimonious descriptions, in which "Entities must not be multiplied beyond necessity" [54]. Additional model complexity in the form of parameters should be pursued only if those additional degrees-of-freedom provide sufficient extra predictive capacity to warrant their inclusion, and various methods have been developed which effectively penalize larger models. Some mathematical approaches are based either on information theory (leading, for example, to the Akaike Information Criterion (AIC) for model selection) or Bayesian statistics (resulting in the Bayesian Information Criterion (BIC)). An excellent recent overview of methods for model selection, with specific application to the sorts of dynamical models of interest in systems biology, can be found in [34].

While the inner loop of parameter estimation is relatively automated and robust (the challenges described above notwithstanding), the process of model refinement can be rather slow, laborious, and require human intervention. This has led some researchers to develop creative new procedures that aim to couple the processes of structural inference, parametric inference, model selection, and model reduction into more synergistic wholes. The automated discovery of model forms highlighted by Francois and colleagues [55,56] integrates parameter estimation directly into the broader mode of structural inference. Kuepfer et al. advocated the role of "ensemble modeling" that examines not just sets of parameters within a single model structure, but more broadly ensembles of model structures [57]. Sunnaker et al. have combined exploration of parameter space with simplication of models, recognizing that quantitative changes in some parameters that act as edge weights connecting different components can lead to qualitative and topological changes in reaction networks with fewer edges [58].

A promising new model reduction procedure (the manifold boundary approximation method), recently introduced by Transtrum and Qiu [59], makes use of insights into the hierarchical hyperribbon structure of model manifolds in complex models. These high-dimensional manifolds, which map from parameter space to data space, are typically bounded by lower-dimensional surfaces (facets, edges, corners, etc.) that represent simpler models with fewer parameters. The interior of the manifold is characterized by a number of sloppy modes with small but not strictly zero eigenvalues. The manifold boundaries, on the other hand, are associated with zero modes in the full model. The model reduction procedure involves flowing along geodesics on the manifold until a boundary is reached, and inspecting the resulting zero mode that separates out from the spectrum. The associated eigenvector describes a relationship among a subset of parameters that can be used for parameter removal. For example, the binding-unbinding kinetics in the Epo-EpoR model described above can be simplified—in the limit that the rates k_{on} and k_{off} are much faster than other rates—by a single parameter, the dissociation constant $K_D = k_{off}/k_{on}$. This simplification of the model corresponds to a bounding facet of the manifold with one fewer parametric degree-of-freedom than the original model. This procedure can be repeated, leading to smaller and smaller models, as depicted schematically in Figure 8.3(b); the process is terminated when all effective parameters in the model can be identified from the available data and any further reductions lead to a loss of predictive power. Not only can complex models be considerably simplified, but the effective parameters that result through such a procedure are themselves functions of the underlying bare parameters that were introduced in the original model [60].

8.3.3 THE MANY FACES OF SYSTEMS BIOLOGY

Systems biology is a field of study that is broadly interested in understanding how the vast array of genomic and molecular components that make up living organisms are organized to produce the bewildering variety of phenotypic behaviors exhibited by those systems; in short, how genotype is mapped to phenotype. Perhaps not surprisingly for a field with such lofty goals, the manner in which different people seek to reach those goals vary considerably. For some, the ability to gather large amounts of data through the use of various high-throughput experimental techniques is the dominant theme, with the hope that insights can come from mining patterns in those data. Although in many cases, such analyses do little more than apply relatively simple statistical techniques to identify or confirm interesting trends in the data without digging down into the mechanistic layers that are responsible for producing phenotype from genotype. For others, systems biology suggests the ability to move beyond molecular "parts lists" to construct cellular "wiring diagrams," complex dynamical descriptions that can be investigated to characterize the emergent phenomena that drive living systems. Others motivated to understand such emergence, however, are deeply skeptical of such models, in large part because so many parameters are unknown: for them, characterizing the phenomenology of living systems is paramount, even if the resulting models might be more difficult to link directly to the sorts of data generated by high-throughput assays and the sorts of microscopic manipulations that are in the molecular biologist's toolbox. Still others aim to develop mechanistic models within other mathematical frameworks that do not rely on the proliferation of unknown parameters characteristic of chemical kinetic networks. These include Boolean models that discretize state spaces and transition rules [61], and in the arena of metabolic modeling, constraint-based models that compute flux distributions consistent with a set of stoichiometric and flux-bound constraints [62].

Model parameterization and parameter estimation are on the front lines of these sorts of debates. Complex wiring diagrams are easy to construct yet difficult to parameterize. For some, a model with nonidentifiable parameters is a nonstarter, although as noted above, it is still possible to have predictive models with poorly characterized parameters. Rather than simply rejecting overly complicated models in favor of parsimonious phenomenological models, insights into sloppiness in complex biological systems allow us to migrate along this spectrum, identifying model structures with lower effective dimensionality that can help point the way toward phenomenological models. Model reduction procedures that retain the full underlying parameter space in effective parameters allow bridges to be built between mechanism and phenomenology [60].

In addition, top-down statistical inference from large data sets can potentially make use of machine learning techniques focused on dimensionality reduction: Big Data are not always as big as they seem, but often reside on lower-dimensional subspaces. Developing better methods for incorporating prior information about mechanistic processes into statistical inferences from system-wide datasets remains a big challenge for the field, but perhaps bridges could be built from mechanism to inference by integrating our insights about low-dimensional subspaces in mechanistic models with discovery of reduced-dimensional statistical descriptions of large datasets.

As prosaic as the parameter estimation process is, it sits in many ways on a knife edge that cuts across many important themes in the modern world of quantitative biology. Appreciating both the mechanics of parameter estimation and its place in the larger realm of modeling, experimental design, and interpretation of data are keys to making further progress in this area.

ACKNOWLEDGMENTS

This review would not be possible were it not for the work I have been fortunate to carry out over several years along with a number of collaborators: Kevin Brown, Josh Waterfall, Ryan Gutenkunst, Fergal Casey, Bryan Daniels, Yan-Jiun Chen, Ben Machta, Mark Transtrum, Rick Cerione, and Jim Sethna. In addition, I acknowledge support from NSF grant IOS-1127017.

ENDNOTES

1. Erythropoietin is also known as Epo, probably best known to the world through its surreptitious abuse by the cyclist Lance Armstrong and others interested in enhancing aerobic performance.
2. In some cases, however, one can relate parametric variation to global environmental parameters, such as temperature. In [26], we modeled temperature compensation in bacterial circadian oscillation networks, modulating chemical activation barriers exponentially with temperature according to the Arrhenius activation law. Even though the model was manifestly dependent on temperature, there exist extended regions of parameter space where the system dynamics is effectively independent of temperature, resulting in a circadian clock unaffected by temperature variation.

REFERENCES

1. Pirsig, R.M. (1974). *Zen and the Art of Motorcycle Maintenance: An Inquiry into Values*. William Morrow.
2. Transtrum, M.K., Machta, B., Brown, K.B., Daniels, B.C., Myers, C.R., and Sethna, J.P. (2015). Perspective: Sloppiness and Emergent Theories in Physics, Biology, and Beyond. *The Journal of Chemical Physics 143*(1), 010901.
3. Singh, S., Schneider, D.J., and Myers, C.R. (2014). Using multitype branching processes to quantify statistics of disease outbreaks in zoonotic epidemics. *Physical Review E 89*(3), 032702.
4. Gillespie, D.T. (1977). Exact stochastic simulation of coupled chemical reactions. *The Journal of Physical Chemistry*.
5. Mannakee, B.K., Ragsdale, A.P., and Transtrum, M.K., and Gutenkunst R.N. (2016). Sloppiness and the geometry of parameter space. In L. Geris and D. Gomez-Cabrero (Eds.), *Uncertainty in Biology: A Computational Modeling Approach* (271–299). Cham: Springer International Publishing.
6. Toni, T., and Stumpf, M.P.H. (2010). Parameter inference and model selection in signaling pathway models. *Methods in Molecular Biology 673*, 283–295.
7. Rawlings, J.S. (2004). The JAK/STAT signaling pathway. *Journal of Cell Science 117*(8), 1281–1283.
8. Aaronson, D.S. (2002). A Road Map for Those Who Don't Know JAK-STAT. *Science 296*(5573), 1653–1655.
9. Laub, M.T., and Goulian, M. (2007). Specificity in Two-Component Signal Transduction Pathways. *Annual Review of Genetics 41*(1), 121–145.
10. Qi, Y.F., Huang, Y.X., Wang, H.Y., Zhang, Y., Bao, Y.L., Sun, L.G., Wu, Y., Yu, C.L., Song, Z.B., Zheng, L.H., Sun, Y., Wang, G.N., and Li, Y.X. (2013). Elucidating the crosstalk mechanism between IFN-gamma and IL-6 via mathematical modelling. *BMC Bioinformatics 14*, 41.
11. Shannon, C.E. (1948). A mathematical theory of communication. *Bell System Technical Journal 27*, 379–656.
12. Itzkovitz, S., Tlusty, T., and Alon, U. (2006). Coding limits on the number of transcription factors. *BMC Genomics 7*(1471–2164), 239.
13. Myers, C.R. (2008). Satisfiability, sequence niches and molecular codes in cellular signalling. *IET Systems Biology 2*(5), 304–312.
14. Swameye, I., Müller, T.G., Timmer, J., Sandra, O., and Klingmuller, U. (2003). Identification of nucleocytoplasmic cycling as a remote sensor in cellular signaling by databased modeling. *Proceedings of the National Academy of Sciences of the United States of America 100*(3), 1028–1033.
15. Timmer, J., Müller, T.G., Swameye, I., and Sandra, O. (2004). Modeling the nonlinear dynamics of cellular signal transduction. *International Journal of Bifurcation and Chaos in Applied Sciences and Engineering*.
16. Zi, Z., and Klipp, E. (2006). SBML-PET: A Systems Biology Markup Language-based parameter estimation tool. *Bioinformatics 22*(21), 2704–2705.
17. Gutenkunst, R.N., Atlas, J.C., Casey, F.P., Daniels, B.C., Kuczenski, R.S., Waterfall, J.J., Myers, C.R., and Sethna, J.P. (2007). SloppyCell. http://sloppycell.sourceforge.net.

18. Myers, C.R., Gutenkunst, R.N., and Sethna, J.P. (2007). Python Unleashed on Systems Biology. *Computing in Science and Engineering 9*(3), 34–37.

19. Raue, A., Steiert, B., Schelker, M., Kreutz, C., Maiwald, T., Hass, H., Vanlier, J., Tönsing, C., Adlung, L., Engesser, R., Mader, W., Heinemann, T., Hasenauer, J., Schilling, M., Höfer, T., Klipp, E., Theis, F., Klingmuller, U., Schöberl, B., and Timmer, J. (2015). Data2Dynamics: A modeling environment tailored to parameter estimation in dynamical systems. *Bioinformatics 31*(21), 3558–3560.

20. Raue, A., Kreutz, C., Maiwald, T., Bachmann, J., Schilling, M., Klingmuller, U., and Timmer, J. (2009). Structural and practical identifiability analysis of partially observed dynamical models by exploiting the profile likelihood. *Bioinformatics 25*(15), 1923–1929.

21. Vanlier, J., Tiemann, C.A., Hilbers, P.A.J., and van Riel, N.A.W. (2012). A Bayesian approach to targeted experiment design. *Bioinformatics*, 28(8), 1136–1142.

22 Skoge, M.L., Endres, R.G., and Wingreen, N.S. (2006). Receptor-Receptor Coupling in Bacterial Chemotaxis: Evidence for Strongly Coupled Clusters. *Biophysical Journal 90*(12), 4317–4326.

23. Becker, V., Schilling, M., Bachmann, J., Baumann, U., Raue, A., Maiwald, T., Timmer, J., and Klingmüller, U. (2010). Covering a broad dynamic range: Information processing at the erythropoietin receptor. *Science 328*(5984), 1404–1408.

24. Casey, F.P., Baird, D., Feng, Q., Gutenkunst, R.N., Waterfall, J.J., Myers, C.R., Brown, K.S., Cerione, R.A., and Sethna, J.P. (2007). Optimal experimental design in an epidermal growth factor receptor signalling and down-regulation model. *IET Systems Biology 1*(3), 190–202.

25. Data2Dynamics. http://data2dynamics.org.

26. Daniels, B., Chen, Y., Sethna, J.P., Gutenkunst, R.N., and Myers, C.R. (2008). Sloppiness, robustness, and evolvability in systems biology. *Current Opinion in Biotechnology 19*(4), 389–395.

27. Raue, A., Schilling, M., Bachmann, J., Matteson, A., Schelker, M. Schelke, M., Kaschek, D., Hug, S., Kreutz, C., Harms, B.D., Theis, F.J., Klingmüller, U., and Timmer, J. (2013). Lessons learned from quantitative dynamical modeling in systems biology. *PLoS ONE 8*(9), e74335.

28. Cedersund, G., Samuelsson, O., Ball, G., Tegnér, J., and Gomez-Cabrero, D. (2016). Optimization in Biology Parameter Estimation and the Associated Optimization Problem. In L. Geris and D. Gomez-Cabrero (Eds.), *Uncertainty in Biology: A Computational Modeling Approac* (177–197). Cham: Springer International Publishing.

29. Transtrum, M.K., Machta, B.B., and Sethna, J.P. (2011). Geometry of nonlinear least squares with applications to sloppy models and optimization. *Physical Review E 83*(3 Pt 2), 036701.

30. Brown, K.S. and Sethna, J.P. (2003). Statistical mechanical approaches to models with many poorly known parameters. *Physical Review E 68*(2 Pt 1), 021904.

31. Chis, O.-T., Banga, J.R., and Balsa-Canto, E. (2011). Structural identifiability of systems biology models: A critical comparison of methods. *PLoS ONE 6*(11), e27755.

32. Raue, A., Becker, V., Klingmüller, U., and Timmer, J. (2010). Identifiability and observability analysis for experimental design in nonlinear dynamical models. *Chaos 20*(4), 045105.

33. Box, G.E.P. (1976). Science and statistics. *Journal of the American Statistical Association 71*(356), 791–799.

34. Sunnåker, M., and Stelling, J. (2016). Model Extension and Model Selection. In L. Geris and D. Gomez-Cabrero, (Eds.), *Uncertainty in Biology: A Computational Modeling Approach* (213–241). Springer International Publishing, Cham.

35. Gutenkunst, R.N., Waterfall, J.J., Casey, F.P., Brown, K.S., Myers, C.R., and Sethna, J.P. (2007). Universally Sloppy Parameter Sensitivities in Systems Biology Models. *PLoS Computational Biology 3*(10), e189 EP.

36. Erguler, K., and Stumpf, M.P.H. (2011). Practical limits for reverse engineering of dynamical systems: A statistical analysis of sensitivity and parameter inferability in systems biology models. *Molecular BioSystems 7*(5), 1593–1602.

37. Liepe, J., Kirk, P., Filippi, S., Toni, T., Barnes, C.P., and Stumpf, M.P.H. (2014). A framework for parameter estimation and model selection from experimental data in systems biology using approximate Bayesian computation. *Nature Protocols 9*(2), 439–456.

38. Keeling, M.J., and Ross, J.V. (2008). On methods for studying stochastic disease dynamics. *Journal of The Royal Society Interface 5*(19), 171–181.

39. Wilkinson, D.J. (2011). *Stochastic Modelling for Systems Biolog* (2d ed.) *(Chapman & Hall/CRC Mathematical and Computational Biology)*. CRC Press.

40. Ionides, E.L., Bretó, C., and King, A.A. (2006). Inference for nonlinear dynamical systems. *Proceedings of the National Academy of Sciences 103*(49), 18438–18443.

41. Toni, T., Welch, D., Strelkowa, N., Ipsen, A., and Stumpf, M.P.H. (2009). Approximate Bayesian computation scheme for parameter inference and model selection in dynamical systems. *Journal of the Royal Society, Interface / the Royal Society 6*(31), 187–202.

42. King, A.A., Ionides, E.L., Bretó, C.M., Ellner, S., and Kendall, B. (2010). *pomp: Statistical inference for partially observed Markov processes (R package)*. http://pomp. r-forge. r- . . . .

43. Golightly, A., and Wilkinson, D.J. (2011). Bayesian parameter inference for stochastic biochemical network models using particle Markov chain Monte Carlo. *Interface Focus 1*(6), 807–820.

44. Waterfall, J.J., Casey, F.P., Gutenkunst, R.N., Brown, K.S., Myers, C.R., Brouwer, P.W., Elser, V., and Sethna, J.P. (2006). Sloppy-model universality class and the Vandermonde Matrix. *Physical Review Letters 97*(15), 150601.

45. Brown, K.S., Hill, C.C., Calero, G.A., Myers, C.R., Lee, K.H., Sethna, J.P., and Cerione, R.A. (2004). The statistical mechanics of complex signaling networks: Nerve growth factor signaling. *Physical Biology 1*(3), 184.

46. Machta, B.B., Chachra, R., Transtrum, M.K., and Sethna, J.P. (2013). Parameter space compression underlies emergent theories and predictive models. *Science 342*(6158), 604–607.

47. Gutenkunst, R.N., Casey, F.P., Waterfall, J.J., Myers, C.R., and Sethna, J.P. (2007). Extracting Falsifiable Predictions from Sloppy Models. *Annals of the New York Academy of Sciences 1115*(1), 203–211.

48. Silk, D., Kirk, P.D.W., Barnes, C.P., Toni, T., and Stumpf, M.P.H. (2014). Model selection in systems biology depends on experimental design. *PLoS Computational Biology 10*(6), e1003650.

49. Transtrum, M.K., and Qiu, P. (2012). Optimal experiment selection for parameter estimation in biological differential equation models. *BMC Bioinformatics 13*, 181.

50. Lee, E., Salic, A., Krüger, R., Heinrich, R., and Kirschner, M.W. (2003). The roles of APC and axin derived from experimental and theoretical analysis of the Wnt pathway. *PLoS Biology 1*(1), e10.

51. Tönsing, C., Timmer, J., and Kreutz, C. (2014). Cause and cure of sloppiness in ordinary differential equation models. *Phys Rev E 90*, 023303.

52. Apgar, J.F., Witmer, D.K., White, F.M., and Tidor, B. (2010). Sloppy models, parameter uncertainty, and the role of experimental design. *Molecular BioSystems 6*(10), 1890.

53. Hagen, D.R., White, J.K., and Tidor, B. (2013). Convergence in parameters and predictions using computational experimental design. *Interface Focus 3*(4), 20130008.

54. Occam's razor. https://en.wikipedia.org/wiki/Occam%27s_razor.

55. Francois, P., and Siggia, E.D. (2010). Predicting embryonic patterning using mutual entropy fitness and in silico evolution. *Development 137*(14), 2385–2395.

56. François, P., Hakim, V., and Siggia, E.D. (2007). Deriving structure from evolution: Meta-zoan segmentation. *Mol Syst Biol 3*.

57. Kuepfer, L., Peter, M., Sauer, U., and Stelling, J. (2007). Ensemble modeling for analysis of cell signaling dynamics. *Nature Biotechnology 25*(9), 1001–1006.

58. Sunnåker, M., Zamora-Sillero, E., Dechant, R., Ludwig, C., Busetto, A.G., Wagner, A., and Stelling, J. (2013). Automatic generation of predictive dynamic models reveals nuclear phosphorylation as the key msn2 control mechanism. *Science Signaling 6*(277), ra41.

59. Transtrum, M.K., and Qiu, P. (2014). Model reduction by manifold boundaries. *Physical Review Letters 113*(9), 098701.

60. Transtrum, M.K., and Qiu, P. (2015). Bridging mechanistic and phenomenological models of complex biological systems. *PLoS Computational Biology 12*(5), 1–34.

61. Thakar, J., and R Albert, R. (2010). Boolean models of within-host immune interactions. *Current Opinion in Microbiology*.

62. Bogart, E., and Myers, C.R. (2016). Multiscale Metabolic Modeling of C4 Plants: Connecting Nonlinear Genome-Scale Models to Leaf-Scale Metabolism in Developing Maize Leaves. *PLoS ONE 11*(3), e0151722.

Spatial kinetics in immunological modeling

DANIEL COOMBS AND BYRON GOLDSTEIN

9.1 INTRODUCTION

Many situations in immunology require us to solve problems involving spatiotemporal dynamics. For example, T cells of the immune system are mobile within a lymph node, where they must make direct contact with an antigen-presenting cell (APC) in order to detect an antigenic stimulus. Alternatively, we might wish to study the rate of binding of T cell receptors (TCR) to sparse peptide-major-histocompatibility-complexes (pMHC) on the APC surface. Or perhaps we want to know the rate of delivery of a secreted cytokine travelling from one cell to another across the immunological synapse. These three examples (illustrated in Figure 9.1) represent fundamentally important processes in the immune response but also show some essential aspects of spatial dynamic problems that we will examine in detail in this chapter:

1. *Dimensionality.* How many spatial dimensions must we consider? T cells move around in a three-dimensional lymph node. However, TCR are restricted to the cell membrane—essentially a two-dimensional domain. Cytokine molecules diffusing in the immunological synapse represent an interesting case: they inhabit a three-dimensional volume, but it is extremely narrow in one direction and so we might want to simplify and model the situation in two dimensions only.

2. *Scales of random motion.* For molecular-scale objects such as TCRs or cytokines, we have reasonably good evidence that their motion obeys the law of chemical diffusion, also known as Brownian motion or thermal motion. For larger objects such as cells, which actively control their mobility, it might initially seem that we should develop rather complicated models to describe their motion. However, for some particular questions—such as how long a T cell might take to find a particular APC within a

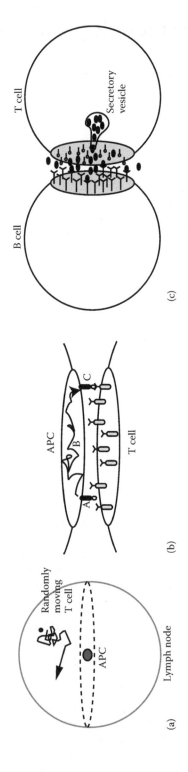

Figure 9.1 Three examples of immunological situations where spatial effects are important. **(a)** A T cell, initially at an arbitrary point inside a lymph node, moves diffusively to locate a particular antigen-presenting cell (APC). **(b)** At the immunological synapse between an APC and a T cell, sparse peptide-MHC diffuse in the membrane of the APC and (potentially) serially bind to T cell receptors. **(c)** A T cell delivers cytokines to a B cell at the immunological synapse. Secretory vesicles fuse with the T cell membrane, releasing a cargo of diffusing molecules (black ellipses) into the synapse volume, where they can bind to specialized receptors on the B cell surface).

lymph node—we actually find that a diffusive model of motion is an extremely useful tool. Of course for some questions, using a detailed and complicated model is inescapable!

3. *How many mobile objects are there?* It could be that only one T cell in the lymph node has receptors that will recognize a particular antigen, itself present on a single APC. In this case, we might want to ask with what probability will the T cell find the APC? (and if so, how long might that take?) On the other hand, a single T cell can have 50,000 or more identical TCR on its cell surface, each of which can bind to pMHC that can also be present at fairly high densities. Because of this high density we might prefer to work with the local surface density of TCR rather than trying to model individual receptors.

In this chapter, we will begin by describing chemical diffusion, and why it can be a useful approximation for objects that are not undergoing true Brownian motion (such as mobile T cells). We will then outline how diffusion-based modeling can be applied to model particular scenarios arising in cell- and tissue-scale immunology.

9.2 BROWNIAN MOTION AND DIFFUSION

Consider a tiny particle such as a biomolecule in solution. The solvent molecules surrounding it are in constant thermal motion and so the particle is continuously jostled about. Brown observed this in 1827 while looking at organelles ejected from pollen grains under a microscope. This observation remained mysterious until Einstein published a physical explanation of Brownian motion in 1905 as one of the *Annus Mirabilis* papers (this historical statement may only be approximately true). We will not go through the derivation of all the properties of Brownian motion or diffusion—there are many books and review papers on that topic for the interested reader. A great starting point for reading about diffusive models is Berg's book (Berg, *Random Walks in Biology*, 1993). However, here are the essential facts that you should know.

1. *The theory of diffusion can be formally derived from consideration of a particle undergoing infinitesimal accelerations (due to bumps by solvent molecules) occurring infinitely often.* Does that make sense? Why does the particle move at all, since the accelerations are infinitesimal? On the other hand, why does it not accelerate to an infinite velocity, since it is bumped at an infinite rate? In the mathematical derivation, we must be careful to avoid both these problems and this is done through a delicate process. Suppose that the change in position of the particle during a small time dt is dx. When we take the limit $dt \to 0$ (as in the derivation of the derivative from calculus), we must simultaneously enforce that dx^2/dt approaches a finite constant, or equivalently, that the jumps in space are proportional to the square root of the time step, provided that the time step is sufficiently small.

2. *The assumptions needed for the mathematical theory are physically reasonable.* The main assumptions we need are that the particle is bombarded by solvent molecules at a very high rate, and that the bombardment is spatially uniform—that is, it comes from all directions uniformly. These assumptions are certainly good approximations for a study of particles in water at room temperature, provided the time scales we are considering are not ridiculously small.

3. *There is only ONE parameter governing the particle motion.* We call this parameter the diffusion coefficient D and it can be estimated using the famous Einstein relation (Einstein, 1956):

$$D = k_B T / \zeta$$

Here, T is the temperature and k_B is the Boltzmann constant. Together, $k_B T$ describes the energy available for moving the particle due to thermal motion of the solvent. ζ is the drag coefficient due to friction of the particle, describing resistance to motion. When we calculate the dimension of D, it turns out to have units of length^2 per time (so it is measured in m^2/s or more commonly in cell biology, μm^2/s). The Einstein relation also tells us that the diffusion coefficient should scale linearly with temperature. The Stokes drag law of fluid mechanics predicts that the drag coefficient ζ is proportional to the particle size. So we predict that larger particles should diffuse more slowly.

4. *The mean-square displacement of the particle is proportional to time.* This means that if we perform many experiments where the particle is free to move from a starting position for some time t, the mean of the square of the total displacement over that time $<dx^2> = 2\,n\,D\,t$ where n is the dimension we are working in. For instance a particle moving in a membrane is effectively in dimension $n = 2$, while a particle diffusing in solution is in dimension $n = 3$. Notice also that the diffusion coefficient D shows up here as a constant of proportionality. Equivalently, as we shall see below, the standard deviation of the particle position is proportional to the square root of time.

5. *The probability distribution of particle displacement after a fixed time t is a Normal (aka Gaussian) distribution with mean zero and variance 2 n D t.* This probability distribution can be expressed as the function plotted in Figure 9.2.

$$p(r,t) = \frac{1}{s^n} \frac{1}{(2\pi)^{n/2}} e^{-r^2/(2s^2)} \text{where } s = \sqrt{2Dt},$$

In these points, we have emphasized the random behavior of a single particle and in particular, we have the probability distribution function for changes in the particle position as we step forward in time. By sampling from this distribution, one can generate simulated particle trajectories (Figure 9.2).

Now let's consider situations where there are lots of particles, so it makes sense to build our model around the particle density. Temporarily focusing on the one-dimensional case, we imagine that every particle is equally likely to move left or right, so the net flow of particles will be down concentration gradients.

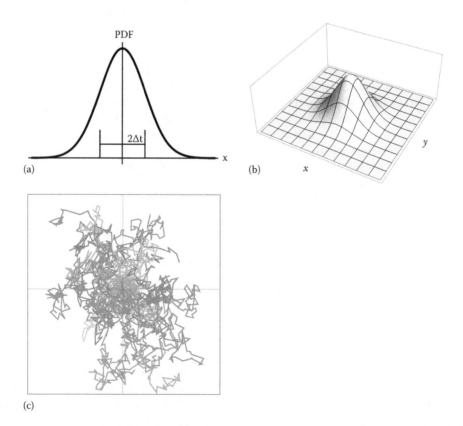

Figure 9.2 Gaussian probability distributions of steps in Brownian motion. **(a)** During a time Δt, a particle undergoing one-dimensional Brownian motion takes a step sampled from a Gaussian distribution with mean zero and standard deviation $2\Delta t$. **(b)** In two dimensions, movement steps are sampled from a two-dimensional Gaussian function. **(c)** 20 simulated two-dimensional tracks, all starting at the origin, are plotted.

This simple concept is called Fick's law, and it can (in one dimension) be written as an equation for the flux J in terms of the density profile $u(x, t)$:

$$J(x,t) = -D\frac{\partial u}{\partial x}.$$

The interpretation of D at this point is as a simple proportionality constant, but we shall see below that it is indeed the diffusion coefficient defined above. Now we can use the transport law $\partial u/\partial t = -J(x, t)$ to find the famous *diffusion equation*

$$\frac{\partial u}{\partial t} = D\frac{\partial^2 u}{\partial x^2}.$$

In two or three dimensions, this equation becomes

$$\frac{\partial u}{\partial t} = D\left(\frac{\partial^2 u}{\partial x^2} + \frac{\partial^2 u}{\partial y^2}\right) \text{ or}$$

$$\frac{\partial u}{\partial t} = D\left(\frac{\partial^2 u}{\partial x^2} + \frac{\partial^2 u}{\partial y^2} + \frac{\partial^2 u}{\partial z^2}\right) \text{ respectively.}$$

We can also write the equation in cylindrical coordinates (r, θ, z) or spherical coordinates (r, θ, ϕ):

$$\frac{\partial u}{\partial t} = D\left(\frac{1}{r}\frac{\partial}{\partial r}\left(r\frac{\partial u}{\partial r}\right) + \frac{1}{r^2}\frac{\partial^2 u}{\partial \theta 2} + \frac{\partial^2 u}{\partial z^2}\right)$$

$$\frac{\partial u}{\partial t} = D\left(\frac{1}{r^2}\frac{\partial}{\partial r}\left(r^2\frac{\partial u}{\partial r}\right) + \frac{1}{r^2 \sin\theta}\frac{\partial}{\partial \theta}\left(\sin\theta\frac{\partial u}{\partial \theta}\right) + \frac{1}{r^2 \sin^2\theta}\frac{\partial^2 u}{\partial \phi^2}\right).$$

Suppose that we have N particles all at position $x = 0$ at time $t = 0$. This is represented by the density function $u(x) = N\delta(x)$ where $\delta(x)$ is a Dirac delta function based at $x = 0$. What will the density function look like at some later time t? Intuitively, we know that the density must become more spread out as particles diffuse away from the origin. We can also imagine that the shape of the function will be symmetric, but with a peak at the origin. Alternatively, we can consider each particle forming the density individually. We know from above that the probability density function for the position of every particle at a later time is a Gaussian function, and since the particles are identical and move independently, the N particle distribution function must also be a Gaussian (written here for $n = 1$ dimension):

$$u(x,t) = \frac{N}{\sqrt{4\pi Dt}}e^{-x^2/(4Dt)}$$

This is exactly the solution to the diffusion equation, and can be checked by taking the partial derivatives. The higher dimensional analogues work too.

An important observation here is that the probability distribution of position for N identical independent Brownian particles can be calculated by solving a corresponding diffusion equation. This interpretation also allows us to find the probability distribution function for a particle constrained by a boundary (in the above description, the particles was implicitly completely unconstrained). The most common forms of the boundary conditions, expressed here as a boundary at $x = L$ in a one dimensional form, are:

1. $u(L) = 0$. (Dirichlet or absorbing boundary, any particle that reaches $x = L$ is permanently removed from the system)
2. $\partial u / \partial x \, (L) = 0$. (Neumann or reflecting boundary, particles may not cross $x = L$)
3. $u(L) + k \, \partial u / \partial x \, (L) = 0$. (Robin or partially absorbing boundary. The density flux into the boundary is proportional to the density at the boundary)

Analogues of these conditions for two- and three-dimensional problems can be applied by replacing the derivative term $\partial u / \partial x$ with the directional derivative taken at the boundary in question.

9.3 IS BROWNIAN MOTION/DIFFUSION ALWAYS THE RIGHT MODEL TO APPLY?

The diffusion model is relatively simple and stands on a solid physical footing. It is quick and easy to parameterize (there is only a single parameter!) and has been applied to model an enormous array of scientific situations. However, there are situations in which we should use a different model of particle mobility, even when we believe the motion is random or has a random component.

An important thing to remember is that the derivation of the diffusion equation requires that the motion be structured in the same way over all time and length scales. If the motion of the particle deviates from this universal behavior, we should think about whether pure diffusion is an appropriate model. Often, one can still use a relatively simple diffusion model but at least with an understanding of the limits of validity of the approximation. We now present some illustrative examples from immunological problems to hopefully make this point more clear.

1. *Immune cell surface receptor mobility.* Surface receptors on immune cells, include the fundamental units of the adaptive response: T cell receptors and B cell receptor. These are known to be mobile on the cell surface. Understanding their motion (and how this relates to cell signaling and activation) is a very active part of cellular immunology research. Since receptors are known to encounter barriers to motion on the cell surface, their motion is certainly not diffusive. However, the diffusion model is often applied to cell surface data. How is this justifiable? The answer is that it depends on the downstream application. Over long time-scales (exceeding a few seconds), receptor motion seems to be approximately diffusive, and in any case this model reduces the number of parameters that must be fit. For these reasons, models of receptor dynamics at the immunological synapse usually take the receptor motion as diffusive.
2. *Secreted molecules within the immunological synapse.* When molecules (for example cytokines) are released into the volume of an immunological synapse between two cells (such as a T cell and an antigen-presenting cell), they would be expected to diffuse freely in the volume. However, recent work has suggested that the dense assembly of adhesion molecules and other cell-surface receptors present in the synapse significantly hinders their diffusive motion (Woodsworth, Dunsing, & Coombs, 2015). The simplest way to handle hindered diffusion is to reduce the diffusion coefficient by a factor reflecting the loss of available volume for diffusion.
3. *T cell motion within a lymph node.* Cells are much larger than the diffusing molecules described so far, and their motion due to thermal noise would be extremely slow. So we cannot justify applying a diffusion model from pure physics. However, it has been experimentally established via two-photon microscopy that T cell motion is not purely diffusive. Rather, they exhibit short-term persistence of motion and this is probably due to the fact that they preferentially attach to, and move on, an array of filamentous cell structures within the lymph node (Bajenoff, Glaichenhaus, & Germain, 2008). Nonetheless, the motion of motile T cells within the lymph node has been established to be consistent with underlying random walk behavior when reasonably long time scales (greater than a few minutes) are considered

(Cahalan, Parker, Wei, & Miller, 2003; Meyer-Hermann & Maini, 2005). Indeed, a network-based model of T cell motion can be reduced to Brownian motion over medium- to long-time scales (Donovan & Lythe, 2012). For long-time situations, a pure diffusion model has many benefits: it is simple and well defined, and requires only one parameter estimate. However, the diffusive model of T cell motion should always be regarded as a convenient large-scale approximation, which loses validity if we ask questions at the scale of a single cell.

9.4 HOW CAN WE ESTIMATE THE DIFFUSION COEFFICIENT?

As described above, the Einstein relation is the official starting point for estimating D. In particular, when we consider three dimensional diffusion, there is a simple formula for the drag coefficient of a spherical particle of radius a:

$$D = \frac{k_B T}{6\pi\mu a}$$

Working in MKS units at 20°C, the Boltzmann factor $k_B T = 4 \times 10^{-21}$ J and the dynamic viscosity of water is $\mu = 10^{-3}$ kg m^{-1} s^{-1}. Therefore, a spherical particle of radius 2nm (roughly a small protein) would have $D = 7 \times 10^{-11}$ m^{2}s^{-1} or perhaps more usefully we can express this as $D = 700$ μm^{2}s^{-1}. Recall from above that we can estimate the root mean square average of the distance travelled by this protein as $L = \sqrt{2\,n\,D\,t}$. Here, the dimension $n = 3$ and if we set $t = 1$s we find L = 20 μm, which is a little more than the typical diameter of a lymphocyte (10 μm). This typical displacement shows that unimpeded proteins are expected to rapidly propagate across cells or within tissues.

For particles diffusing in three dimensions, the Einstein relation gives a reasonable starting estimate. Comparing to experimental data it is usually found to be a little too fast. This may be because proteins carry with them a shell of water molecules that effectively increases the radius and therefore their susceptibility to hydrodynamic drag.

In two dimensions, such as when we are estimating the diffusion coefficient of a cell surface-bound receptor, the Stokes Einstein relation still applies, but the calculation of the relevant drag coefficient becomes challenging. Saffman and Delbruck presented the relevant theory in 1975 where they derived the following equation for the frictional drag on a membrane-embedded protein, valid when the drag force is primarily due to membrane viscosity:

$$D = \frac{k_B T}{4\pi\eta h}\left(\frac{\eta h}{\eta' a} - \gamma\right)$$

where η is the membrane viscosity, h is the membrane thickness, η' is the viscosity of the solvent external to the membrane, and γ is a numerical constant approximately equal to 0.577 (Saffman & Delbruck, 1972).

A key parameter in the Saffman-Delbruck equation is the effective viscosity of the cell membrane, which can change rapidly over only a small temperature range. For this reason, it is preferable to obtain the diffusion coefficient for a receptor of interest directly from experiments conducted at 37°C. Experimental techniques for experimental determination of membrane protein diffusion coefficients include Fluorescence Recovery After Photobleaching (FRAP), Fluorescence Correlation Spectroscopy (FCS), and Single Particle Tracking (SPT). The details of estimation in each case involve fitting the data to a model of pure diffusion (Coombs, Das, & Morrison, 2011; Phillips, 2012).

In most cases, typical diffusion coefficients for membrane proteins are around .02–0.1 μm^2 s^{-1}. For a typical protein, this value is approximately 10^4 times slower than for diffusion in three dimensions, reflecting the strong viscous drag arising from the cell's lipid membrane.

9.4.1 EFFECTIVE DIFFUSION COEFFICIENTS

As discussed above, sometimes we would like to apply the simple diffusion model to the motion of cells over sufficiently long time- and space-scales, or even to model the motion of larger objects. For example, the diffusion model is often used in ecology to describe the random motion of animals or seed dispersal from trees. In this case, we cannot appeal to the Einstein relation and must instead allow experiments to guide us. A reasonable approach is to estimate the mean-square displacement from experimental data and then set this value equal to $2nDt$ where n is the dimension. Typical estimates for motile lymphocytes in a lymph node are in the vicinity of $60\ \mu m^2\ min^{-1}$ (Donovan & Lythe, 2012).

9.5 DIFFUSIVE TRANSPORT AND DIFFUSION-LIMITED BINDING

We are now ready to investigate the impact of diffusive transport on kinetics. Let's consider a fundamental question in immunology related to the rate of arrival of T cells to antigen-presenting cells (APCs) in a lymph node. One approach to this problem would be to set up an array of APCs in a three dimensional domain, and then solve a diffusion problem where T cells diffuse around at a given rate D until they hit an APC (an absorbing boundary). This approach would lead to a numerical solution of a partial differential equation. We will instead consider an approximation to this full problem that nonetheless gives us a lot of insight into the problem (Lauffenburger & Linderman, 1996).

Let's define T to be the density of free T cells in the lymph node, and A to be the fixed density of APCs. Since we are only modeling the rate of arrival of T cells at APCs (for now), we can suppose that the number of APCs is constant. Then a simple model for the generation of T cell – APC pairs (defined as $P(t)$) could be written as the differential equations

$$\frac{dP}{dt} = k_+ AT \text{ and}$$

$$\frac{dT}{dt} = -(k_+ AT) \text{ or equivalently, } k_+ = -\frac{1}{T}\frac{1}{A}\frac{dT}{dt}.$$

We have replaced the whole spatial problem with a much simpler ODE, and importantly, all the complicated dynamics of T cell motion that would be explicitly captured in a PDE formulation have been replaced by a single rate constant k_+. We call this the diffusion-limited forward rate constant, and it has units of $\mu m^3\ s^{-1}$. The way to calculate k_+ in this context is to calculate the flux of T cells into a single APC, and then divide this by the concentration of T cells (T). The trick that makes this possible is to calculate the flux assuming that the system is at equilibrium, where new free T cells are being created at a rate that balances the loss of free T cells as they bind to APCs. There may be more than one way to establish this equilibrium—and the answer that you find may depend on how you set up the equilibrium! This is the price that sometimes has to be paid in order to build a simple theory. If you need a more precise answer to a problem, you may need to attack it in a more laborious way.

Let's start by modeling a single APC as a perfectly absorbing sphere of radius a in an otherwise empty (and infinite) volume. After this calculation, we will develop corrections to account for the presence of other APC. Since there is only one sphere, we can work in radially symmetric spherical coordinates centered on that sphere and the diffusion equation for the spatial concentration of T cells, $T(r,t)$ becomes

$$\frac{dT}{dt} = D\left(\frac{1}{r^2}\frac{d}{dr}r^2\frac{dT}{dr}\right).$$

We need to calculate a steady state flux, so we set $dT/dt = 0$ and integrate twice to obtain

$$T(r) = A_1 + \frac{A_2}{r}.$$

To find A_1 and A_2 we apply the boundary conditions $T(r = a) = 0$ (meaning that the APC is perfectly absorbing) and $T(r \to \infty) = T_0$ (meaning that the concentration of T cells far from the trap remains at a constant background concentration). This gives us the steady state solution

$$T(r) = T_0 \left(1 - \frac{a}{r} \right),$$

from which we can calculate the total flux into the sphere

$$4\pi a^2 D \frac{dT}{dr}_{(r=a)} = 4\pi D a T_0,$$

and therefore (for this one-APC problem), we have found

$$k_+ = 4\pi D a.$$

This is the flux per T cell into a single immobile APC of radius a. We could also derive the same result by imposing a fixed flux of T cells into the "lymph node" at infinity. This would lead to a steady state where the flux of T cells meeting the APC would be the same as the flux of T cells into the lymph node, and the background concentration of T cells would be proportional to the flux. This problem should be attempted as an exercise!

This result was originally derived by Smoluchowski and is referred to as the "dilute limit"—meaning that the targets (APCs in our context) are infinitely far apart (von Smoluchowski, 1916). We will now derive a correction when there is a nonzero density of APCs for the T cells to bind to. We focus attention on a single APC of radius a as before, but we treat the effect of all the other APCs by smearing them out over all space, i.e., we treat them as a uniform field of competing APCs. This is called a mean field approximation. To achieve a steady state situation, we create T cells uniformly in space at a rate S. Our steady state diffusion equation now becomes

$$0 = S + \frac{D}{r^2} \frac{d}{dr} \left(r^2 \frac{dT}{dr} \right) - k_+ T A.$$

In this equation, A is the background density of APC. These are treated no differently than the focal APC — T cells arrive at them at the same rate k_+. We solve this equation by successively rearranging and integrating. After applying the boundary condition that $T(r = a) = 0$ and requiring that T remains finite as $r \to \infty$, we find the solution

$$T = \frac{S}{k_+ A} \left(1 - \frac{a}{r} e^{-(r-a)/\lambda} \right).$$

Here, $\lambda = \sqrt{\dfrac{D}{k_+A}}$ is a characteristic length corresponding to the distance a T cell typically travels before it reaches an APC. The concentration far from the focal APC is $T_0 = \dfrac{S}{k_+A}$ and so it follows that

$$k_+ = 4\pi a^2 \frac{D}{T_0}\frac{dT}{dr_{(r=a)}} = 4\pi Da\left(1+\frac{a}{\lambda}\right).$$

Let's use this to look at a particular biological situation now. Suppose a lymph node is a sphere of radius $L = 1$mm and contains 100 APC bearing a particular pathogenic antigen. This corresponds to an APC density of about 2.4×10^{-8} cells per μm^3. We know that APC typically have a dendritic shape that is not close to a sphere, so we must assign an effective radius to each. Suppose this is $a = 20\ \mu m$. Now suppose there are 10^3 T cells within the lymph node that have the ability to recognize the particular antigen, and suppose their effective diffusion coefficient is $D = 10\ \mu m^2/min$. Plugging the numbers in and solving a quadratic equation, we obtain $k_+ = 2.6 \times 10^3\ \mu m^3/min$ and $\lambda = 400\ \mu m$. To convert k_+ to a rate of T cell – APC encounters, we must multiply by (AT) and the volume of the lymph node:

$$\text{Rate of encounters} = k_+TA\,\frac{4}{3}\pi L^3 = 0.063\,/\,min.$$

So according to our model, we might expect it to take on the order of $(1/0.063) = 16$ min for one T cell out of 1000 to find any of 100 APC, within a single lymph node. This would be an important parameter to know in developing a model of an initial immune response. We also found an estimate of the typical distance a cell must travel before an encounter, $\lambda = 400\ \mu m$. This is a substantial fraction of the radius of a lymph node.

To find these results from the model, we had to make a number of assumptions. We replaced the dendritic structure of the APC with a sphere. We ignored the potential crowding effect, where a T cell might have difficulty reaching an APC due to other T cells already being bound to it. We did not consider the possible effects of local cytokine signaling by APCs to attract T cells. We also ignored the known structural network of reticular cells that pervade the lymphoid tissue, and along which T cells are known to preferentially migrate. However, the calculation was quick and simple and gave us a reasonable answer. In summary, this example nicely illustrates the power of diffusion-limited reaction rates as a tool for solving spatial problems.

9.6 EFFECTIVE RATE CONSTANT MODELING OF TRANSPORT ACROSS THE IMMUNOLOGICAL SYNAPSE

When lymphocytes meet antigen-presenting cells, they form a region of tight contact called the immunological synapse. Among its many important functions, this allows for the directed secretion of signaling molecules from one cell to another. Molecules are released from one cell and diffuse across the short distance to the second cell, where they may bind to receptors and potentially be internalized. The two cells are held together by adhesion molecules of a given length. We can ask, what is the effect on the efficiency of delivery of signaling molecules of the length of the adhesion molecules? One way to assess this is to examine the flux of molecules hitting the target cell, as well as the diffusion limited rate constant for binding. See Coombs and Goldstein, 2005 for more discussion and details about these calculations.

We set up our mathematical model as follows. Let the immunological synapse region be a wide, short cylinder of radius a and height d. Suppose that signaling molecules are released from the cell at the base of the cylinder with a constant, spatially uniform rate of release S, and that these molecules diffuse with diffusion coefficient D. To calculate the rate of arrival of molecules at the top of the cylinder (corresponding to the target cell in this scenario), we solve the steady state diffusion problem for $u(r, z)$ assuming radial symmetry:

$$D\left(\frac{1}{r}\frac{d}{dr}r\frac{du}{dr}+\frac{d^2u}{dz^2}\right)=0 \text{ with boundary conditions}$$

$$-D\frac{du}{dz}_{(r,z=0)} = S, \quad u(r,z=d)=0 \quad \text{and} \quad u(r=a,z)=0.$$

The absorbing boundary condition at $r = a$ indicates that particles reaching the outside edge of the synapse volume are lost.

To solve this equation requires the technique of separation of variables and involves a simple Bessel function series. The solution can also be found in (for instance) (Carslaw & Jaeger, 1959):

$$u = \sum_{n=1}^{\infty} A_n \, J_0(\alpha_n \, r) \sinh \alpha_n(d-z),$$

where we must choose the eigenvalues α_n as solutions to $J_0 (\alpha_n \, a) = 0$. Therefore, the form of the solution matches the diffusion equation and the two absorbing boundary conditions. The coefficients A_0 are chosen to satisfy the nonzero boundary condition $-D \, du/dx(r,z = 0) = S$, leading to the overall solution

$$u = \sum_{n=1}^{\infty} \frac{2S}{Da\alpha_n^2} \frac{J_0(\alpha_n \, r)}{J_0(\alpha_n \, a)} \frac{\sinh \alpha_n(d-z)}{\cosh \alpha_n d}. \tag{9.1}$$

Finally, we can determine the net flux of molecules reaching the target cell by integrating over the whole top surface:

$$\text{flux} = \sum_{n=1}^{\infty} \frac{4\pi S \, a^2}{\hat{\alpha}_n^2 \cosh \hat{\alpha}_n(d/a)} = \pi S a^2 f_1(d/a). \tag{9.2}$$

The dimensionless function $f_1(d/a)$ encodes the fraction of secreted molecules that hit the target cell as a function of the aspect ratio of the cylindrical immunological synapse. Plotting this function shows that leakage of the molecules through the edges of the synapse is not a big effect for realistic synapses with diameters in the range of μm and heights in the range of tens of nm.

We can also calculate the average concentration of secreted molecules at the target cell, as a function of the secretion rate S and the synapse geometry. This calculation is performed by averaging $u(d,r)$ over the target cell surface in the synapse, whereby we obtain

$$\bar{u} = \frac{4Sa}{D} \sum_{n=1}^{\infty} \frac{1}{\hat{\alpha}_n^3 \sinh \hat{\alpha}_n(d/a)}.$$

By setting this concentration $\bar{u}$ equal to the dissociation constant for the binding reaction between the signaling molecule and the target cell surface receptors, we can estimate the secretion rate S that will lead to substantial receptor occupancy.

Let's now use this to look at the transmission of the cytokine IL-4 from T cells to B cells across the immunological synapse. IL-4 binds to the surface receptor IL-4Rα on the B cell, leading to intracellular signaling.

We estimate $D = 10^2 \mu m/s$ and use the measured dissociation constant for the molecular binding, $K_D = 100$ pM (Wang, Shen, & Sebald, 1997). This molar quantity can be converted to $6 \times 10^{-2} \mu m^{-3}$ for ease of use. Let's define the height of the synapse to be $d = 40$ nm (the length of an adhesion molecule pair) and the radius to be $a = 2\mu m$, as observed in fluorescence microscopy experiments. Inserting these specific numbers into the equation $\bar{u} = K_D$, we find that a total release rate of around six molecules per second is sufficient to occupy half of the IL-4Rα on the B cell, at steady state.

9.7 COMBINING DIFFUSIVE TRANSPORT WITH CHEMICAL BINDING

So far, we have looked at problems where we are only interested in the rate of arrival of diffusing objects to a defined region. In the first example, the diffusing objects were T cells, and we were interested in the rate of arrival at an antigen-presenting cell within a lymph node. In the second example, the diffusing objects were cytokines diffusing from one cell to another in the immunological synapse, and we wanted to know what release rate would be able to saturate a cytokine receptor on the target cell. In both cases, we did not explicitly consider binding and unbinding of the diffusing object once it had reached its target. To allow for this to happen (and thus study diffusion-limited kinetics), we can extend the theory in the following way. We will first explain the theory in the context of a soluble ligand diffusing to and binding with a spherical cell and then consider the geometry of the immunological synapse as in the second example just above.

Consider a cytokine diffusing in three dimensions that can bind to and unbind from a spherical cell. Suppose the cell has surface area A, decorated with a finite number of receptors for the cytokine, and suppose that the cytokine binds to these receptors monovalently. We will assume that the cytokine (concentration L_0) is present in excess, so that its concentration far from the cell remains unchanged. Let the number of unbound receptors be AR, so the concentration of receptors is R. When the cytokine is present, we expect some of the receptors will become bound. Call that number AB so the concentration of bound receptors is B. Under the usual well-mixed chemical kinetics, we would expect the concentration of receptor-cytokine pairs to follow a rule of the type

$$\frac{dB}{dt} = k_{on} \, RL - k_{off} \, B,$$

where k_{on} and k_{off} are the forward and reverse rate constants for the reaction respectively. If this reaction reaches equilibrium, we find that $B = (k_{on}/k_{off}) \, RL$, allowing us to interpret k_{on}/k_{off} as the affinity of the reaction (or equivalently, $K_D = k_{off}/k_{on}$ is the usual dissociation constant). However, in this situation neither species is well mixed. The receptors are confined to the cell surface, while the cytokine molecules will transiently be less abundant close to the cell, as they bind the receptor. Eventually we would expect the cytokines to be uniform in space, but in the spirit of the previous sections, we are aiming for an ordinary differential equation description of the binding dynamics rather than determining the dynamics of the cytokine density over space. For that we would need to resort to numerical solution of a partial differential equation with a reactive boundary at the cell surface.

In order for binding to occur, the cytokines must approach the cell very closely and the rate of this approach is governed by diffusion. In the previous sections, we saw how to calculate the rate of approach, $k_+ = 4\pi D a$ where a is the radius of the cell and D is the diffusion coefficient of the cytokine molecules. We would therefore like to write an equation for the concentration of cytokines that are sufficiently close to the cell that they can bind available receptors in a form like:

$$\frac{dL}{dt} = k_+ L_0 - k_- L - k_{on} LR + k_{off} B.$$

Here L is the concentration of free cytokines in the region close to the cell. Free cytokines enter this region either by diffusion-limited arrival from outside (rate k_+) or by unbinding from a receptor (rate k_{off}). Free cytokines may be lost from the region due to binding (rate k_{on}) or by diffusing away. The new parameter k_- governs the rate at which cytokines exit the region. To calculate k_- requires a brief calculation in the spirit of the calculation of k_+. We are interested in the rate at which unbound particles move away from the cell. Therefore, set up a steady state where there is a fixed concentration of particles S at the cell surface, and a concentration of zero far away from the spherical cell. Mathematically, this is encoded in the following boundary value problem in spherical coordinates:

$$0 = \frac{D}{r^2}\frac{d}{dr}\left(r^2 \frac{dL}{dr}\right) \text{ subject to } L(r=a)=L_0 \text{ and } L(\infty)=0.$$

The solution is found as $L(r) = L_0\, a/r$. The diffusion-limited reverse rate constant k_- is then the flux of molecules exiting the cell surface divided by the concentration of cytokine at the cell surface, $k_- = 4\pi D \dfrac{L_0 a}{L_0} = 4\pi Da$. Surprisingly, the diffusion limited forward and reverse rates are the same for this geometry. In fact this is quite often the case, but in the next section when we re-visit secretion and absorption at the immunological synapse, we will find that they are not the same.

The final step in the derivation of the diffusion-limited kinetics is to assume that the concentration of cytokines in the region close to the cell (L) reaches equilibrium rapidly. This allows us to write

$$L(t) = L = \frac{k_+ L_0 + k_{off} B}{k_- + k_{on} R}$$

and finally, after inserting this expression into the basic chemical kinetics equation for B, we get

$$\frac{dB}{dt} = k_f R\, L_0 - k_r B,$$

where we have introduced the **effective** forward and reverse rate constants

$$k_f = \frac{k_{on}}{\left(1 + \dfrac{k_{on} R}{k_+}\right)} \quad \text{and} \quad k_r = \frac{k_{off}}{\left(1 + \dfrac{k_{on} R}{k_+}\right)}.$$

Here we have exploited the fact that $k_+ = k_-$ in this problem to simplify the equations.

We can make several interesting observations at this point.

1. The equilibrium number of bound receptors is $\dfrac{k_{on}}{k_{off}} L_0$, which is the same as when the system is well mixed and we do not worry about diffusive transport to the cell.
2. If diffusion is fast, k_+ is big and the rate constants approach their well-mixed analogues. On the other hand if diffusion is very slow then the effective rate constants can be much smaller.
3. In the limit of high k_{on}, the maximum possible forward rate is $\dfrac{k_+}{R}$ and we call the process *diffusion-limited*. In the opposite case, when k_{on} is small, the forward rate is approximately governed by k_{on} alone and we call the process *reaction-limited*.
4. The diffusion-limitation for weakly binding reactions can be mitigated by increasing the number of surface receptors on the cell (high R). In order for the effective forward rate constant to be equal to half its maximum value, we require $k_{on} R = k_+$. For some "typical" parameters, $D = 10^2\ \mu m^2/s$, $a = 5\ \mu m$,

and $k_{on} = 10^{-7}\,M^{-1}s^{-1} = 1.66 \times 10^{-2}\,\mu m^3$, it can be calculated that the total number of receptors achieving this k_f is only 3800. As Berg and Purcell pointed out, *it takes surprisingly few receptors distributed over the cell surface to raise the effective forward rate constant to half its maximal value* (Berg & Purcell, Physics of chemoreception, 1977). There is plenty of room on the cell surface for many different populations of receptors to be displayed in sufficiently high numbers to capture their ligands effectively.

5. The difference between k_{off} and k_r is entirely due to dissociation and rapid re-binding of cytokines. In fact, the ratio k_r/k_{off} is equal to the probability that a dissociated cytokine escapes from the cell periphery rather than rebinding to a receptor.

6. The given derivation is only valid in three dimensions. In two dimensions, it becomes much more difficult to set up the steady state, and beyond the scope of this chapter (Goldstein, Griego, & Wofsy, 1984; Lauffenburger & Linderman, 1996).

9.8 DIFFUSION-LIMITED REACTIONS OF SECRETED MOLECULES IN THE IMMUNOLOGICAL SYNAPSE

Let us return to the example of IL-4 diffusion across the helper T cell – B cell immunological synapse. We will calculate k_+ for this situation and use this to estimate the degree of competition among IL-4 receptors, as well as the degree to which diffusion might limit dissociation of IL-4 from its receptor. For the synapse geometry, k_+ is obtained by setting up a steady state and calculating the mean flux into the target cell, assuming that it is perfectly absorbing. We have already solved for the concentration of IL-4 at steady state (equation 9.1 above) and calculated the flux of molecules into a perfectly absorbing target (equation 9.2). The diffusion-limited forward rate constant k_+ is computed as the ratio of "flux" (equation 9.2) to the mean concentration at $z = 0$ (equation 9.1) averaged over the contact area:

$$k_+ = \text{flux} / \left(\pi a^2 \sum_{n=1}^{\infty} \frac{4aS \tanh\left(\hat{\alpha}_n (d/a) \right)}{D\hat{\alpha}_n^3} \right).$$

Using the same parameters as above, $a = 2\,\mu m$, $d = 40$ nm, $D = 10^2\,\mu m^2 s^{-1}$, we find $k_+ \approx 3 \times 10^{-8}\,cm^3 s^{-1}$. From the definition of k_f, we see that transport will have a big influence on the kinetics when $k_{on}R/k_+ > 1$. Since we know k_{on} and k_+, we can calculate the relevant number of receptors that would have to be in the contact area: $R \approx 9 \times 10^5$ per contact area. The number of IL-4 receptors expressed on B cells has been found to be in the range of 50–5000 receptors on the whole cell, so we can see that transport by diffusion is rapid and the binding reaction occurs as if the system were well mixed. However, if the secretion of IL-4 is switched off and we look at dissociation, transport effects are rather important, as we will now discuss.

Consider the reverse reaction, where secretion of IL-4 by the T cell is turned off. IL-4 will begin to dissociate from its receptor and diffuse away. Because the volume in which this happens is so confining, a diffusing ligand that dissociates from a receptor will usually return to the B cell surface many times before it exits the synapse. The un-binding reaction is described by

$$\frac{dB}{dt} = k_f R\, L - k_r B,$$

and we expect that, over time, L will decay to zero as ligands escape. The effective rate constants have the same form as in the previous section, except that the diffusion-limited forward rate constant k_+ must be replaced by the diffusion-limited rate constant for leaving the surface k_-. The effective dissociation rate constant is

$$k_r = \frac{k_{off}}{1 + R k_{on}/k_-},$$

where k_- is the diffusion-limited rate constant for leaving the surface, averaged over the area of the target cell within the contact. The quantity $R\,k_{on}/k_-$ controls the reduction in the off-rate constant due to rebinding (Berg & Purcell, Physics of chemoreception, 1977; Goldstein & Dembo, 1995). When $R\,k_{on}/k_- \geq 1$, rebinding plays a significant role in slowing dissociation.

To calculate k_-, we set up a steady state where there is a fixed flux of molecules entering the cylinder through its base (corresponding to the B cell), no molecules can enter the T cell (at $z = d$), and molecules escaping the cylinder through its sides are lost. These boundary conditions are encoded mathematically as

$$-D\frac{\partial u}{\partial z}\bigg|_{(z=0)} = S, \quad \frac{\partial u}{\partial z}\bigg|_{(z=d)} = 0 \text{ and } u(r = a, z) = 0.$$

This is identical to the mathematical problem considered in the previous section, so we can see that the flux leaving the cylinder through its sides is just the total inward flux minus the flux computed in equation 9.2. This quantity ($\pi S a^2$ – flux) must then be divided by the averaged concentration at $z = 0$ (from equation 9.1 above). Note that this reverse rate constant is certainly *not* the same as the forward rate constant k_+. The full calculations for this case are given elsewhere (Coombs & Goldstein, 2005).

Using the parameters given above, we find that having 381 IL-4 receptors in the contact area is enough to achieve equality in this relation. Even though the numbers of IL-4 receptors are small on B cells, if they move to the contact region when a synapse is established, the half-life for dissociation of an IL-4 molecule from the contact volume will be significantly increased. Because of the confined geometry of the synapse, diffusion limitation during binding can be negligible but this may produce a significant effect during dissociation. This reflects the fact that a large fraction of diffusive paths that start on one surface lead directly to the second surface without ever encountering the side of the cylinder whereas only a small fraction of paths that start on one surface and end by reaching the side of the cylinder do so without returning to the starting surface many times. Compounding this effect, in recent theoretical work it was proposed that diffusion in the synaptic volume is significantly hindered by the density of adhesion and other membrane proteins that are present (Woodsworth, Dunsing, & Coombs, 2015). This result serves to emphasize the importance of the immunological synapse in promoting efficient delivery of signaling proteins from one cell to another.

9.9 THE MEAN FIRST PASSAGE TIME FOR DIFFUSIVE PROBLEMS

The diffusion-limited rate constants we have seen so far are based on differential equations and as such, carry an implicit assumption that the number of objects we are modeling is quite large. Under many circumstances in immunology, we might be interested in small numbers of particles or rare events. For example, a particular T cell might be stimulated only by a rare antigenic peptide presented at very low densities on a given antigen-present cell. Experimental evidence indicates that extremely few (single digits) of these antigenic signatures can be sufficient for a measurable response *in vitro*. In this section we will briefly discuss an approach to calculating the probability distributions of times to events for diffusing particles and show how this can be related to the theory of diffusion-limited reactions as described above.

To motivate this approach, let's look at the following simple case. Imagine a spherical lymph node of radius R, containing a single stationary antigen-presenting cell of interest. For simplicity, place this at the center of the lymph node, and suppose that it has radius a. Now, imagine a T cell located at an arbitrary position (x, y, z) within the lymph node and suppose it is moving diffusively with diffusion coefficient D. We will try to calculate the mean (average) time it will take for the T cell to reach its target. To do this we also have to impose a boundary condition at the outer boundary of the lymph node. The simplest case is to suppose that the T cell motion will reflect at the boundary but we can consider other possible behaviors—such as a boundary where the T cell exits the lymph node if it reaches the boundary.

Working with the outer reflective boundary, let's define $T(x, y, z)$ as the mean first passage time for the T cell to reach the APC. This is the average over all possible diffusive paths from (x, y, z) to the sphere $r = a$. It can be shown (Karlin & Taylor, 1981; Goldstein, Griego, & Wofsy, 1984; Gardiner, 2009) that

$$D\Delta T(x, y, z) = -1.$$

Here, Δ represents the Laplacian operator in the relevant coordinates (rectilinear, spherical, cylindrical, etc.) for the problem we are working on. This is a boundary value problem, so we must have enough boundary information. When the T cell is at $r = a$, it has already found the target, so we can set $T(r = a) = 0$. At the outer boundary, we already said that the particle will not exit. This corresponds to a no-flux boundary condition $\dfrac{\partial T}{\partial n}\Big|_{(r=R)} = 0$. We can now solve the problem (using the spherical coordinate Laplacian) to obtain

$$T(r) = \frac{r - a}{3D}\left(\frac{R^3}{ar} - \frac{a + r}{2} \right).$$

Averaging this formula over all points in the volume between the antigen-presenting cell ($r = a$) and the outer boundary ($r = R$), we obtain an averaged mean first passage time $\overline{T} = \dfrac{5R^6 - 9aR^5 + 5a^3R^3 - a^6}{15aD\left(R^3 - a^3\right)}$. Dimensionless forms of these expressions are shown in Figure 9.3a. If we suppose that a T cell diffuses with an effective diffusion constant of $60\ \mu\mathrm{m}^2\mathrm{min}^{-1}$, then within a lymph node of radius 0.5mm and assuming an effective target radius of $20\ \mu\mathrm{m}$, we find $\overline{T} \sim 537$ hours. This may seem high, but it is clearly an overestimate

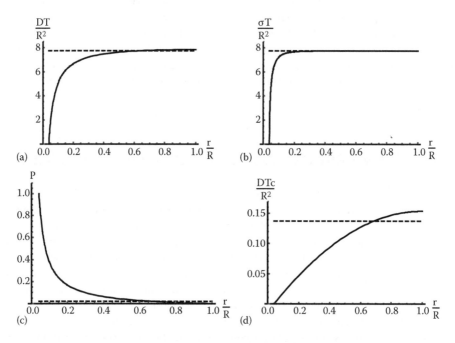

Figure 9.3 Calculations related to the first passage time. **(a)** The dimensionless mean first passage time for a diffusing T cell (diffusion constant D) to reach a centrally located spherical target cell of radius $0.05R$ in a spherical lymph node of radius R is plotted against the dimensionless starting position r/R. In this case the outer boundary of the lymph node is reflecting. **(b)** The dimensionless variance of the first passage time is plotted against starting position again with a reflecting outer boundary. **(c)** The probability of reaching the target cell is plotted against the starting position, in a situation where the outer boundary absorbs the searching cell. **(d)** The conditional dimensionless mean first passage time is plotted against the starting position. **(a-d)** In each panel, the dashed line indicates the spatial average over all possible starting positions of the T cell.

for the time for a T cell response to begin to a particular pathogen for several reasons: (1) there will likely be more than one antigen-presenting cell in a given lymph node; (2) there may be more than one lymph node containing antigen; (3) there may be several potential reactive T cells available; and (4) the motion of the T cell may not be entirely random—it is believed that T cells preferentially track along a branched network of reticular cells, which may lead to a higher rate of encounters with antigen-presenting cells. See (Donovan & Lythe, 2012; Delgado, Ward, & Coombs, 2015) and references therein for more discussion of these issues.

It is also possible to calculate the higher moments of the escape time distribution by solving some slightly more complicated equations that form a recursion in the order of the moments. The general formula is that

$$D\Delta T_j = - i\, T_{j-1},$$

where T_j is the j'th moment of the exit time distribution (Karlin & Taylor, 1981). So for the spherical lymph node case that we are considering, we can compute the second moment via $D\Delta T_2 = -2T$ and thus the variance of the time distribution $V(r) = T_2 - T^2$. The details of this calculation are left as an exercise. Using the parameters given above, the averaged standard deviation is found to be $\sigma \sim 537$ hours. We observe that the averaged standard deviation is very close to the mean and therefore the mean is not a great descriptor of the behavior of the time distribution, which is approximately exponential (Figure 9.3b).

Let us also consider the variation of this problem where the diffusing T cell will permanently leave the lymph node if it reaches the outer boundary before the antigen-presenting cell. We can now see that we must solve for the probability, $P(x, y, z)$ that a cell initially located at (x, y, z) will diffuse to the central antigen-presenting cell *before* it reaches the outer boundary. This probability is calculated by solving Laplace's equation,

$$\Delta P(x,y,z)=0$$

subject to the boundary conditions that $P(r = a) = 1$ (the T cell has reached the target cell) and $P(r = R) = 0$ (the T cell has exited the lymph node). The solution of this in our spherical geometry is easily found to be

$$P(r) = \frac{a(R-r)}{r(R-a)}.$$

(Plotted in Figure 9.3c). We can apply this result to calculate the *conditional first passage time* for the T cell to reach the target cell. This is the average duration of all diffusive paths from the initial point to the target cell, conditioned on not hitting the outer boundary. This quantity, which we denote by T_C, satisfies the following problem:

$$D\Delta\big(T_C(r)\, P(r)\big)= -P(r); \quad T_C(r=a)=0; \quad T_C(r=R)P(r=R)=0.$$

This is solved in this geometry to give $T_C(r) = (r - a)\,(2R - r - a)/(6D)$. Again averaging over all possible starting and positions and using the parameter estimates from above, we find $\bar{T}_C \approx 9.5$ hours which is an order of magnitude below the averaged first passage time we found when the outer boundary was impermeable to the T cell (Figure 9.3d). The difference here is the conditioning: the vast majority of diffusing cells will exit the lymph node rather than reaching the central target! We can validate this by calculating the averaged probability (over all starting positions) of ever reaching the target, $\bar{P} = \dfrac{a(2a+R)}{2(a^2 + aR + R^2)} \approx 0.0004$ for these parameters. When we condition on this highly unlikely event, only tracks that reach the central target are considered, and these usually reach the target rapidly.

Similar first passage time calculations can be made for more complicated geometries, partially absorbing boundaries, and multiple traps (Bressloff & Newby, 2013; Delgado, Ward, & Coombs, 2015). However, one should question the importance of calculations of the mean first passage time when the number of events (e.g., arrivals) may be very small and poorly described by the mean. In these cases, it might be more worthwhile to study the full distribution of event times via partial differential equations, or to apply a spatial stochastic simulation algorithm. In the latter case, the software Smoldyn is recommended as a relatively simple and robust application (Andrews, 2012).

9.10 SUMMARY

In this chapter we have developed some basic ideas of diffusion and diffusion-limited reactions in immunological modeling. The methods and examples we have discussed are almost infinitely extensible to situations arising in immunology but in particular related to cell signaling and immune cell motion. Although it is often tempting to go directly to simulation, building an understanding of the space and time scales of the immunological situation via diffusion-limited reaction theory and first passage times almost always yields important insights into the problem and can be used to benchmark simulation approaches if and when those are eventually applied.

9.11 ACKNOWLEDGMENTS

This work was partially supported by a grant from the Simons Foundation and was written at the Isaac Newton Institute during the program "Stochastic Dynamical Systems in Biology".

REFERENCES

Andrews, S. (2012). Spatial and stochastic cellular modeling with the Smoldyn simulator. *Methods in Molecular Biology 804*, 519–542.

Bajenoff, M., Glaichenhaus, N., and Germain, R. (2008). Fibroblastic reticular cells guide T lymphocyte entry into and migration within the splenic T cell zone. *J. Immunol. 181*, 3947–3954.

* Berg, H. C. (1993). *Random Walks in Biology*. Princeton, NJ: Princeton University Press. *Classic introduction to statistical physics concepts for biologists and biophysicists.*

* Berg, H. C., and Purcell, E. M. (1977). Physics of chemoreception. *Biophys. J. 20*, 193–219. *One of the most influential papers in biophysics. Underlines the importance of diffusive transport to biological modelling.*

* Bressloff, P., and Newby, J. (2013). Stochastic models of intracellular transport. *Rev. Modern Phys. 85*, 135–196. *Thorough, modern mathematical approach to stochastic models for intracellular processes.*

Cahalan, M., Parker, I., Wei, S., and Miller, M. (2003). Real-time imaging of lymphocytes in vivo. *Curr. Opin. Immunol. 15*, 372–377.

Carslaw, H., and Jaeger, J. (1959). *Conduction of heat in solids*. Glasgow: Oxford University Press.

Coombs, D., and Goldstein, B. (2005). Effects of the geometry of the immunological synapse on the delivery of effector molecules. *Biophys. J. 87*, 2215–2220.

Coombs, D., Das, R., and Morrison, J. (2011). Modeling membrane domains. In I. Nabi (Ed.), *Membrane Domains* (71–84). Hoboken, NJ: Wiley.

Delgado, M., Ward, M., and Coombs, D. (2015). Conditional mean first passage times to small traps in a 3-D domain with a sticky boundary: Applications to T cell searching behaviour in lymph nodes. *SIAM Multiscale Modeling and Simulation 13*, 1224–1258.

Donovan, G., and Lythe, G. (2012). T-cell movement on the reticular network. *J. Theor. Biol. 295*, 59–67.

* Einstein, A. (1956). *Investigations on the theory of the Brownian movement*. Mineola, NY: Dover Publications. *Reprint of the original paper. Very readable and thought-provoking.*

* Gardiner, C. W. (2009). *Stochastic Methods: A Handbook for the Natural and Social Sciences* (4th ed.). Berlin Heidelberg: Springer. *Bible of probabilistic methods for applications.*

Goldstein, B., and Dembo, M. (1995). Approximating the effects of diffusion on reversible reactions at the cell surface: Ligand-receptor kinetics. *Biophys. J. 68*, 1222–1230.

Goldstein, B., Griego, R., and Wofsy, C. (1984). Diffusion-limited forward rate constants in two dimensions: Application to the trapping of cell surface receptors by coated pits. *Biophys. J. 46*, 573–583.

* Karlin, S., and Taylor, H. (1981). *A second course in stochastic processes.* San Diego: Academic Press. *Essential handbook for applied mathematicians working with stochastic models.*

* Lauffenburger, D., and Linderman, J. (1996). *Receptors: Models for Binding, Trafficking, and Signaling.* New York: Oxford University Press. *Excellent introductory book includes a thorough chapter on diffusion-limited reactions.*

Meyer-Hermann, M., and Maini, P. (2005). Interpreting two-photon imaging data of lymphocyte motility. *Phys. Rev. E 71*, 061912.

Phillips, R. K. (2012). *Physical Biology of the Cell.* New York: Garland Science.

Saffman, P., and Delbruck, M. (1972). Brownian motion in biological membranes. *Proc. Natl. Acad. Sci. USA 72*, 3111–3113.

von Smoluchowski, M. (1916). Drei Vorträge über Diffusion, Brownsche Bewegung und Koagulation von Kolloidteilchen. *Physik Z. 16*, 557–585.

Wang, Y., Shen, B., and Sebald, W. (1997). A mixed-charge pair in human interleukin 4 dominates high-affinity interaction with the receptor a chain. *Proc. Natl. Acad. Sci. USA 94*, 1657–1662.

Woodsworth, D., Dunsing, V., and Coombs, D. (2015). Design parameters for granzyme-mediated cytotoxic lymphocyte target-cell killing and specificity. *Biophys. J. 109*, 477–488.

Analysis and modeling of single cell data

DERYA ALTINTAN, JASCHA DIEMER, AND HEINZ KOEPPL

10.1 INTRODUCTION

Understanding dynamic processes inside a single cell can be considered as the first step to understanding the dynamics of an entire multicellular organism. Even if cells are seemingly identical in the cell population of interest, their dynamical behaviors can be very different from each other. Ignoring this cellular heterogeneity leads to inaccurate models on the single cell level that in turn produce inappropriate descriptions of dynamics of the whole organism. Bulk measurements giving average information about the cell population of interest may be insufficient to explain the dynamical behavior of a cell in the environment under consideration.

This chapter is devoted to giving an overview of single cell technologies, modeling of reaction systems, the contribution of extrinsic and intrinsic noises to the cellular heterogeneity, and inference methods that reconstruct the unknown states or parameters by using the given observed data.

Single cell technologies make it possible to categorize individual cells depending on their metabolomics, proteomic, and transcriptomic properties, which in turn will increase our capacity to understand the underlying dynamics of the immune system (Satija and Shalek, 2014), tumor cells (Navin et al., 2011), variability of stem-cells (Tang et al., 2010), and many other processes in prokaryotic and eukaryotic cells (Nachman et al., 2007). The criterium to conduct single cell experiments is detection of small amounts of molecules. The steadily increasing sensitivity of devices enables scientists to perform measurements with volumes in the dimensions of cells and below. But sensitivity alone is not enough. The cell consists of hundreds of thousands of different molecules, which make reliable molecular markers absolutely essential. For applications that rely on light detection, like microscopy and flow cytometry, fluorescent proteins and markers are widely used today to introduce selective visibility and high contrast.

Biochemical reactions in cells are stochastic processes. Single cell measurements reveal that isogenous cells, grown in the same environment, expose different dynamics, which is the result of stochasticity.

The variance of, for example, protein expression within a cell population is one of the most important examples of cell-to-cell variability (Altschuler and Wu, 2010). If we consider the expression of a particular gene, the abundance of the protein varies from cell to cell. Even in the same cell, the protein concentration may change when measured at different time points. The sources of this variability can be separated into two categories: intrinsic noise and extrinsic noise. In a few words, intrinsic noise refers to inherent randomness hidden in the particular cellular process, while extrinsic noise explains the effects of other cellular components on the reaction system under consideration. All interactions between species in a single cell are described by biomolecular systems, defined as a combination of consumed and produced species. Depending on the representation of the abundance of species in a reaction system, different modeling strategies are developed, such as stochastic modeling or deterministic modeling.

Another problem in single cell analysis is to estimate the unknown or partially known quantities by using different types of the data obtained by single cell technologies. Bayesian inference can be used to construct posterior probability distributions and provide knowledge about the reaction inside of cells.

Models of single cell data are necessary to get information that would otherwise remain hidden from the eye of the experimentalist. Based on the nature of experiments and the methods used, some quantities cannot be read out directly or simultaneously by the operating device. Advances in computational methods have the power to complete and further predict data for experiments that are not executable today (Schoeberl et al., 2014). Such approaches and studies are utterly relevant in drug treatment and therapy because diseases like cancer are highly diverse and the effects of a drug differ on each patient (Niepel et al., 2009, Niepel et al., 2014).

In Section 10.2, we give an overview about the most common technologies that derive data from single cells. Section 10.3 will explain how we can measure intrinsic and extrinsic noise based on dual color experiments (Swain et al., 2002). Section 10.4 is devoted to introducing the basic concepts of these approaches. Section 10.5 explains the use of Bayesian inference. Finally, in Section 10.6, we explained how we can use the posterior probability distributions to identify the unknown quantities.

10.2 SINGLE CELL ANALYSIS

The tools to study differences on the single cell level have continuously improved their sensitivity and increased their throughput. A well-known single cell method is flow cytometry, which measures optical features of single cells, see Figure 10.1a. Cells in solution are directed in a steady stream to the detector. Since the stream is tapered, the cells pass the laser-based system for fluorescence and scatter values one after another. This technique is now divided into flow cytometers and fluorescence activated cell sorting (FACS) with the presence of a droplet generator (Fulwyler, 1965). To sort the cells, FACS uses electrical charge to manipulate the flight direction of the droplet. In comparison, a flow cytometer has no droplet generator and is therefore not capable of sorting cells. Although the single cell data from FACS experiments can be used to discover population distributions, the method provides no further tracking of individual cells. It can be used to search for or to enrich rare cells types (Kling, 2015). While the time to measure one cell is on the order of microseconds, the throughput of this method is limited by the available optical markers to select for features. One attempt to bypass this limitation is to combine flow cytometry with mass spectrometry (so called mass cytometry). This can push the limit up to 50 different molecule markers in a single experiment for diverse cellular features in one experimental iteration (Ornatsky et al., 2010, Spitzer and Nolan, 2016). The most prominent targets for this method are metabolites and proteins (Xue et al., 2015). Mass cytometry is sensitive enough to detect the difference in concentration of small molecules between two single cells, which would have been hidden in the populations average (Heinemann and Zenobi, 2011, Onjiko et al., 2015). It is an important tool to investigate signaling pathways in cells, where proteins occur depending on the previous signal molecules and are often drug targets (Shi et al., 2012, Lun et al., 2017).

Another steadily advancing field is the area of DNA sequencing. Huge steps in quantity and quality have led to reduced prices, making it feasible to sequence the genome of a single cell (Kolodziejczyk et al., 2015). But, this has some drawbacks. As the sequencing methods rely on multiplying the sequence with PCR based techniques, errors and sequence bias can be introduced or amplified. Another drawback is the potential lack

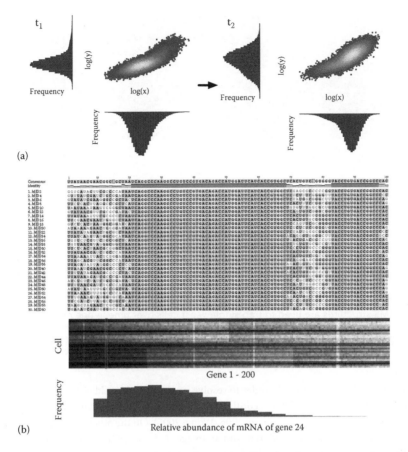

Figure 10.1 Examples of single cell technologies. **(a)** Simulated data for a flow cytometry experiment. Each cell was scanned for two optical features, i.e., fluorescence intensity of two different fluorophores. The axes of the scatter plot show the log of their respective intensities. The histograms for the two optical features on both time points give insights in the evolution of the cell population. Gating can be used with a FACS to gather cells with specified features and enrich for rare cell types. The data collected are *distribution data*. **(b)** Synthetic example for single cell mRNA sequence alignment of one gene. On a first analysis, conserved and unconserved regions can be distinguished. Depending on the function of the corresponding protein the conserved sequence may represent a catalytic domain. Besides the sequence, transcript sequencing is able to estimate the abundance of mRNAs in single cells. A heat map is often used to demonstrate the abundance of mRNA for a set of genes on the cellular level. Along each column a histogram gives insights into the distribution of mRNAs in a given population. Further bioinformatic analysis like correlation and clustering enable us to describe and reveal functions on the process of transcription. The data collected are *distribution data*.

(Continued)

of coverage of the DNA template. The nucleotide composition of a given gene has an influence on the quantity of replicates and can result in a loss of information (Nawy, 2013). However, genomes are not the only target for sequencing methods. Studies of the transcriptome are a powerful tool in the characterization of single cells (Pollen et al., 2014) and have the advantage that common transcripts are present at a higher copy number (approximately 50 molecules per cell) (Eberwine et al., 2013). This method is an important step to understand the dynamics of single cells (Figure 10.1b), especially for multicellular organisms. Improving bioinformatic methods and decreasing costs for a sequencing run are steadily reducing the limitation in this field.

The oldest and still one of the most powerful instruments to investigate a single cell is the microscope. Technical advances in physics and material science influence the resolution and sensitivity and help to bypass the diffraction limit of the microscope (Hess et al., 2006, Klar and Hell, 1999). Since the discovery of the green fluorescent protein, considerable effort has been put into the development of new techniques to tag and target all kinds of intracellular molecules. Now, it is possible to follow single molecules in the cell. One disadvantage

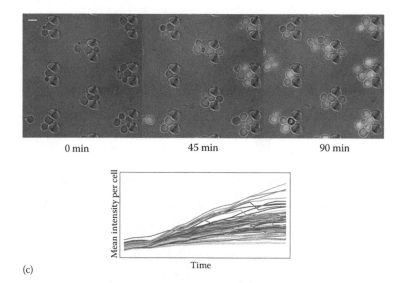

(c)

Figure 10.1 (Continued) Examples of single cell technologies. **(c)** Images from microfluidic experiments with yeast. PDMS structures are used to trap single yeast cells over time in one position and gene expression is induced by raising the concentration of sodium chloride in the medium. For each time point every cell is segmented and the intensity is calculated. The plot shows the mean intensity for each cell over 90 min. The cell-to-cell variability can be calculated and noise can be estimated. The data collected are *trajectory data*.

of the microscope is the throughput. In order to resolve single cells, the field of view is limited to a few hundred micrometers. On the one hand, the recording of cells has to be automated in order to record hundreds or thousands of cells (Pepperkok and Ellenberg, 2006, Wong, 2006). On the other hand, the temporal resolution is limited to the time step that is needed to record an image at every position. Depending on the process that is studied, this can limit the number of cells that can be observed.

Recent developments have taken place in the design and fabrication of microfluidic devices for biological samples (Yin and Marshall, 2012). Droplet-based and continuous flow systems have both learned to deal with the demands of single cell measurements. The droplet-based approach can generate micro environments for single cells, which enable high-throughput screening for protein engineering and for directed evolution (Agresti et al., 2010). Charged-based selection can be used to keep the most promising candidates with the desired feature. Oil-water emulsions, for example, provide good control over single droplets and generally exclude the cross-talk between cells in a suspension cell line (Hu et al., 2015). Continuous flow devices can be used to culture suspension cells as well as adherent cell lines. Depending on the organisms' size and characteristics, different designs are required to keep track of cells over time. For example, steric traps can be used to capture and keep single yeast cells in a constant flow (Crane et al., 2014, Jo et al., 2015). The main advantage of microfluidic systems over flow cytometry and sequencing is the spatial resolution. Since most devices are monitored under a microscope, a time-lapsed image sequence of the single cells during the experiment can be easily recorded (Figure 10.1c).

All these technologies have enabled us to study the processes of life on the single cell level (de Vargas Roditi and Claassen, 2015). In all those experimental findings, noise plays a pivotal role. The following section will give an introduction into the mathematical description of this problem.

10.3 CELL-TO-CELL VARIABILITY

Single cell measurements reveal that the dynamics of isogenic cells can be very different from each other even if they have a common ancestor and the environment they are growing in is exactly the same (Altschuler and Wu, 2010, Snijder and Pelkmans, 2011). This variability indicates that ensemble or bulk measurements may be insufficient to explain the dynamical behavior of an individual cell in the environment of interest.

To determine the sources of this variability, one approach is to mathematically model this variability and to design dedicated experiments that can help to dissect different sources of variability.

As biomolecular measurements are always concerned with a specific cellular process (e.g., a particular signaling pathway), a cell population is said to exhibit variability if the measurement of this process is different across this population. Consequently, one can generally distinguish two sources that contribute to this variability. First, cells exhibit differences because the process of interest itself is random, for instance, due to the intrinsic randomness of biomoecular reactions. This source of variability is usually called *intrinsic noise*. Second, the measurement can differ across cells, because factors that are considered extrinsic to the process of interest vary across cells. This contribution, which is best defined by the variability that remains after removal of the intrinsic noise contribution, is usually called *extrinsic noise* (Bowsher and Swain, 2012, Swain et al., 2002). For instance, for a specific gene-expression system of interest, the global cellular level of ATPs or ribosomes may be considered extrinsic to the process of interest. Nevertheless, differences in those levels across cells will also cause variability in the measurement of the gene expression system of interest. The differences in those extrinsic quantities may themselves arise due to randomness, for instance, in their synthesis process or through randomness in cell division, where daughter cells may inherit different amounts of those extrinsic factors. For processes comprising biochemical reactions, such variability in extrinsic factors can often be approximately accounted for by introducing stochasticity in rate constants for the respective reactions. Whether such stochasticity involves temporal fluctuations or whether it suffices to introduce time-invariant heterogeneity for those quantities depends on the cellular process of interest and in particular on the relative time-scales of intrinsic and extrinsic processes.

To dissect intrinsic from extrinsic contributions to the measured variability, so-called dual color experiments were proposed (Swain et al., 2002) that are reminiscent of classical twin studies (Bouchard et al., 1990). They are based on the following mathematical analysis. Let X be a stochastic process representing a particular cellular process of interest. Furthermore, let Z be a stochastic process describing all cellular processes that are considered extrinsic to the process of interest but that nevertheless influence it. See Figure 10.2a for the graphical representation of this abstraction.

Generally, we deal with a dynamic cellular environment, and the effect of the history of the extrinsic factors onto the process of interest needs to be accounted for. Throughout the chapter, $Z^{\mathcal{H}}$ denotes the history of the extrinsic factors up to time t (Bowsher and Swain, 2012, Hilfinger and Paulsson, 2011). As an example, we consider a gene expression, where $X(t)$ corresponds to the number of molecules of the expressed protein produced at time t.

As a normalized measure of variability of X we introduce the squared coefficient of variation (CV) $\mu_{tot}^2(t)$, at time t (Swain et al., 2002):

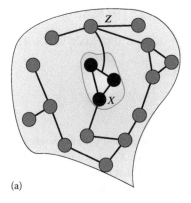
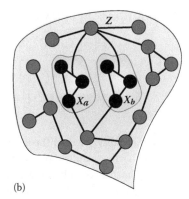

(a)   (b)

Figure 10.2 Separation of the cellular process of interest and modulating components that are extrinsic to the process. **(a)** The process of interest X modulated by its molecular environment Z. **(b)** Twin system comprising identical copies X_a, X_b of the process of interest embedded in the same shared molecular environment Z.

$$\mu_{tot}^2(t) = \frac{\mathbb{V}[X(t)]}{\mathbb{E}[X(t)]^2}, \tag{10.1}$$

where $\mathbb{E}[.]$, $\mathbb{V}[.]$ denote the mean and variance of X at time t, respectively. The law of total variance applied to $X(t)$ for a given history of the dynamic environment $Z^{\mathcal{H}}$ yields:

$$\mathbb{V}[X(t)] = \mathbb{E}\left[\mathbb{V}[X(t)|Z^{\mathcal{H}}]\right] + \mathbb{V}\left[\mathbb{E}[X(t)|Z^{\mathcal{H}}]\right]. \tag{10.2}$$

Accordingly, substituting (10.2) into (10.1) allows us to separate the total normalized variation into two sources,

$$\begin{aligned} \mu_{tot}^2(t) &= \frac{\mathbb{E}\left[\mathbb{V}[X(t)|Z^{\mathcal{H}}]\right]}{\mathbb{E}[X(t)]^2} + \frac{\mathbb{V}\left[\mathbb{E}[X(t)|Z^{\mathcal{H}}]\right]}{\mathbb{E}[X(t)]^2} \\ &\equiv \mu_{int}^2(t) + \mu_{ext}^2(t). \end{aligned} \tag{10.3}$$

Hence, the total variation is the result of both, the fluctuating extrinsic factors and the fluctuations that are intrinsic to the process of interest.

For the case of a time-invariant but random environment, representable by a random variable Z, the conditioning on $Z^{\mathcal{H}}$ in (10.2) naturally reduces to conditioning on Z. This corresponds to the variance decomposition as originally proposed in (Swain et al., 2002).

Based on this decomposition, one may conceive experiments where the two components can be quantified separately. If we consider a cell population, the sample mean and the variance of X can easily be obtained, which in turn allows us to quantify $\mu_{tot}^2(t)$. To determine both sources to the total variation, we set up a twin experiment by ideally incorporating two identical copies of the process of interest (see Figure 10.2b). Naturally, if both copies should be accessible separately, they need to differ at least on their measured readout, i.e., in their reporter. Let us denote the abundance of the two reporters by X_a and X_b. We say that two reporters are conjugate if the following two conditions are satisfied: (i) Given the history of extrinsic noise, $Z^{\mathcal{H}}$, X_a, and X_b are conditionally independent which implies $\mathbb{E}\left[X_a(t)X_b(t)|Z^{\mathcal{H}}\right] = \mathbb{E}\left[X_a(t)|Z^{\mathcal{H}}\right]\mathbb{E}\left[X_b(t)|Z^{\mathcal{H}}\right]$; (ii) $\mathbb{E}\left[X_a(t)|Z^{\mathcal{H}}\right] = \mathbb{E}\left[X_b(t)|Z^{\mathcal{H}}\right]$ and $\mathbb{V}\left[X_a(t)|Z^{\mathcal{H}}\right] = \mathbb{V}\left[X_b(t)|Z^{\mathcal{H}}\right]$. Here, the first condition implies that the fluctuations in the number of molecules X_a doesn't have an effect on the number of molecules of X_b and vice versa.

In order to determine the two noise components in (10.3) we compute the covariance among the two conjugate reporters:

$$\begin{aligned} Cov(X_a(t), X_b(t)) &= \mathbb{E}\left[\mathbb{E}\left[X_a(t)X_b(t)|Z^{\mathcal{H}}\right]\right] - \mathbb{E}\left[\mathbb{E}\left[X_a(t)|Z^{\mathcal{H}}\right]\right]\mathbb{E}\left[\mathbb{E}\left[X_b(t)|Z^{\mathcal{H}}\right]\right] \\ &= \mathbb{E}\left[\mathbb{E}\left[X_a(t)|Z^{\mathcal{H}}\right]\mathbb{E}\left[X_b(t)|Z^{\mathcal{H}}\right]\right] - \mathbb{E}\left[\mathbb{E}\left[X_a(t)|Z^{\mathcal{H}}\right]\right]\mathbb{E}\left[\mathbb{E}\left[X_b(t)|Z^{\mathcal{H}}\right]\right] \\ &= \mathbb{E}\left[\mathbb{E}\left[X_a(t)|Z^{\mathcal{H}}\right]^2\right] - \mathbb{E}\left[\mathbb{E}\left[X_a(t)|Z^{\mathcal{H}}\right]\right]^2 \\ &= \mathbb{V}\left[\mathbb{E}\left[X_a(t)|Z^{\mathcal{H}}\right]\right] = \mathbb{V}\left[\mathbb{E}\left[X_b(t)|Z^{\mathcal{H}}\right]\right] = \mathbb{V}\left[\mathbb{E}\left[X(t)|Z^{\mathcal{H}}\right]\right]. \end{aligned}$$

To obtain the first equality, we used the law of total mean. The second equality holds due to condition (i) while the third and fourth equalities hold due to condition (ii). Since X_b is just a representation, for the sake of simplicity we used X instead of X_b in the last equality. This means that if we measure $Cov(X_a(t), X_b(t))$, we get an estimate of $\mathbb{V}[\mathbb{E}[X[(t)|Z^{\mathcal{H}}]]$ which is the numerator in $\mu_{ext}^2(t)$. Since it is easy to determine its denominator, we can obtain an estimate of the relative extrinsic contribution $\mu_{ext}^2(t)$. Consequently, if we measured $\mu_{tot}^2(t)$ and $\mu_{ext}^2(t)$, then their difference gives an estimate for $\mu_{int}^2(t)$.

Above, we obtained an estimate for $\mu_{ext}^2(t)$ and used it to determine $\mu_{int}^2(t)$. The reverse can also be applied which means that we can determine $\mu_{int}^2(t)$ experimentally and then find the value of extrinsic contribution $\mu_{ext}^2(t)$. To determine $\mu_{int}^2(t)$, we compute the mean squared difference of the two conjugate reporters:

$$
\begin{aligned}
\frac{1}{2}\mathbb{E}[(X_a(t)-X_b(t))^2] &= \frac{1}{2}\mathbb{E}\left[\mathbb{E}\left[X_a^2(t)\big|Z^{\mathcal{H}}\right] - 2\mathbb{E}\left[X_a(t)X_b(t)\big|Z^{\mathcal{H}}\right] + \mathbb{E}\left[X_b^2(t)\big|Z^{\mathcal{H}}\right]\right] \\
&= \frac{1}{2}\mathbb{E}\left[\mathbb{E}\left[X_a^2(t)\big|Z^{\mathcal{H}}\right]\right] - \mathbb{E}\left[\mathbb{E}\left[X_a(t)X_b(t)\big|Z^{\mathcal{H}}\right]\right] + \frac{1}{2}\mathbb{E}\left[\mathbb{E}\left[X_a^2(t)\big|Z^{\mathcal{H}}\right]\right] \\
&= \mathbb{E}\left[\mathbb{E}\left[X_a^2(t)\big|Z^{\mathcal{H}}\right]\right] - \mathbb{E}\left[\mathbb{E}\left[X_a(t)\big|Z^{\mathcal{H}}\right]\mathbb{E}\left[X_b(t)\big|Z^{\mathcal{H}}\right]\right] \\
&= \mathbb{E}\left[\mathbb{E}\left[X^2(t)\big|Z^{\mathcal{H}}\right]\right] - \mathbb{E}\left[\mathbb{E}\left[X(t)\big|Z^{\mathcal{H}}\right]^2\right] = \mathbb{E}\left[\mathbb{V}\left[X(t)\big|Z^{\mathcal{H}}\right]\right].
\end{aligned}
$$

The first equality is just the result of the law of total mean. The second and the third equalities hold because of the conditions (ii) and (i), respectively. For the sake of simplicity, we write again X instead of X_a, X_b and get the fourth equality. As a result, we get an estimate of the numerator of $\mu_{int}^2(t)$, and we also know how to compute its denominator. Finally, we measure the $\mu_{int}^2(t)$. Then, subtracting the intrinsic contribution from the total noise yields an estimate for $\mu_{ext}^2(t)$.

10.4 MODELING INTRINSIC NOISE

In this section, we will discuss how the cellular process of interest, representable in terms of biochemical reactions, can be modeled mathematically. A reaction in a reaction system is a composition of species interacting with each other. Depending on the abundance of the involved species, different mathematical models can be considered.

Let's assume that the process of interest can be abstracted as a well-stirred reaction system involving N species, $S_1, S_2,..., S_N$, interacting through M reaction channels, $R_1, R_2,...,R_M$. The k–th reaction channel has the form

$$
r_1^k S_1 + r_2^k S_2 + r_3^k S_3 + \cdots + r_N^k S_N \xrightarrow{c_k} p_1^k S_1 + p_2^k S_2 + p_3^k S_3 + \cdots + p_N^k S_N,
$$

where $r_j^k, p_j^k \in \mathbb{N}$ represent the reactant and product coefficients, respectively and c_k is the real-valued stochastic reaction rate constant. We specify the state vector of the system at time $t \geq 0$ by $X(t) = (X_1(t), X_2(t),..., X_N(t))^T$ where $X_j(t)$ is the integer abundance of species S_j at time t. One occurrence of the reaction R_k at time t updates the state vector to $X(t^-) + v_k$, where $X(t^-)$ is the state of the system before the jump and v_k represents the stoichiometric vector (the state change vector) whose j-th component, $v_{kj} = p_j^k - r_j^k$, denotes the net change in the number of molecules of S_j. Let $x \in \mathbb{N}^N$ be the given state of the system at time t, the probability of exactly one occurrence of the reaction R_k in the time interval $[t, t + h)$ for sufficiently small h is given by $a_k(x)$ h where $a_k(x)$ denotes the *propensity function*. The mathematical form of this function can be motivated biophysically. The most elementary approach to this is based on the principle of mass-action, which asserts that the propensity of a reaction is proportional to the number of distinct reactant combinations available for execution of this reaction, i.e.:

$$
a_k(x) = c_k \prod_{i=1}^{N} \binom{x_i}{r_i^k}, \tag{10.4}
$$

where the constant of proportionality is the reaction rate constant c_k. Throughout the current section, we will exemplarily consider a model of the gene expression summarized in Table 10.1.

Table 10.1 Reactions, propensity functions, and stoichiometric vectors for the gene expression model

Reaction	Propensity function	Stoichiometric vector
$R_1 : \text{Gene}_{\text{off}} \xrightarrow{c_1} \text{Gene}_{\text{on}}$	$a_1(x) = c_1 x_2$	$v_1 = (1, -1, 0, 0)^T$
$R_2 : \text{Gene}_{\text{on}} \xrightarrow{c_2} \text{Gene}_{\text{off}}$	$a_2(x) = c_2 x_1$	$v_2 = (-1, 1, 0, 0)^T$
$R_3 : \text{Gene}_{\text{on}} \xrightarrow{c_3} \text{Gene}_{\text{on}} + \text{mRNA} \text{ (transcription)}$	$a_3(x) = c_3 x_1$	$v_3 = (0, 0, 1, 0)^T$
$R_4 : \text{mRNA} \xrightarrow{c_4} \text{mRNA} + \text{Protein} \text{ (translation)}$	$a_4(x) = c_4 x_3$	$v_4 = (0, 0, 0, 1)^T$
$R_5 : \text{mRNA} \xrightarrow{c_5} \emptyset \text{ (mRNA degration)}$	$a_5(x) = c_5 x_3$	$v_5 = (0, 0, -1, 0)^T$
$R_6 : \text{Protein} \xrightarrow{c_6} \emptyset \text{ (Protein degration)}$	$a_6(x) = c_6 x_4$	$v_6 = (0, 0, 0, -1)^T$

The state vector of the gene expression model is defined by $X(t) = (\text{Gene}_{\text{on}}, \text{Gene}_{\text{off}}, \text{mRNA}, \text{Protein})^T$. The value of a propensity function only depends on the current amounts of the reactant species. This is the main property of any Markov process, which is based on the idea that future of the system depends on only its current state; in other words, past behavior of the system has no role in predicting the time-evolution of the process. Since biochemical reactions are evolving in continuous-time and discrete state space, the resulting process is a continuous time Markov chains (CTMCs). It is not difficult to see that given initial copy numbers, $X(0)$, the state vector of the process at time t is then determined as

$$X(t) = X(0) + \sum_{k=1}^{M} Y_k(t) v_k, \tag{10.5}$$

where $Y_k(t)$ denotes the number of occurrences of the reaction R_k up to time t. Using the fact that the reaction counting process in Equation (10.5) can be understood as a time-warped homogeneous Poisson process, the state of the reaction system can be described through the random time change model (RTCM) (Anderson and Kurtz, 2011):

$$X(t) = X(0) + \sum_{k=1}^{M} \xi_k \left(\int_0^t a_k(X(s)) ds \right) v_k, \tag{10.6}$$

where ξ_k, $k = 1,...,M$, are now independent unit Poisson processes. Observe that $X_1(t) + X_2(t) = X_1(0) + X_2(0)$ for our running example, which means that the total number of gene copies cannot change during time. This indicates that conservation relations play an important role in constructing the dynamics of a reaction system and can be used to reduce the dimensionality of the dynamics to some lower-dimensional linear manifold (Klipp et al., 2009).

Up to now, we focused on a discrete stochastic process where the amounts of species are considered as integers representing the copy numbers of molecules of the species. However, when the species have high copy numbers, it is permissible and more conducive to approximate the process in terms of real-valued concentrations. Accordingly, the process will now be considered as a continuous-time continuous-state stochastic process, i.e., a general diffusion process. For a given volume Ω of the reaction compartment, we define the concentration of the j–th species as $U_j(t) = \Omega^{-1} X_j(t)$. In case of having unimolecular and bimolecular reactions of species with high copy numbers, we will say $a_k(X(t)) = \Omega \tilde{a}_k(U(t))$, where $\tilde{a}_k$ is computed by using the corresponding deterministic reaction rate constant $\tilde{c}_k$. Then, the system (10.6) can be rewritten as:

$$U(t) = U(0) + \frac{1}{\Omega} \sum_{k=1}^{M} \xi_k \left(\Omega \int_0^t \tilde{a}_k(U(s)) ds \right) v_k. \tag{10.7}$$

For large Ω values, $(\xi_k(\Omega t) - \Omega t)/\sqrt{\Omega}$ converges in distribution to a standard Brownian motion W_k (Anderson and Kurtz, 2011), i.e., $(\xi_k(\Omega t) - \Omega t)/\sqrt{\Omega} \xrightarrow{d} W_k(t)$. Based on this fact the diffusion approximation of (10.7) can be written as:

$$U(t) = U(0) + \sum_{k=1}^{M} v_k \int_0^t \tilde{a}_k(U(s))ds + \frac{1}{\sqrt{\Omega}} \sum_{k=1}^{M} v_k W_k \left(\int_0^t \tilde{a}_k(U(s))ds \right). \tag{10.8}$$

This means that the difference $U(t) - U(0)$ is generated by a deterministic drift term and a stochastic diffusion term represented by the first and the second term in (10.8), respectively. The solution of the integral equation (10.8) agrees in distribution with the solution of the following Ito stochastic differential equation (SDE), i.e., the chemical Langevin equation (CLE) (Gillespie, 2000):

$$dU_j(t) = \sum_{k=1}^{M} v_{kj} \tilde{a}_k(U(t))dt + \frac{1}{\sqrt{\Omega}} \sum_{k=1}^{M} v_{kj} \sqrt{\tilde{a}_k(U(t))} dW_k(t), j = 1, 2, \ldots, N. \tag{10.9}$$

When the number of molecules of species, X, and the system volume both approach to infinity, but the concentration of species, U, remains constant, then the term with $1/\sqrt{\Omega}$ in Equation (10.9) becomes negligible. As a result, in that "thermodynamic limit" case, the process can be described with a set of ordinary differential equations (ODEs) called reaction rate equations (RREs)

$$\frac{dU(t)}{dt} = \sum_{k=1}^{M} v_k \tilde{a}_k(U(t)), \tag{10.10}$$

which is the representation of the time evolution of concentrations of species when the system is modeled by the traditional deterministic approach (Wilkinson, 2006). The hierarchy of the discussed models can be seen in Figure 10.3.

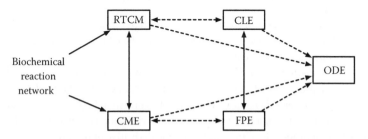

Figure 10.3 The hierarchy of the models. The stochastic approach to modeling biochemical reaction networks starts with a continuous time Markov chain. For the discrete state space of molecule counts $X \in \mathbb{N}^N$, the time evolution of the state is given by RTCM while the time evolution of the corresponding probability distribution is governed by the CME. In the case of a diffusion approximation, leading to continuous state space $X \in \mathbb{R}^N$, the time evolution of the state is given by the CLE and the time evolution of the corresponding probability density function is governed by the FPE. We consider that the reactions take place in a compartment of volume Ω. Then, when $X \to \infty$ and also $\Omega \to \infty$, but the concentration $U = X/\Omega$ remains constant all governing equations converge in this thermodynamic limit to the reaction rate ODE. It gives the time evolution of concentrations of species for infinite volumes. When all propensity functions of the reaction network are affine functions, the time evolution of the mean of X/Ω whose probability distribution satisfies either the CME or the FPE is given by the reaction rate ODE, for any Ω.

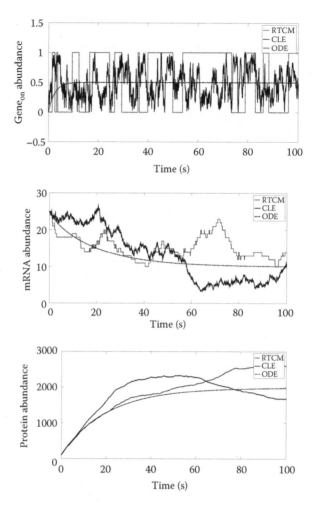

Figure 10.4 Abundances of $Gene_{on}$, mRNA, protein when the dynamics of the reaction system is modeled by RTCM given by Equation (10.6) (dotted line), CLE given by Equation (10.9) (black line), and ODE Equation (10.10) (dashed line). The initial value of the state vector is $X(0) = (0, 1, 25, 100)$ and the parameter values $c_1 = 0.2$ s^{-1}, $c_2 = 0.2$ s^{-1}, $c_3 = 1$ s^{-1}, $c_4 = 4$ s^{-1}, $c_5 = 0.05$ s^{-1} and $c_6 = 0.02$ s^{-1}. For the CLE model, we set $\Omega = 1$.

Figure 10.4 depicts the abundances of $Gene_{on}$, mRNA, Protein for our running example when the system is modeled by the RTCM given by Equation (10.6) (dotted line), the CLE given by Equation (10.9) (black line), and the ODE given by Equation (10.10) (dashed line).

It is apparent that the main difference between the CLE given by Equation (10.9) and the RRE given by Equation (10.10) is a term proportional to $1/\sqrt{\Omega}$. When the system satisfies the conditions of the thermodynamic limit, this term goes to zero, then, the CLE turns to the corresponding RRE. If we assume that the solution of the CLE can be represented by a state vector that is the summation of the solution of the corresponding RRE and a stochastic term proportional to $1/\sqrt{\Omega}$, the time derivative of the stochastic term gives the linear noise approximation (LNA) (Kampen, 1981). Consider the solution of CLE in the form $V(t) = \hat{U}(t) + \dfrac{1}{\sqrt{\Omega}}\eta(t)$, where $\hat{U}(t)$ is the solution of RRE given by Equation (10.10) and $\eta(t)$ represents the state vector of the stochastic process whose time derivative satisfies the LNA. To obtain LNA, we use the first order Taylor expansion of each propensity function:

$$\tilde{a}_k\left(\widehat{U}(t) + \frac{1}{\sqrt{\Omega}}\eta(t)\right) = \tilde{a}_k(\widehat{U}(t)) + \frac{1}{\sqrt{\Omega}}\sum_{n=1}^{N} f_{kn}(t)\eta_n(t) + O(\Omega^{-1}), \qquad (10.11)$$

where $f_{kn}(t) = \frac{\partial \tilde{a}_k(U)}{\partial U_n}\big|_{U=\widehat{U}(t)}$, $k = 1,2,\ldots, M$, and $n = 1, 2, \ldots, N$. Substituting $V(t)$ and Equation (10.11) into CLE given by Equation (10.9) and considering Ω is large enough such that we can neglect all terms proportional to the powers of $1/\sqrt{\Omega}$ gives us the following stochastic differential equation which is called LNA:

$$d\eta(t) = \sum_{n=1}^{N}\left(\sum_{k=1}^{M}v_k f_{kn}(t)\right)\eta_n(t)dt + \sum_{k=1}^{M}v_k\sqrt{\tilde{a}_k\left(\widehat{U}(t)\right)}dW_k(t).$$

If we have Gaussian initial conditions, the solution of this system is a random variable distributed according to a normal distribution with zero mean and covariance $\sigma_{ij}(t)$ satisfying the following differential equation:

$$\frac{d\sigma_{ij}(t)}{dt} = \sum_{n=1}^{N}\left(\sum_{k=1}^{M}v_{ik} f_{kn}(t)\right)\sigma_{nj}(t) + \sum_{n=1}^{N}\left(\sum_{k=1}^{M}v_{jk} f_{kn}(t)\right)\sigma_{ni}(t) + \sum_{k=1}^{M}v_{ik}v_{jk}\tilde{a}_k\left(\widehat{U}(t)\right),$$

subject to the initial condition $\sigma_{ij}(0) = 0$ for all $i,j = 1, 2, \ldots, N$.

Until now, we described the dynamics of biochemical reactions by using their state vector representations, but another way of analyzing these systems is to obtain a time evolution equation for the probability mass function of $X(t)$ given by

$$\mathbb{P}\big[X(t+h) = x + v_k | X(t) = x\big] = a_k(x)h + o(h),$$

where some correction term $f(h)$ is said to be in $o(h)$ if $\lim_{h \to 0}\frac{f(h)}{h} = 0$. Based on the definition of $a_k(x)$, we can write $\mathbb{P}\big(X(t+h) = x\big)$ as follows:

$$\mathbb{P}(X(t+h) = x) = \mathbb{P}(X(t) = x)\left[1 - \sum_{k=1}^{M}a_k(x)h + o(h)\right] + \sum_{k=1}^{M}\mathbb{P}(X(t) = x - v_k)[a_k(x - v_k)h + o(h)] + o(h). \quad (10.12)$$

The first term on the right hand-side of Equation (10.12) represents the situation that the system is in state x at time t, and *no reaction* will fire in $[t, t + h)$. The second term expresses the route that the system is in state $x-v_k$ at time t, and there will be only one occurrence of the reaction R_k. Dividing both sides by h and taking the limit $h \to 0$ results in the famous chemical master equation (CME) (Gillespie, 1992):

$$\frac{d\mathbb{P}(X(t) = x)}{dt} = \sum_{k=1}^{M}\big[a_k(x - v_k)\mathbb{P}(X(t) = x - v_k) - a_k(x)\mathbb{P}(X(t) = x)\big], \quad (10.13)$$

which is the time derivative of the probability function of the path wise representation of X given in (10.6). Although it is possible to obtain analytical solutions of the CME for monomolecular reactions (Jahnke and Huisinga, 2007), when the system consists of multiple reaction channels and multiple species, it will be a diffi-cult task to solve it analytically. Therefore, moment based methods that approximate the solution of the CME by using its moments have been proposed. We refer to (Andreychenko et al., 2015) and the references therein for more details about the moment based methods. Let g: $\mathbb{N}^N \to \mathbb{R}^N$ be any function, then, the time evolution of the mean of $g(X(t))$, $\mathbb{E}\left[g(X(t))\right]$, satisfies the following equation:

$$\frac{d\mathbb{E}\left[g(X(t))\right]}{dt} = \sum_x g(x) \frac{d\mathbb{P}(X(t)=x)}{dt}$$

$$= \sum_{k=1}^{M} \mathbb{E}\left[a_k(X(t))\left(g(X(t)+v_k)-g(X(t))\right)\right],$$

which coincides with the adjoint or backward chemical master equation. We note that for $g(x) = x^n$, with n some multi-index, we obtain the n–th order moment of the probability distribution $\mathbb{P}$.

In case of having zero-th and first order reactions, the moment equations will be in the closed form, i.e., the moment equation for a certain order n will not depend on higher order moments. On the contrary, if the reaction system involves bimolecular reactions the moment equations will include higher-moments leading to an infinite hierarchy of moments equations that cannot be solved. To overcome this problem, moment closure technique that truncates the moments at a fixed order and approximates the higher order moments by using functions of lower moments is proposed in (Hespanha and Singh, 2005).

As mentioned before, if the amount of any species is represented by integers, the time evolution of the state is described by the RTCM given by Equation (10.6) and the time evolution of the corresponding probability distribution function is given by CME (10.13). In case of a diffusion approximation to this discrete-state stochastic process, the time evolution of the state is given by the CLE of Equation (10.9). Then, the time evolution of the corresponding probability distribution function satisfies Fokker Planck Equation (FPE), which can be obtained from the CME given by Equation (10.13). To construct the FPE from the CME, we define the shift operator L_k, $k = 1,2,\ldots, M$, of the form (Ullah and Wolkenhauer, 2011):

$$L_k a_k(x) = a_k(x+v_k).$$

Then, an alternative representation of CME (10.13) can be given as follows:

$$\frac{d\mathbb{P}(X(t)=x)}{dt} = \sum_{k=1}^{M} (L_k^{-1}-1)a_k(x)\mathbb{P}(X(t)=x). \tag{10.14}$$

The Taylor expansion of the inverse operator L_k^{-1} is

$$L_k^{-1} = \sum_{m=0}^{\infty} \frac{1}{m!}\left(-\sum_{i=1}^{N} v_{ki}\frac{\partial}{\partial x_i}\right)^m = 1 - \sum_{i=1}^{N} v_{ki}\frac{\partial}{\partial x_i} + \frac{1}{2}\sum_{i=1}^{N}\sum_{j=1}^{N} v_{ki}v_{kj}\frac{\partial^2}{\partial x_i \partial x_j} + \ldots.$$

By using the fact that propensity functions are smooth functions, we approximate L_k^{-1} in Equation (10.14) with its Taylor series expansion given above. Truncating the Taylor series expansion of L_k^{-1} after $m = 2$ and substituting it into Equation (10.14) gives the following FPE for the probability density function $p(x,t)$ defined by $\mathbb{P}(X(t)\in[x,x+dx]) = p(x,t)dx$:

$$\frac{\partial p(x,t)}{\partial t} = -\sum_{i=1}^{N} \frac{\partial}{\partial x_i}\left[\left(\sum_{k=1}^{M} v_{ki}a_k(x)\right)p(x,t)\right]$$

$$+\frac{1}{2}\sum_{i=1}^{N}\sum_{j=1}^{N} \frac{\partial^2}{\partial x_i \partial x_j}\left[\left(\sum_{k=1}^{M} v_{ki}v_{kj}a_k(x)\right)p(x,t)\right].$$

To simplify notation, we set $\Omega = 1$ into the above equation which results in $U(t) = X(t)$ and $\tilde{a}_k(U(t)) = a_k(X(t))$. Similar to the CME, it is hard to solve FPE analytically. Hence, numerical methods such as finite element and finite difference are used to obtain its approximate solutions (Pichler et al., 2013). When all propensity functions of the system are linear, then the first moment of the solutions of the CME and the FPE satisfies the corresponding ODE system obtained by the traditional deterministic approach given in Equation (10.10).

Another way of analyzing the dynamics of biochemical systems is to simulate their trajectories. Therefore, different algorithms that aim to find the realizations of the state vector of the system of interest have been proposed. Among these algorithms, the stochastic simulation algorithm (SSA) developed by Gillespie provides an exact sampling scheme. There are two versions of the SSA: the direct method and the first reaction method (Gillespie, 2007).

Due to the high computational costs of these simulation-based methods, more efficient versions of the SSA have been developed by several researchers (Cao et al., 2004, Gibson and Bruck, 2000, McCollum et al., 2006). The main downside of these proposed algorithms is still the great computation time required to simulate the system. In order to overcome this problem the τ-leaping method was proposed by (Gillespie, 2001), which is based on the idea that for a small fixed time increment τ the change in the propensities during $[t, t + \tau)$ is negligible and hence reaction counts within τ can be assumed to be Poisson distributed. Different versions of τ-leaping methods can be found in (Cao et al., 2005, Chatterjee et al., 2005).

Hybrid algorithms that combine deterministic and stochastic approaches are considered as an alternative to pure algorithms. Various types of hybrid models that partition the reactions into two or more subgroups such that the dynamical behavior of the species with high copy number of molecules can be modeled through a deterministic approach, while Markov chains are used to model the dynamics of species with low concentrations, as proposed in (Ganguly et al., 2015, Jahnke and Kreim, 2012).

10.5 MEASUREMENT PROCEDURES AND THE BAYESIAN PARADIGM

In Section 10.2, we gave an overview of single cell technologies that are used to demonstrate cellular differences experimentally, and in Section 10.3, we broke down the sources of the total variability into two components, namely, intrinsic and extrinsic noise. Additionally, in Section 10.4, we explained what kind of approximations exist to describe the dynamics of a given reaction system. In general, biological processes are poorly characterized in terms of parameters and states. That's why the mathematical models given in Section 10.4 involve hidden quantities. Therefore, inferring unknown states or reaction rates by using experimental data is an essential problem. The current section is devoted to explain the basics of Bayesian inference, which has a crucial importance for obtaining the unknown quantities by using all available data.

Depending on the data provided by the single cell technology, it is possible to separate the tools given in Section 10.2 into two categories: *distribution methods*, such as flow cytometry and sequencing, and *trajectory methods*, which mainly consist of fluorescence microscopy (see [Godfrey et al., 2005, Huang, 2009] and the references therein for detailed explanation of the measurement methods).

Flow cytometry is a tool that measures a specific feature, say ϕ, of a cell such as the abundance of a protein or a typical reaction's constant by providing snapshots of cell states from the entire cell population of interest. It produces a histogram that represents the distribution frequency of ϕ. If we observe a cell population consisting of K cells at L different time points, $t_1, t_2, \ldots, t_L$ the flow cytometry produces the data $D = (d_1^1, \ldots, d_1^K, \ldots, d_L^1, \ldots, d_L^K)$ where $d_l^k, k = 1, 2, \ldots, K$, $l = 1, 2, \ldots, L$ represents the measurement of the k-th unique cell at time point t_l. In the present chapter, this type of data is refereed as *distribution data*. In flow cytometry, we use a different cell population at each measurement time.

Fluorescence microscopy provides another type of data. Unlike flow cytometry, fluorescence microscopy measures temporal behavior of ϕ in a single cell by using time-lapsed records (Bronstein et al., 2015). The main drawback of this method is the provided number of measured cells compared with flow cytometry: this limitation leads to insufficient data for ensemble measurements. The data set produced with fluorescence microscopy can be represented by $D = (\mathbf{d}^1, \mathbf{d}^2, \ldots, \mathbf{d}^K)$ where $\mathbf{d}^k$, $k = 1, 2, \ldots, K$, is a vector whose l-th component shows the measurement for the k–th cell at time point t_l, $l = 1,2,...,L$. We refer to this type of data as *trajectory data*.

If we consider distribution data for a cell population consisting of K cells, the cell state has the form $\mathbf{X} = \left(x_1^1, x_1^2, ..., x_1^K, ..., x_L^1, x_L^2, ..., x_L^K \right)$, whose component, $x_l^k, k = 1,2,..., K$ and $l = 1,2,...,L$ corresponds to the state of the system for the k–th cell of the environment under consideration at discrete time point t_l. Similarly, for the trajectory data, we represent the state of the cell population by $\mathbf{X} = (\mathbf{x}^1, \mathbf{x}^2, ..., \mathbf{x}^K)$ where $\mathbf{x}^k, k = 1, 2, ...,K$, is the vector of the state obtained at different time points for the k–th cell.

Although there are various ways to estimate unknown quantities from a given data, the Bayesian inference can be considered as the most prominent approach (Boys et al., 2008, Bretthorst, 1990, Golightly and Wilkinson, 2005). Let's consider we have a finite set of unknowns (called hypotheses in [Wilkinson, 2006]) $\Theta_1, \Theta_2, ..., \Theta_S$ together with observed data set D. Bayesian inference aims to obtain the *posterior probability distribution* or *posterior* in short, $\mathbb{P}(\Theta_i | D)$, with the help of the probability function named as *prior probability distribution* or *prior* in short, $\mathbb{P}(\Theta_i)$, by using the following Bayes formula

$$\mathbb{P}(\Theta_i | D) = \frac{\mathbb{P}(D | \Theta_i) \mathbb{P}(\Theta_i)}{\displaystyle\sum_{j=1}^{S} \mathbb{P}(D | \Theta_j) \mathbb{P}(\Theta_j)}, i = 1,2,...,S. \tag{10.15}$$

Here, $\mathbb{P}(D | \Theta_i)$ is the *likelihood function*. It is considered as a function of Θ_i for the observed data D. Our prior information, obtained through mathematical models that describe the behavior of the system or previous experiments, is used to construct the prior distribution.

Since the summation in the bottom of Equation (10.15) is not a function of Θ_i, it can be considered as a constant. As a result, we obtain the relation

$$\mathbb{P}(\Theta_i | D) \propto \mathbb{P}(D | \Theta_i) \mathbb{P}(\Theta_i),$$

which says that "the posterior is proportional to prior times likelihood" (Wilkinson, 2006).

10.6 INFERENCE

Inferring unknown quantities such as intrinsic and extrinsic factors or hidden states is one of the most challenging problems in system biology. Naturally, depending on the provided data and the quantities that need to be estimated the posterior distribution will change. In the following sections, we aim to explain how we can construct the posterior for the trajectory and the distribution data and how these distributions can be used to infer the hidden quantities based on studies (Zechner et al., 2014, Zechner et al., 2012).

In Section 10.3, we mentioned that the extrinsic factors have an important role in cellular heterogeneity. In order to take into account the fact that extrinsic factors can fluctuate during the time scale of interest, we condition on the histories of them and represent it by $Z^{\mathcal{H}}$. In the following sections, we assume that we have a particular modulating environment such that $Z^{\mathcal{H}}$ is fixed as a random vector, i.e., $Z^{\mathcal{H}} = Z$, distributed according to a probability distribution $p(z | \alpha)$, where z denotes a realization of Z and α represents the extrinsic statistics which we assume to be identical across cells in the population of interest.

It is apparent that the presence of extrinsic factors increases the number of unknowns in a cell population. To avoid this complexity, the trajectories of the process can be marginalized over the extrinsic factors that differ from cell to cell, which in turn reduce the problem of inferring extrinsic factors into a problem of inferring extrinsic statistics that are the same through all cells in the environment under consideration. Therefore, in the following Sections 10.6.1 and 10.6.2, our goal is to construct posterior probability distributions after extrinsic factors of the process under consideration are marginalized out to estimate extrinsic statistics and intrinsic factors that are shared among the cells in the cell population of interest by using trajectory and distribution data based on the papers (Zechner et al., 2014, Zechner et al., 2012), respectively.

Based on the result given in Section 10.5, it is trivial that the computation of posterior has a close relation with the computation of likelihood functions. Modeling dynamics of reaction systems specifies the cost of the computation of the likelihood function. If we use CTMCs to model the dynamical behavior of the process, the likelihood function corresponds to the probability distribution whose time evolution is represented by CME. Similarly, if we use CLE to model the system, we must solve the corresponding FPE to obtain the likelihood function.

For the rest of the chapter, we consider a reaction system involving N species whose abundances at time $t \geq 0$ are denoted by $X(t) \in \mathbb{Z}_{\geq 0}^N$. The system consists M reactions $R_1, R_2, ..., R_M$ with corresponding reaction rates $C = \{C_k : k = 1, 2, ..., M\}$. We model the system by using CTMCs. Therefore, the time evolution of the corresponding probability distribution satisfies the CME given in Equation (10.13). The propensity function of the k–th reaction at state $X(t) = x$ is separated into two parts such that $a_k(x) = C_k g_k(x)$ where g_k is a function of x determined by the law of mass action.

10.6.1 INFERENCE FOR TRAJECTORY DATA

In this section, we will assume that we were given trajectory data obtained from the measurement of a cell population. Different algorithms are proposed to infer the hidden quantities of the process at interest such as reaction rates and states of the system in case of having this type of data. For example, in (Boys et al., 2008), the main steps of the Bayesian inference for estimating reaction rates of a process by using complete data, discrete data, and partially observed data are explained. In this study, the authors first considered an example in which we were given a complete data set over the time interval of interest. It is unrealistic to have such complete data, therefore, after explaining the main principles of the Bayesian inference for this perfect data scenario, different strategies are proposed to infer the hidden quantities of the process in case of having data observed at discrete time points and having partially observed data. We then complete the hidden parts of these incomplete paths by using a Markov chain Monte Carlo (MCMC) method based on reversible jump or block updating method. Then, kinetic rate constants can be inferred by using the complete path produced by MCMC methods.

In (Golightly and Wilkinson, 2011), the authors showed that particle methods can be very efficient to estimate the kinetic parameters of systems modeled by SDEs. An approximate Bayesian inference method based on the properties of the posterior distribution was proposed in (Beaumont et al., 2002). In (Hey et al., 2015), a stochastic switch model based on LNA or a new method called birth death approximation (BDA) was proposed to infer unknown quantities in an extended gene expression model. Another method that uses LNA to obtain the likelihood function was proposed in (Komorowski et al., 2010). In (Golightly et al., 2014), the authors presented a new MCMC algorithm that avoids the computation of the marginal likelihood by proposing an approximation to it, which uses approximate methods such as LNA or CLE. When the proposed approximation is accepted, sequential Monte Carlo (SMC) methods are used to estimate the marginal likelihood distribution of the original model.

In (Skilling et al., 2006), the authors proposed a new Bayesian method called *nested sampling* to obtain the evidence (marginal likelihood) by transforming the multidimensional integral of the likelihood function over unknown parameters to a one-dimensional integral over the unit interval. This method is used to estimate unknown parameters of biological processes and to make a comparison between the models that fit for the available data.

Finally, in (Zechner et al., 2014), the authors proposed a new method to infer the unknown molecular states and the reaction rates in the presence of a trajectory data for a heterogeneous cell population. The method separates reaction rates into two subgroups: the first group involves the reaction rates that are identical for all cells and called intrinsic factors, while the second group includes the reaction rates that change from cell to cell and leads extrinsic noise. Based on marginalization of the extrinsic factors, a new marginal process is obtained. The posterior distribution of this new process is used to estimate the unknown quantities that are identical across the cells. The details of the method will be explained in the rest of this section.

First, we will discuss how we can infer the unknown reaction rates of the biochemical process whose general properties are given above when the complete path of the process is given, then we extend concepts that are used to infer reaction rates of a complete path in a single cell to estimate unknown quantities in a heterogeneous cell population.

For the rest of the section, $\mathbf{x}_{[a,b]}$ represents the complete path in between a and b, i.e., $\mathbf{x}_{[a,b]} = \{X(t) : t \in [a, b]\}$ and $\mathbf{x} \equiv \mathbf{x}_{[0,T]}$. Consider that biochemical reaction system of interest is observed in the time interval $[0, T]$ and we have the complete path $\mathbf{x}$. Let us define a vector $\rho = (\rho_1, \rho_2,..., \rho_M)$ where ρ_j represents the number of firings of the j–th reaction channel in $[0, T]$. Total number of reactions fired in the interval under consideration is represented by $n = \sum_{j=1}^{M} \rho_j$ The index of the reaction fired at time t_j, $j = 1, 2,...,n$, is represented by η_j and $t_0 = 0, t_{n+1} = T$.

Based on the fact that Gillespie's SSAs are exact algorithms, given complete paths can be considered as trajectories obtained by the direct method. Therefore, the likelihood function of the system can be represented by the joint probability distribution of random variables η_j and t_j as follows:

$$\mathbb{P}(\mathbf{x}|C) = \left(\prod_{j=1}^{n} a_{\eta_j}(X(t_{j-1})) \exp\left(-a_0(X(t_{j-1}))[t_j - t_{j-1}]\right) \right) \exp\left(-a_0(X(t_n))[T - t_n]\right)$$

$$= \prod_{j=1}^{n} a_{\eta_j}(X(t_{j-1})) \exp\left(\sum_{j=1}^{n+1} -a_0(X(t_{j-1}))[t_j - t_{j-1}] \right).$$

By using the fact that $a_0(x)$ is a piece-wise constant function, we can represent the likelihood function of the system in the following form:

$$\mathbb{P}(\mathbf{x}|C) = \prod_{j=1}^{n} C_{\eta_j} g_{\eta_j}(X(t_{j-1})) \exp\left(-\int_0^T a_0(X(s))ds \right)$$

$$\propto \prod_{j=1}^{M} C_j^{\rho_j} \exp\left(-\int_0^T C_j g_j(X(s))ds \right) \tag{10.16}$$

$$= \prod_{j=1}^{M} \mathbb{P}^j(\mathbf{x}|C_j),$$

where $\mathbb{P}^j(\mathbf{x}|C_j) = C_j^{\rho_j} \exp\left(-\int_0^T C_j g_j(X(s))ds \right)$. According to the Bayesian inference, C's are distributed according to a prior distribution $\mathbb{P}(C)$. If we choose C_j's from independent Gamma distributions such that $Cj \sim \Gamma(a_j, b_j)$ where $\Gamma(a_j, b_j)$ denotes the Gamma distribution with parameters a_j, b_j, then, the prior distribution takes the form $\mathbb{P}(C) = \prod_{j=1}^{M} \Gamma(a_j, b_j)$. Consequently, we have the likelihood function and the prior, so we obtain the posterior as follows (Wilkinson, 2006):

$$\mathbb{P}(C|\mathbf{x}) = \prod_{j=1}^{M} \Gamma\left(a_j + \rho_j, b_j + \int_0^T g_j(X(s))ds \right).$$

We will call ρ_j and $\beta_j = \int_0^T g_j(X(s))ds, j = 1, 2,...,M$, as sufficient statistics for inferring rate constants of the system under consideration for given complete path $\mathbf{x}$.

Heterogeneous Cell Populations

Now, we will consider a cell population consisting of K cells. Naturally, each individual cell in the population has a different extrinsic environment. Therefore, even if we are observing the same particular process in each cell, we must take into account the fact that dynamics of the process will be different for each cell. In this section, we define the effect of extrinsic factors by using the reaction rates that vary from cell to cell. Therefore, we separate the reaction rates into two subgroups such that $S = \{S_i : i = 1,2,...,I\}$ which are identical for all cells and called intrinsic factors and a second group $Z = \{Z_j : j = 1, 2,..., J\}$ called extrinsic factors. Then, we redefine the rate constants $C = (Z_1, Z_2,..., Z_J, S_1, S_2,..., S_I)$ such that $M = J + I$. As a result, propensity functions at state x take the form $a_j(x) = Z_j g_j(x), j = 1, 2,..., J$ and $a_k(x) = S_i g_k(x), i = 1, 2,...,I, k = i + J$.

As discussed before, the extrinsic factors Z are distributed according to the probability distribution $\mathbb{P}(z|\alpha)$. We assume that intrinsic factors and extrinsic statistics are independent from each other, i.e., $\mathbb{P}(S,\alpha) = \mathbb{P}(S)\mathbb{P}(\alpha)$.

Marginalization of extrinsic factors will give a conditional process $X|(S,\alpha)$ which is independent from the extrinsic factors. Now the goal of the inference problem is just to estimate intrinsic factors and extrinsic statics which are shared among the cells. This can be achieved by the theorem innovatied in (Aalen, 1978).

To construct the marginal process $X|(S,\alpha)$, we must redefine the propensity functions by using marginalized extrinsic factors. For the details of the marginalized processes, we refer (Zechner et al., 2014, Zechner and Koeppl, 2014) and the references therein.

Theorem 10.1

The marginal propensity for the j–th, $j = 1,2,...,J$, reaction is

$$a_j(\mathbf{x}_{[0,t]},t) = \mathbb{E}[Z_j | \mathbf{x}_{[0,t]},\alpha] g_j(X(t)), \tag{10.17}$$

where $\mathbb{E}[Z_j | \mathbf{x}_{[0,t]},\alpha]$ represents the conditional mean of Z_j given a complete sample path $\mathbf{x}_{[0,t]}$. The other propensities remain unchanged, i.e., $a_k(x) = S_i g_k(x), i = 1, 2,...,I, k = i + J$.

The conditional mean of the extrinsic factors is defined as follows:

$$\mathbb{E}[Z_j | \mathbf{x}_{[0,t]},\alpha] = \int_{\mathcal{Z}^J} z_j \frac{\mathbb{P}(\mathbf{x}_{[0,t]}|z)\mathbb{P}(z|\alpha)}{\mathbb{P}(\mathbf{x}_{[0,t]}|\alpha)} dz_j,$$

where $\mathcal{Z}^J$ is the support of random variable Z_j and z_j is a realization of Z_j. Then, the marginal propensity function has the form:

$$a_j(\mathbf{x}_{[0,t]},t) = \frac{\mathbb{E}[z_j \mathbb{P}(\mathbf{x}_{[0,t]}|z)|\alpha]}{\mathbb{E}[\mathbb{P}(\mathbf{x}_{[0,t]}|z)|\alpha]} g_j(X(t)).$$

Together with Equation (10.16), this expression can be represented by Laplace transformations as follows:

$$a_j(\mathbf{x}_{[0,t]},t) = -\frac{\mathcal{L}^{\rho_1 \cdots \rho_j+1,\cdots \rho_J}(\beta)}{\mathcal{L}^{\rho_1 \cdots \rho_J}(\beta)} g_j(X(t)),$$

with $\beta = (\beta_1,...,\beta_J) = \left(\int_0^t g_1(X(s))ds, \int_0^t g_2(X(s))ds,..., \int_0^t g_J(X(s))ds\right)$ where ρ_j represents the number of occurrences of the j–th reaction in the time interval of interest while $\mathcal{L}^{\rho_1 \cdots \rho_J}(\beta)$ denotes the partial derivatives of the Laplace transform $\mathcal{L}$ with respect to $\beta_1,..., \beta_J$ taken $\rho_1,..., \rho_J$ times, respectively.

This kind of marginalization makes it possible to involve cell-to-cell variability in the inference problem. Also, marginalizing the extrinsic factors and just being interested in inferring the extrinsic statistics decreases the complexity of the problem. In (Zechner et al., 2014), the authors proposed a method called dynamic prior propagation (DPP) that combines the marginal process with sequential Monte Carlo (SMC) methods to infer the unknown quantities of a particular process from trajectory data. For small systems, posterior distributions over latent states can also be obtained through the respective conditional master equation (Huang et al., 2016).

Assume that we have trajectory data obtained from a heterogeneous cell population involving K cells. We want to estimate the unknown cell states between observation times in time interval $[0, T]$, intrinsic factors S, and extrinsic statistics α. Then, the posterior distribution has the form:

$$\mathbb{P}\left(\mathbf{x}^1, \mathbf{x}^2, \ldots, \mathbf{x}^K, S, \alpha \middle| \mathbf{d}^1, \mathbf{d}^2, \ldots, \mathbf{d}^K\right) \propto \left[\prod_{k=1}^K \prod_{l=1}^L \mathbb{P}\left(\mathbf{d}_l^k \middle| \mathbf{x}_{[t_l, t_l]}^k\right)\right] \mathbb{P}\left(\mathbf{x}^1, \mathbf{x}^2, \ldots, \mathbf{x}^K \middle| S, \alpha\right) \mathbb{P}(S) \mathbb{P}(\alpha),$$

where $\mathbf{x}_{[a,b]}^k, k = 1, 2, \ldots, K$, represents the complete path for the k–th cell in the time interval $[a, b]$ and $\mathbf{x}^k \equiv \mathbf{x}_{[0,T]}^k$. Since the conditional probability of each path given the intrinsic and extrinsic factors are independent from each other, this factorization can be done. Sampling from this posterior distribution is not an easy task, therefore, the authors propose using a recursive Bayesian inference that makes it possible to construct the posterior distribution at a given observation point, t_l, by using the posterior distribution given at the previous step t_{l-1}, as follows:

$$\mathbb{P}\left(\mathbf{x}_{[0,t_l]}^1, \mathbf{x}_{[0,t_l]}^2, \ldots, \mathbf{x}_{[0,t_l]}^K, S, \alpha \middle| \mathbf{d}^1, \mathbf{d}^2, \ldots, \mathbf{d}^K\right)$$

$$\propto \left[\prod_{k=l}^K \mathbb{P}\left(\mathbf{d}_l^k \middle| \mathbf{x}_{[t_l, t_l]}^k\right) \mathbb{P}\left(\mathbf{x}_{[t_{l-1}, t_l]}^k \middle| \mathbf{x}_{[0,t_{l-1}]}^k, S, \alpha\right)\right] \mathbb{P}\left(\mathbf{x}_{[0,t_{l-1}]}^1, \mathbf{x}_{[0,t_{l-1}]}^2, \ldots, \mathbf{x}_{[0,t_{l-1}]}^K, S, \alpha \middle| \tilde{\mathbf{d}}^1, \tilde{\mathbf{d}}^2, \ldots, \tilde{\mathbf{d}}^K\right)$$

$$= \left[\prod_{k=1}^K \mathbb{P}\left(\mathbf{d}_l^k \middle| \mathbf{x}_{[t_l, t_l]}^k\right) \mathbb{P}\left(\mathbf{x}_{[t_{l-1}, t_l]}^k \middle| \mathbf{x}_{[t_{l-1}, t_{l-1}]}^k, \beta_{l-1}^k, \rho_{l-1}^k, S, \alpha\right)\right] \mathbb{P}\left(\mathbf{x}_{[0,t_{l-1}]}^1, \mathbf{x}_{[0,t_{l-1}]}^2, \ldots, \mathbf{x}_{[0,t_{l-1}]}^K, S, \alpha \middle| \tilde{\mathbf{d}}^1, \tilde{\mathbf{d}}^2, \ldots, \tilde{\mathbf{d}}^K\right)$$
$$\tag{10.18}$$

where $\tilde{\mathbf{d}}^k$ is a vector whose s–th component $\tilde{\mathbf{d}}_s^k$ denotes the measurement for the k–th cell at time points t_s, $s = 1, 2, \ldots, l - 1$ and $\rho_{l-1}^k, \beta_{l-1}^k$ represents the sufficient statistics calculated by using the path $\mathbf{x}_{[0,t_{l-1}]}^k$. The second line in Equation (10.18) is just a general decomposition that is always possible. Although the original model is Markovian, the marginalized model is not Markovian. That is why, instead of conditioning on the current state of the given path, we condition on the whole history of the path, i.e., $\mathbb{P}\left(\mathbf{x}_{[t_{l-1}, t_l]}^k \middle| \mathbf{x}_{[0,t_{l-1}]}^k, S, \alpha\right)$. Using sufficient statistics we can condition on the current state of the system, which produces the third line. We refer to (Bronstein et al., 2015, Zechner et al., 2014) for the details and applications of the method explained in the current section.

10.6.2 INFERENCE FOR DISTRIBUTION DATA

In this section, we will explain how the distribution data can be used to infer unknown quantities based on the study (Zechner et al., 2012). It is well-known that estimating the hidden parameters of a cell population involving large number of cells measured by distribution methods requires solving high dimensional CME or FPE that correspond to the time derivative of the probability distribution function of the state vector that are represented by RTCM or CLE, respectively. To avoid this curse of dimensionality, various methods have been proposed to estimate hidden quantities of a cell population from the distribution data.

For example, in (Hasenauer et al., 2011b), the authors presented a method that models the dynamics of each cell in the cell population by using SDEs. Intrinsic noise is represented by Wiener processes, while extrinsic noise is considered as the result of differences in parameter values and the initial conditions through the cells. Properties of the extrinsic noise and the SDE modeling are used to construct a partial differential equation (PDE) corresponding to the time evolution of the population density, which is a joint probability distribution of parameters leading to extrinsic noise and the state variables. The probability distribution of the measured output and the population density is approximated by kernel density estimators. Then, L_2 norm of the differences between these two distributions is minimized to infer unknown reaction rates. In (Hasenauer et al., 2011a), the authors proposed a new inference method that can be used to estimate the parameters of a heterogeneous cell population from the provided sparse and noisy data. Differently than (Hasenauer et al., 2011b), (Hasenauer et al., 2011a) uses ODEs to describe the dynamics of each single cell in the environment of interest, and, similar to (Hasenauer et al., 2011b), cell-to-cell variability is considered as the result of differences in parameters distributed according to a parameter density function. The method is based on parametrization of the parameter density that produces a parametrized posterior distribution whose samples are obtained by the Metropolis Hastings algorithm (MHA). In (Munsky et al., 2009), the authors used CTMCs to model the gene expression model. One norm difference between the measured distribution and the solution of the corresponding CME is obtained as a function of unknown parameters, and the parameter values that minimize this function are considered the optimal parameter set. In (Neuert et al., 2013), single cell experiments and CTMC models were combined to find the best model to describe the dynamics of the osmotic stress response in a yeast.

In (Zechner et al., 2012), the authors proposed a moment-based method that estimates S, α values, which were described in the previous section. We devote the rest of this section to explaining this method. Although extrinsic factors Z were considered as a subgroup of reaction rates in the previous section, they are random variables in the current section that represent a constant extrinsic component. If we consider a cell population involving K cells, the posterior distribution that is used to estimate extrinsic statistics and intrinsic factors is as follows:

$$\mathbb{P}\left(S,\alpha\middle|d_1^1,d_1^2,...,d_1^K,...,d_L^1,d_L^2,...,d_L^K\right). \tag{10.19}$$

When the number of cells in the environment under consideration increases, it becomes difficult to analyze the given posterior distribution. To avoid this disadvantage, in (Zechner et al., 2012), the authors proposed a moment-based inference method that uses moment closure method to obtain a system of equations of lower moments.

As mentioned previously, the stochastic process of interest is modeled by CTMCs, therefore, the probability distribution of the state vector of the system satisfies the corresponding CME whose moments can be approximated by the moment closure techniques (Hespanha and Singh, 2005). Time derivative of the approximate moments of the CME for each single cell depends on the extrinsic factors, which are different for each cell, and the intrinsic factors, which are identical for all cells. Due to the differences in extrinsic factors between cells, naturally, we will obtain different differential equations. To obtain the moments of cell population, we must average approximate moments of CMEs for each cell, which requires a high computational cost. In (Zechner et al., 2012), the authors obtained the time derivative of the population-moments by marginalizing the time derivative of moments with respect to extrinsic variable Z. Then, the obtained moment equations are closed by replacing the higher order moments, say E, by functions of the moments with lower order than E. As a result, the following system of equations for the approximate population moments is obtained:

$$\frac{d\tilde{\mu}}{dt} = A(S)\tilde{\mu} + B(S)\tilde{\mu}_{x,z} + D(S)\alpha + F(S)g(\tilde{\mu},\tilde{\mu}_{X,Z},\alpha)$$
$$\frac{d\tilde{\mu}_{X,Z}}{dt} = H(S)\tilde{\mu}_{X,Z} + R(S)\alpha + T(S)h(\tilde{\mu},\tilde{\mu}_{X,Z},\alpha), \tag{10.20}$$

where $\tilde{\mu}$ represents the moments of species up to order E and $\tilde{\mu}_{X,Z}$ involves the cross moments of species and the extrinsic statistics given up to order E. $A(S)$, $B(S)$, $D(S)$, $F(S)$, $H(S)$, $R(S)$, $T(S)$ are functions of intrinsic parameters shared among the cells, and g and h are functions obtained by the moment closure techniques.

The method proposes using the following posterior instead of the posterior distribution given in Equation (10.19):

$$\mathbb{P}\left(S,\alpha\big|\hat{\mu}_1^1,\ldots,\hat{\mu}_1^E,\ldots,\hat{\mu}_L^1,\ldots,\hat{\mu}_L^E\right), \tag{10.21}$$

where $\hat{\mu}_l^e$ represents the empirical moment of order E at time point t_l. To simplify the notation, let's define a vector: $\hat{\mu}^e = \left\{\hat{\mu}_l^e : l = 1,2,\ldots,L\right\}, e = 1,2,\ldots,E$.

Since each cell is measured at different time points and different data sets are used to obtain moment estimates for each order, the posterior distribution is given by:

$$\mathbb{P}(S,\alpha\big|\hat{\mu}^1,\hat{\mu}^2,\ldots,\hat{\mu}^E) \propto \prod_{l=1}^{L}\prod_{e=1}^{E}\mathbb{P}\left(\hat{\mu}_l^e\big|S,\alpha\right)\mathbb{P}(S,\alpha).$$

For the purpose of cleaner representation, let's consider only a single species is measured; the extension to more than one species is straightforward. The E–th order empirical moments at time point t_l satisfies the following equation

$$\hat{\mu}_l^e = \begin{cases} \dfrac{1}{K}\sum_{k=1}^{K}x_l^k, & e=1, \\[3mm] \dfrac{1}{K}\sum_{k=1}^{K}\left(x_l^k - \hat{\mu}_l^1\right)^e, & e=2,3,\ldots,E. \end{cases}$$

When we have a large system, the central moment theorem says that the experimental moments are normally distributed, i.e., $\hat{\mu}_l^e \sim \mathcal{N}\left(\mu_l^e,(\tilde{\sigma}_l^e)^2\right)$ where μ_l^e represents the exact e–th moment at time point t_l and its corresponding variances are denoted by $\left(\sigma_l^e\right)^2$. Here, it must be noted that $\mu_l^e,\left(\sigma_l^e\right)^2$ is approximated by Equation (10.20). Then, the posterior distribution is proportional to:

$$\mathbb{P}(S,\alpha\big|D) \propto \mathbb{P}(S)\mathbb{P}(\alpha)\prod_{l=1}^{L}\left\{\frac{1}{\sqrt{2\pi|\mathcal{A}|}}\exp\left\{\frac{-1}{2}\left(\gamma_l^1 - \hat{\gamma}_l^1\right)^T\mathcal{A}^{-1}\left(\gamma_l^1 - \hat{\gamma}_l^1\right)\right\}\right\}, \tag{10.22}$$

where $\mathcal{A}$ represents the covariance matrix whose components are computed by Equation (10.20) while $\gamma_l^1 = \left(\mu_l^1,\left(\sigma_l^1\right)^2\right), \hat{\gamma}_l^1 = \left(\hat{\mu}_l^1,\left(\hat{\sigma}_l^1\right)^2\right)$ (Bronstein et al., 2015). More complicated priors than the independence prior, $\mathbb{P}(S,\alpha) = \mathbb{P}(S)\mathbb{P}(\alpha)$, assumed here can be used if respective prior information is available.

At this point, we can use MHA to sample from the posterior distribution. Since MHA plays an important role in this chapter, we will provide a brief summary. Suppose we want to draw samples θ from the target probability distribution $p(\theta)$, MHA generates samples by using a proposed probability distribution $q(\theta)$ and accepts or rejects these samples by using the following algorithm:

(1) Set $j = 1$ and sample $\theta^0 \sim q(\theta)$.
(2) Generate a candidate sample $\theta_{cand}^j \sim q\left(\theta_{cand}^j\big|\theta^{j-1}\right)$.
(3) Compute the *acceptance probability*

$$\beta\left(\theta_{cand}^j\big|\theta^{j-1}\right) = \min\left\{1,\frac{q\left(\theta^{j-1}\big|\theta_{cand}^j\right)p\left(\theta_{cand}^j\right)}{q\left(\theta_{cand}^j\big|\theta^{j-1}\right)p\left(\theta^{j-1}\right)}\right\}.$$

(4) Accept the candidate sample and set $\theta^j = \theta^j_{cand}$ with probability $\beta\left(\theta^j_{cand}\big|\theta^{j-1}\right)$ or reject it with probability $1 - \beta\left(\theta^j_{cand}\big|\theta^{j-1}\right)$ and set $\theta^j = \theta^{j-1}$

(5) Set $j = j + 1$ and go to step (2).

In our model, we want to infer S and α values which means that $\theta = (S,\alpha)$. Our target distribution is the posterior, so $p(S,\alpha) = \mathbb{P}\left(S,\alpha\big|\hat{\mu}^1, \hat{\mu}^2, \ldots, \hat{\mu}^E\right)$. Finally, we can use the prior distribution as a proposal distribution $q(S,\alpha) = \mathbb{P}(S,\alpha)$. Applications of the method can be found in (Bronstein et al., 2015, Zechner et al., 2012).

ACKNOWLEDGMENTS

Derya Altıntan acknowledges support from the Scientific and Technological Research Council of Turkey (TÜBİTAK), Program no: 3501 Grant no. 115E252.

REFERENCES

Aalen, O. (1978). Nonparametric inference for a family of counting processes. *Ann. Statist. 6*, 701-726.

Agresti, J.J., Antipov, E., Abate, A.R., Ahn, K., Rowat, A.C., Baret, J.C., Marquez, M., Klibanov, A.M., Griffiths, A.D., and Weitz, D.A. (2010). Ultra high-throughput screening in drop-based microfluidics for directed evolution. *PNAS 107*, 4004-4009.

Altschuler, S.J., and Wu, L.F. (2010). Cellular heterogeneity: Do differences make a difference? *Cell 141*, 559-563.

Anderson, D.F. and Kurtz, T.G. (2011). Continuous time Markov chain models for chemical reaction networks. In H. Koeppl, G. Setti, M.D. Bernardo, and D. Densmore (Eds.), *Design and Analysis of Biomolecular Circuits.* Springer-Verlag.

Andreychenko, A., Mikeev, L., and Wolf, V. (2015). Model reconstruction for moment-based stochastic chemical kinetics. *ACM Trans. Model. Comput. Simul. 25.*

Beaumont, M.A., Zhang, W., and Balding, D.J. (2002). Approximate Bayesian computation in population genetics. *Genetics 162*, 2025-2035.

Bouchard, T.J., Lykken, D.T., McGue, M., Segal, N.L., and Tellegen, A. (1990). Sources of human psychological differences: The Minnesota study of twins reared apart. *Science 250*, 223-228.

Bowsher, C.G. and Swain, P.S. (2012). Identifying sources of variation and the flow of information in biochemical networks. *PNAS 109*, E1320-E1328.

Boys, R.J., Wilkinson, D.J., and Kirkwood, T. (2008). Bayesian inference for a discretely observed stochastic kinetic model. *Statistics and Computing 18*,125-135.

Bretthorst, G.L. (1990). *Maximum Entropy and Bayesian Methods* (53-79). Springer Netherlands.

Bronstein, L., Zechner, C., and Koeppl, H. (2015). Bayesian inference of reaction kinetics from single-cell recordings across a heterogeneous cell population. *Methods 85*, 22-35.

Cao, Y., Gillespie, D.T., and Petzold, L.R. (2005). Avoiding negative populations in explicit Poisson tau-leaping. *J. Chem. Phys. 123*, 054104.

Cao, Y., Li, H., and Petzold, L.R. (2004). Efficient formulation of the stochastic simulation algorithm for chemically reacting system. *J. Chem. Phys. 121*, 4059-4067.

Chatterjee, A., Vlachos, D.G., and Katsoulakis, M.A. (2005). Binomial distribution based tau-leap accelerated stochastic simulation. *J. Chem. Phys. 122*, 024112.

Crane, M.M., Clark, I.B.N., Bakker, E., Smith, S., and Swain, P.S. (2014). A microfluidic system for studying ageing and dynamic single-cell responses in budding yeast. *PloS one 9*, e100042.

de Vargas Roditi, L., and Claassen, M. (2015). Computational and experimental single cell biology techniques for the definition of cell type heterogeneity, interplay and intracellular dynamics. *Curr. Opin. Biotechnol. 34*, 9-15.

Eberwine, J., Sul, J.Y., Bartfai, T., and Kim, J. (2013). The promise of single-cell sequencing. *Nat. Methods 11*, 25-27.

Fulwyler, M.J. (1965). Electronic separation of biological cells by volume. *Science 150*, 910-911.

Ganguly, A., Altıntan, D., and Koeppl, H. (2015). Jump-diffusion approximation of stochastic reaction dynamics: Error bounds and algorithms. *Multiscale Model Simul. 13*, 1390-1419.

Gibson, M.A. and Bruck, J. (2000). Efficient exact stochastic simulation of chemical systems with many species and many channels. *J. Chem. Phys. A 104*, 1876-1889.

Gillespie, D.T. (1992). A rigorous derivation of the chemical master equation. *Physica A 188*, 404-425.

Gillespie, D.T. (2000). The chemical Langevin equation. *J. Chem. Phys. 113*, 297-306.

Gillespie, D.T. (2001). Approximate accelerated stochastic simulation of chemically reacting systems. *J. Chem. Phys. 115*, 1716-1733.

Gillespie, D.T. (2007). Stochastic simulation of chemical kinetics. *Annu. Rev. Phys. Chem. 58*, 35-55.

Godfrey, W.L., Hill, D.M., Kilgore, J.A., Buller, G.M., Bradford, J.A., Gray, D.R., Clements, I., Oakleaf, K.D., Salisbury, J.J., Ignatius, M.J., and Janes, M.S. (2005). Complementarity of flow cytometry and fluorescence microscopy. *Microsc. Microanal. 11*, 246-247.

Golightly, A., Henderson, D.A., and Sherlock, C. (2014). Delayed acceptance particle MCMC for exact inference in stochastic kinetic models. *Statistics and Computing 25*, 1039-1055.

Golightly, A., and Wilkinson, D.J. (2005). Bayesian inference for stochastic kinetic models using a diffusion approximation. *Biometrics 61*, 781-788.

Golightly, A. and Wilkinson, D.J. (2011). Bayesian parameter inference for stochastic biochemical network models using particle Markov chain Monte Carlo. *Interface Focus 1*, 807-820.

Hasenauer, J., Waldherr, S., Doszczak, M., Radde, N., Scheurich, P., and Allgöwer, F. (2011a). Identification of models of heterogeneous cell populations from population snapshot data. *BMC Bioinformatics 12*, 125.

Hasenauer, J., Waldherr, S., Doszczak, M., Scheurich, P., Radde, N., and Allgöwer, F. (2011b). Analysis of heterogeneous cell populations: A density-based modeling and identification framework. *J Process Control 21*, 1417-1425.

Heinemann, M., and Zenobi, R. (2011). Single cell metabolomics. *Curr. Opin. Biotechnol. 22*, 26-31.

Hespanha, J.P., and Singh, A. (2005). Stochastic models for chemically reacting systems using polynomial stochastic hybrid systems. *Int. J. Robust Nonlinear Control 15*, 669-689.

Hess, S.T., Girirajan, T.P.K., and Mason, M.D. (2006). Ultra-high resolution imaging by fluorescence photoactivation localization microscopy. *Biophys. J. 91*, 4258-4272.

Hey, K.L., Momiji, H., Featherstone, K., Davis, J.R.E., White, M.R.H., Rand, D.A., and Finkenstädt, B. (2015). A stochastic transcriptional switch model for single cell imaging data. *Biostatistics 655-669*.

Hilfinger, A., and Paulsson, J. (2011). Separating intrinsic from extrinsic fluctuations in dynamic biological systems. *PNAS 108*, 12167-12172.

Hu, H., Eustace, D., and Merten, C.A. (2015). Efficient cell pairing in droplets using dual-color sorting. *Lab On a Chip 15*, 3989-3993.

Huang, L., Pauleve, L., Zechner, C., Unger, M., Hansen, A.S., and Koeppl, H. (2016). Reconstructing dynamic molecular states from single-cell time series. *J Roy Soc Interface 13*, 20160533.

Huang, S. (2009). Non-genetic heterogeneity of cells in development: More than just noise. *Development 136*, 3853-3862.

Jahnke, T., and Huisinga, W. (2007). Solving the chemical master equation for monomolecular reaction systems analytically. *J Math Biol 54*, 1-26.

Jahnke, T., and Kreim, M. (2012). Error bound for piecewise deterministic process modelling stochastic reaction systems. *Multiscale Model Simul 10*, 1119-1147.

Jo, M.C., Liu, W., Gu, L., Dang, W., and Qin, L. (2015). High-throughput analysis of yeast replicative aging using a microfluidic system. *Proc Natl Acad Sci U S A 112*, 9364-9369.

van Kampen, N.G. (1981). *Stochastic processes in physics and chemistry*. Elsevier North-Holland.

Klar, T.A. and Hell, S.W. (1999). Subdiffraction resolution in far-field fluorescence microscopy. *Opt. Lett. 24*, 954.

Kling, J. (2015). Cytometry: Measure for measure. *Nature 518*, 439-443.

Klipp, E., Liebermeister, W., Wierling, C., Kowald, A., Lehrach, H., and Herwig, R. (2009). *Systems Biology: A Textbook*. WILEY - VCH Verlag GmbH & Co. KGaA.

Kolodziejczyk, A.A., Kim, J.K., Svensson, V., Marioni, J.C., and Teichmann, S.A. (2015). The Technology and Biology of Single-Cell RNA Sequencing. *Mol. Cell 58*, 610-620.

Komorowski, M., Finkenstädt, B., and Rand, D. (2010). Using a single fluorescent reporter gene to infer half-life of extrinsic noise and other parameters of gene expression. *Biophys J. 98*, 2759-2769.

Lun, X.-K., Zanotelli, V.R.T., Wade, J.D., Schapiro, D., Tognetti, M., Dobberstein, N., and Bodenmiller, B. (2017). Influence of node abundance on signaling network state and dynamics analyzed by mass cytometry. *Nat. Biotech. 35*, 164-172.

McCollum, J.M., Peterson, G.D., Cox, C.D., Simpson, M.L., and Samatova, N.F. (2006). The sorting direct method for stochastic simulation of biochemical systems with varying reaction execution behavior. *Comput. Biol. Chem. 30*, 39-49.

Munsky, B., Trinh, B., and Khammash, M. (2009). Listening to the noise: random fluctuations reveal gene network parameters. *Mol. Syst. Biol. 5*, 318.

Nachman, I., Regev, A., and Ramanathan, S. (2007). Dissecting timing variability in yeast meiosis. *Cell 131*, 544-556.

Navin, N., Kendall, J., Troge, J., Andrews, P., Rodgers, L., McIndoo, J., Cook, K., Stepansky, A., Levy, D., Esposito, D., Muthuswamy, L., Krasnitz, A., McCombie, W.R., Hicks, J., and Wigler, M.S. (2011). Tumour evolution inferred by single-cell sequencing. *Nature 472*, 90-94.

Nawy, T. (2013). Single-cell sequencing. *Nat. Methods 11*, 18.

Neuert, G., Munsky, B., Tan, R.Z., Teytelman, L., Khammash, M., and van Oudenaarden, A. (2013). Systematic identification of signal-activated stochastic gene regulation. *Science 339*, 584-587.

Niepel, M., Hafner, M., Pace, E.A., Chung, M., Chai, D.H., Zhou, L., Muhlich, J.L., Schoeberl, B., and Sorger, P.K. (2014). Analysis of growth factor signaling in genetically diverse breast cancer lines. *BMC Biology 12*, 20.

Niepel, M., Spencer, S.L., and Sorger, P.K. (2009). Non-genetic cell-to-cell variability and the consequences for pharmacology. *Curr Opin Biotechnol 13*, 556-561.

Onjiko, R.M., Moody, S.A., and Nemes, P. (2015). Single-cell mass spectrometry reveals small molecules that affect cell fates in the 16-cell embryo. *PNAS 112*, 6545-6550.

Ornatsky, O., Bandura, D., Baranov, V., Nitz, M., Winnik, M.A., and Tanner, S. (2010). Highly multiparametric analysis by mass cytometry. *J. Immunol. Methods 361*, 1-20.

Pepperkok, R. and Ellenberg, J. (2006). High-throughput fluorescence microscopy for systems biology. *Nat. Rev. Mol. Cell Biol. 7*, 690-696.

Pichler, L., Masud, A., and Bergman, L.A. (2013). Numerical solution of the Fokker-Planck equation by finite difference and finite element methods – A comparative study. In M. Papadrakakis, G. Stefanou, and V. Papadopoulos (Eds.), *Computational Methods in Stochastic Dynamics*, Computational Methods in Applied Sciences (69-85). Springer Netherlands.

Pollen, A.A., Nowakowski, T.J., Shuga, J., Wang, X., Leyrat, A.A., Lui, J.H., Li, N., Szpankowski, L., Fowler, B., Chen, P., Ramalingam, N., Sun, G., Thu, M., Norris, M., Lebofsky, R., Toppani, D., Kemp, D.W., Wong, M., Clerkson, B., Jones, B.N., Wu, S., Knutsson, L., Alvarado, B., Wang, J., Weaver, L.S., May, A.P., Jones, R.C., Unger, M.A., Kriegstein, A.R., and West, J.A.A. (2014). Low-coverage single-cell mRNA sequencing reveals cellular heterogeneity and activated signaling pathways in developing cerebral cortex. *Nature Biotechnol 32*, 1053-1058.

Satija, R. and Shalek, A.K. (2014). Heterogeneity in immune responses: From populations to single cells. *Trends Immunol. 35*, 219-229.

Schoeberl, B., Harms, B., Gibbons, F., Fitzgerald, J., Onsum, M., Nielsen, U., and Kubasek, W. (2014). Methods and systems for predicting response of cells to a therapeutic agent. U.S. Patent 8,623,592.

Shi, Q., Qin, L., Wei, W., Geng, F., Fan, R., Shin, Y.S., Guo, D., Hood, L., Mischel, P.S., and Heath, J.R. (2012). Single-cell proteomic chip for profiling intracellular signaling pathways in single tumor cells. *Proc Natl Acad Sci U S A 109*, 419-424.

Skilling, J. et al. (2006). Nested sampling for general Bayesian computation. *Bayesian Analysis 1*, 833-859.

Snijder, B.L. and Pelkmans, L. (2011). Origins of regulated cell-to-cell variability. *Nat Rev Mol Cell Biol 12*, 119-125.

Spitzer, M.H. and Nolan, G.P. (2016). Mass cytometry: Single cells, many features. *Cell 165*, 780-791.

Swain, P.S., Elowitz, M.B., and Siggia, E.D. (2002). Intrinsic and extrinsic contributions to stochasticity in gene expression. *PNAS 99*, 12795-12800.

Tang, F., Barbacioru, C., Bao, S., Lee, C., Nordman, E., Wang, X., Lao, K., and Surani, M.A. (2010). Tracing the derivation of embryonic stem cells from the inner cell mass by single-cell RNA-Seq analysis. *Cell Stem Cell 6*.

Ullah, M. and Wolkenhauer, O. (2011). *Stochastic approaches for systems biology*. Springer, New York.

Wilkinson, D.J. (2006). *Stochastic modelling for systems biology*. Boca Raton, FL: Taylor & Francis.

Wong, S.T.C. (2006). Informatics challenges of high-throughput microscopy. *IEEE Signal Process Mag. 23*, 63-72.

Xue, M., Wei, W., Su, Y., Kim, J., Shin, Y.S., Mai, W.X., Nathanson, D.A., and Heath, J.R. (2015). Chemical methods for the simultaneous quantitation of metabolites and proteins from single cells. *J. Am. Chem. Soc. 137*, 4066-4069.

Yin, H. and Marshall, D. (2012). Microfluidics for single cell analysis. *Curr. Opin. Biotechnol. 23*, 110-119.

Zechner, C. and Koeppl, H. (2014). Uncoupled analysis of stochastic reaction networks in fluctuating environments. *PLoS Comput. Biol. 10*, e1003942.

Zechner, C., Ruess, J., Krenn, P., Pelet, S., Peter, M., Lygeros, J., and Koeppl, H. (2012). Moment-based inference predicts bimodality in transient gene expression. *PNAS 109*, 8340-8345.

Zechner, C., Unger, M., Pelet, S., Peter, M., and Koeppl, H. (2014). Scalable inference of heterogeneous reaction kinetics from pooled single-cell recordings. *Nat. Methods 11*, 197-202.

Quantifying lymphocyte receptor diversity

THIERRY MORA AND ALEKSANDRA M. WALCZAK

11.1 INTRODUCTION

To protect its host against pathogens, the adaptive immune system of jawed vertebrates expresses a large repertoire of distinct receptors on its B and T lymphocytes. These receptors must recognize a wide range of pathogens to trigger the response of the adaptive immune system. Since each receptor is specialized in recognizing specific pathogens, a very diverse repertoire of receptors is required to cover all possible threats. While one can now sequence the repertoires of individuals with some depth, it remains unclear how to quantify or even define their diversity and what aspects of this diversity are relevant for recognition. These fundamental questions are further obscured by the purely technical but important issue of reliably sampling immune repertoires.

The actual number of lymphocytes varies from species to species, but in all cases is large. Estimates of the number of T cells in humans are of the order of $3 \cdot 10^{11}$ cells [1]. Each cell expresses only one type of receptor. Cells proliferate and form clones, so that many distinct cells may share a common receptor. As we will discuss further, the number of unique distinct receptors is very hard to estimate. However, even a conservative lower bound of 10^6 unique receptors [2,3] is much larger than the total number of genes in the human genome (~ 20,000). This broad diversity of receptors is not hard-coded, but is instead generated by a unique gene rearrangement process that couples a combinatoric choice of genomic templates with additional randomness.

Each receptor is made up of two arms: B cell receptors (BCR) have a light and a heavy chain, while T cell receptors (TCR) have analogous α and β chains. Each chain is composed of three segments called V, D, and J in the case of heavy or β chains, and two segments V and J in the case of light or α chains. These segments are combinatorically picked out of several genomic templates for each type, in a process called V(D)J recombination [4], as schematized in Figure 11.1a. This recombination is achieved by looping DNA and excising the template genes that lie between the selected gene segments. In the case of heavy or β chains, the D-J junction is assembled first, followed by the V-D junction. The precise number of templates for each segment differs from species to species, but generally results in a combinatoric diversity of ~ 1000 for each chain. This combinatoric assortment is followed by stochastic nucleotide deletions and insertions at the junctions between

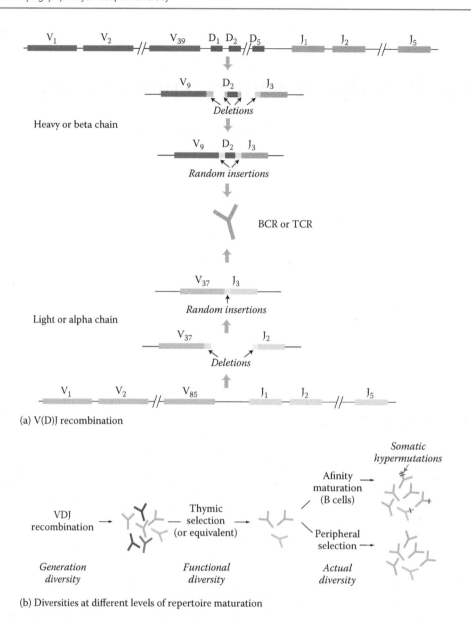

(a) V(D)J recombination

Heavy or beta chain

Light or alpha chain

(b) Diversities at different levels of repertoire maturation

Figure 11.1 **(a)** V(D)J recombination of T and B cell receptors (TCR and BCR). TCRs and BCRs are made of two chains, one shorter and one longer, called the α and β chains for TCRs, and the light and heavy chains for BCRs. Each chain is obtained by a gene rearrangement process called V(D)J recombination, by which two (for the shorter chain) or three (for the longer chain) segments are assembled together from palettes of templates encoded in the genome. At each of the junction between these segments, further diversity is added by stochastic deletions and insertions of random, non-templated nucleotides. **(b)** Evolution of repertoires of TCR and BCR. After their generation by V(D)J recombination, receptors first pass a selection process, called thymic selection for TCRs, whereby nonfunctional and self-reactive receptors are discarded. They are then released into the periphery, where they may divide, die, proliferate, and differentiate as a function of the signals they receive from antigens or other immune cells. In addition, BCRs are subject to somatic hypermutations as B cells mature in germinal centers following an infection.

the newly assorted V-D and D-J fragments (or V-J fragment for the shorter chain), forming what is termed junctional diversity. This stochastic step largely increases the repertoire diversity, as we will show in detail. As a result of this procedure the receptor DNA may be out of frame, or the encoded protein may not be functional or correctly folded. The newly assembled β chain sequences then are tested with a surrogate α chain for their binding and expression properties. If they pass this selection step, the second chain is assembled and the whole receptor undergoes a similar round of selection against proteins that are natural to the organism, or self proteins. Receptors that do not bind any self-protein or bind too strongly to self-proteins are discarded. If a receptor fails these tests, the cell may attempt to recombine its second chromosome.

The processes of recombination and selection are stochastic, and therefore are characterized by their own intrinsic diversity, which we may view as a statistical or potential diversity. It is distinct from the diversity realized in a given individual at a given time, with its finite number of recombined receptors, much like the potential diversity of the English language is distinct from—and much larger than—the diversity of texts found in a single library. While most previous discussions, with the exception of [5], have focused on the realized rather than potential diversity of receptors, in this chapter we will discuss both.

After generation and selection, B and T cells feed the naive repertoire where they attempt to recognize foreign antigens (Figure 11.1b). The dynamics of lymphocytes vary widely between B and T cells, as well as between species. However, a common feature is that cells whose receptors successfully bind to antigens proliferate, producing either identical offspring (T cells) or that differ by somatic point hypermutations (B cells). A fraction of the cells that have undergone proliferation are kept in what is called the memory repertoire, while cells that have not received a proliferation signal stay in the naive repertoire. Cells that share a common receptor, or "clonotype," define a clone. The clonal structure of the lymphocyte repertoire is one of the characteristics of repertoire diversity.

The diversity of lymphocyte receptors can be studied with the help of repertoire high-throughput sequencing experiments [2,6–8], which have been developing rapidly over the last few years [9–14]. These experiments focus on the region of the chain that encompasses the junctions between the recombined segments, allowing for the complete identification of the receptor chain. This region includes the Complementarity Determining Region 3 (CDR3), defined from roughly the end of the V segment to the beginning of the J segment, which is believed to play an important role in recognition. Because sequence reads can only cover one of the two chains making up the receptor, most studies have focused on the diversity of one chain at a time. However, new techniques make it possible to pair the two chains together [15–17], opening the way for the analysis of repertoires of complete receptors. In general, a tissue (blood, lymph node, thymus, germinal center, etc.) sample is taken and the mRNA or DNA of the lymphocytes of interest are sorted out. Different technologies have been developed for DNA and mRNA. Data are usually clustered and error-corrected for PCR and sequencing errors [18]. Many recent experiments use unique molecular barcodes associated to each initial mRNA molecule, which help correct for PCR amplification noise [19–21], and allow for the direct measurement of relative clone sizes using sequence counts. Unless an error occurred in the first round of PCR, barcodes can reliably pick up even very rare sequences, as long as they are present in the sample. The output of these experiments is a list of sequences of receptor chains. If unique molecular barcodes were used, the number of RNA molecules in the initial sample can be evaluated from the number of distinct barcodes with the same receptor sequence. This information is the starting point for the analysis of repertoire diversity.

In this chapter we discuss approaches for estimating repertoire diversity from the datasets generated by these new technologies. We first review and discuss the different definitions of diversity—species richness, entropy, and other diversity indices—and their relation to the distribution of clonotype frequencies. We also emphasize the need to distinguish the different levels at which diversity may be evaluated: recombination diversity, post-selection potential diversity, actual diversity realized in a particular individual, in a particular tissue, with a particular phenotype, etc. We review recent efforts to calculate accurately the diversity of receptors generated by V(D)J recombination using high-throughput sequencing data. We discuss the challenges of estimating diversity when the clonal structure is scale-free, as is generically the case in many reported cases. We conclude by discussing the importance of sequence diversity and contrast it with more biologically relevant but elusive notion of functional diversity.

11.2 A FAMILY OF DIVERSITY MEASURES

A number of different diversity measures have been proposed to quantify the vastness of lymphocyte repertoires [22–24]: the Shannon entropy [25], the Simpson index [26], and most commonly the total number of clonotypes or species richness [2,3,27–29]. These diversity measures are taken from ecology where they are used to quantify the diversity of species. They are all related to a generalized family of diversity measures called the Rényi entropy [30], parametrized by β and defined as:

$$H_\beta = \frac{1}{1-\beta}\ln\left[\sum_s p(s)^\beta\right],$$ (11.1)

where $p(s)$ is the probability, frequency, or abundance of a given receptor sequence or clonotype s. For $\beta \to 1$ we recover Shannon's entropy:

$$H_1 = -\sum_s p(s)\ln p(s).$$ (11.2)

The exponential of the Rényi entropy defines a generalized class of diversity indices called Hill diversities [31]:

$$D_\beta = \exp[H_\beta].$$ (11.3)

This index can be interpreted as an effective number of clonotypes in the data. For $\beta = 1$, it is simply the exponential of Shannon's entropy, and we will refer to it as Shannon's diversity. For $\beta = 2$, it reduces to the inverse of Simpson's diversity index, $D_2 = 1/\sum_s p(s)^2$. The Simpson index gives the probability that two sequences drawn at random from the distribution are identical, and is related to a common measure of inequality, the Gini-Simpson index, defined as $1 - 1/D_2$. D_0 is the species richness, while $D_\infty = 1/\max_s p(s)$ is the inverse of the Berger-Parker index.

Each of these diversity indices is a summary statistics of the information contained in the distribution of clonotype frequencies, i.e., the distribution of values of $p(s)$ themselves. This frequency distribution may in fact be viewed as the most complete description of the diversity of the repertoire. Conversely, the whole spectrum of Rényi entropies H_β is sufficient to reconstruct the full clonotype frequency distribution. In other words, the functions H_β, D_β, and the distribution of frequencies carry the exact same information [32]. The choice of a single diversity measure D_β, rather than the full frequency distribution, is often useful to make comparisons between individuals, tissues, experiments, etc. When β is large enough, it may also be less sensitive to experimental noise than the frequency distribution.

It is possible to get a rough estimate of Hill diversities by simple inspection of the frequency distribution, represented as a rank-frequency graph with a double logarithmic scale [32]. A simple geometric construction, illustrated by Figure 11.2, helps understand the meaning of the various indices, what properties of the underlying cumulative clone size distribution they are most likely to capture, and where one should stop trusting them because of insufficient sampling. The intersection of the the tangents of slope –1 and $-\beta^{-1}$ to the rank-frequency curve gives the Hill diversity index D_β. This construction emphasizes the fact that different diversity measures focus on sequences of various frequencies: large values of β tend to favor very common

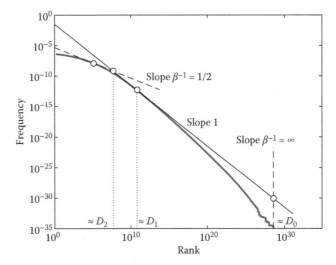

Figure 11.2 Geometric construction of Hill diversities from a rank-frequency curve. The Hill diversity of order β, $D_\beta = [\sum_s p(s)^\beta]^{1/(1-\beta)}$, can be approximated from the intersection between the tangents of slope -1 and $-1/\beta$. D_0 is the total number of types or species richness, D_1 is the exponential of Shannon's entropy, and D_2 is the inverse of Simpson's diversity index. The rank-frequency curve was created from a generative model of random TRB (T cell receptor beta chains) inferred in Murugan et al. (From Murugan, A. et al., *Proc Natl Acad Sci*, *109*, 16161–16166, 2012.)

clonotypes, while low values favor rare ones. Geometrically, tangents of small slopes (large β, e.g., Simpson's index or Shannon's entropy) osculate the rank-frequency curve at high frequencies, while large slopes do so at low frequencies. Thus, diversity indices D_β with a small β rely very strongly on correctly capturing the tail of rare clonotypes. This is particularly true for D_0, the species richness, which is very hard to estimate as it requires estimating the number of unseen clonotypes. This observation warns us against the pitfalls of estimating diversity when dealing with incomplete samples. The larger the β, the more reliable the Hill index D_β should be. In general, estimates of the species richness D_0 should be taken with extreme caution, as we will further discuss in concrete examples.

11.3 QUANTIFYING V(D)J RECOMBINATION

The repertoire is a dynamic ensemble of receptors that evolves somatically, by cell division, cell death, and hypermutations in the case of B cells. As the repertoire is shaped, its diversity changes significantly. Repertoires at different functional stages, from generation to memory, show different levels of potential and realized diversity. By analyzing unique receptors from high-throughput sequencing data, one can track these changes. We start by describing the diversity of the initial stochastic recombination of receptors.

Each cell has two sets of chromosomes. If the first V(D)J rearrangement results in a non-functional receptor, the second one recombines [33]. When this second rearrangement is successful, the cell expresses the functional receptor but keeps the rearranged nonfunctional DNA. This nonfunctional receptor is expressed at a basal, leaky level despite allelic exclusion, especially for α chains, and may also be captured by genomic DNA sequencing. These out-of-frame receptors offer unique insight into the raw generation process because they were never selected for, as they owe their survival to the gene expressed from the other chromosome. We can therefore use these sequences to gain insight into the generation process and analyze the *potential* diversity of recombination, i.e., the statistics of unique receptors that can ever be formed as a result of V(D)J recombination. As already noted, this diversity of the generation process should not be confused with the actually realized diversity in a given individual, which is generically smaller.

As the numbers will show, the recombination probability of each generated sequence is so small that it is hopeless to sample their distribution by simply counting how often we observe them. Besides, this counting number is not expected to reflect the frequency of generation alone, because of lymphocyte population dynamics. As we pointed out, cell proliferation is independent of the identity of the out-of-frame sequence of interest, and the limit of infinite data should not in principle affect such an estimate. However, for any dataset coming from a single individual, these heterogeneities in the clone size completely dominate the sequence counts. For this reason, it is suitable to count each unique sequence only once to remove these possible biases. Starting with a dataset of unique realizations of the recombination process, we need a model to describe their probability distribution. This model is based on what we know about the recombination process: choice of V(D)J segments, stochastic number of deletions of each gene segments, and stochastic number and identities of inserted nucleotides at each junction. Thus, taking the simpler case of α or light chains, the probability of a given recombination scenario r can be written as:

$$P_{\text{rearr}}(r) = P(V, J)P(\text{del}V|V)P(\text{del}J|J)P(\text{ins}), \tag{11.4}$$

where $\text{del}V$ and $\text{del}J$ denote the number of deletions at the V and J ends, and "ins" is the list of inserted nucleotides. A very similar expression accounting for three genes and two junctions can be written for the β or heavy chains. The form of the model is motivated by biophysical considerations: the number of deletions of the J end does not depend on the choice of the V segment, the number and identities of insertions does not depend on the gene choice and follows a Markov chain. These assumptions, however, should and can be checked consistently by verifying that no correlations in the data remain unaccounted for by the model [34].

The parameters of the generation model (11.4) cannot be directly read off the sequences, because it is impossible in general to assign with certainty a recombination scenario to a given sequence as many distinct scenarios can lead to the same sequence through convergent recombination [35]. As we will quantify below, this effect is very significant and cannot be ignored. Importantly, it forces us to think of scenarios or sequence annotation in a probabilistic manner, rather than try to select the most probable one as is often done in annotation software [36–38]. The generation parameters can be inferred using a standard implementation of the Expectation-Maximization algorithm, an iterative procedure that maximizes the likelihood of the data. The algorithm works by collecting summary statistics about the elements of the recombination scenarios to build the model distribution (11.4). The recombination scenarios are themselves assigned probabilistically using the previous iteration of the model. The algorithm, which relies on the enumeration of all plausible scenarios giving rise to each sequence, is computationally heavy but can be significantly sped up after mapping the problem onto a hidden Markov model and using standard dynamic programming tools [39].

Once a recombination model such as Eq. 11.4 has been inferred, it can be used to generate and analyse sequences with the same statistical properties as the original data. It can also be used to quantity the various types of diversity indices discussed in the previous section. Note that, because of convergent recombination, the diversity of generated sequences is expected to be smaller than the diversity of the scenarios that produce them. The generation probability of a sequence s is given by the sum of the probabilities of all scenarios that could have given rise to this sequence:

$$P_{\text{gen}}(s) = \sum_{r \to s} P_{\text{rearr}}(r). \tag{11.5}$$

The diversity measures calculated from P_{gen} and P_{rearr} are therefore distinct.

Recombination models have been inferred for T cell β [34] and α [39] chains, as well as for B cell heavy chains [40]. In all these cases, the distributions inferred from different individuals were found to be surprisingly similar, with some variability in the gene segment usage, but very reproducible deletion and insertion profiles, consistent with a common biophysical mechanism of enzyme function. The entropy H_1 of sequences and recombination scenarios obtained from these models are reported in Figure 11.3a. Because the distribution of scenarios (11.4) is a product of its various elements (gene choice, deletions, insertions), its entropy can also be broken up into their respective contributions. The entropy difference between recombination events and sequences, is the entropy of convergent recombination, which quantifies the diversity of scenarios

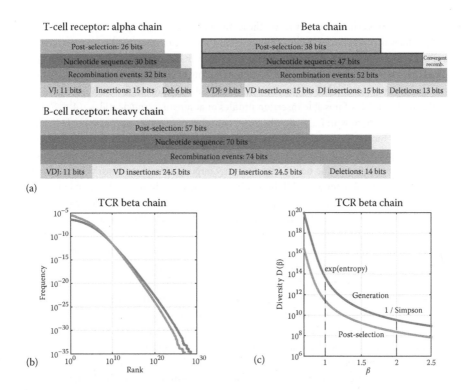

Figure 11.3 Entropies and diversity indices of the receptor generation and selection process. **(a)** Entropy of the V(D)J recombination process in TCR α and β chains and in BCR heavy chains. The entropy of recombination events can be decomposed into contributions for the choice of the V(D)J genes, the number and identity of insertions, and deletions. The sequence entropy is slightly smaller than the recombination entropy because several recombination events can lead to the same sequence (convergent recombination). Following thymic selection, or the B cell counterpart, the entropy is further (light gray). **(b)** Rank-frequency curves of TCR β chain sequences, upon generation (dark gray), and following thymic selection. **(c)** Hill diversities for the same statistical ensembles. The Shannon diversity $D(1)$ is the exponential of the entropies shown in black boxes in **(a)**.

resulting in the same sequence. For example, it is five bits for TCR β chains, corresponding to a fairly large Shannon diversity number, $D_1 \sim 30$. Note that the total number of possible scenarios for a given sequence, D_0 is much larger, but its precise definition depends on the cutoff we impose on the possible number of deletions and insertions.

Diversity in the heavy chain of B cells is larger than that of T cells. This difference can be attributed to longer CDR3 regions due to many more insertions at the junctions between the genes. The receptor generation process is characterized by an entropy of ~ 70 bits for BCR heavy chains and ~ 43 bits for TCR β chains. These numbers correspond to a Shannon diversity index $D_1 \sim 10^{21}$ and $\sim 10^{14}$, respectively.

Although most studies have focused on the Shannon diversity index D_1, the full diversity spectrum of the generation process can be calculated. In Figure 11.3b we show the rank-frequency curve of human TCR β chains, taken from [32] based on the model of [34]. As explained in the previous section, the full range of diversity indices D_β can be calculated from that curve, and are shown in Figure 11.3c. In addition to the Shannon diversity D_1 already discussed, of special interest is the inverse of the Simpson index, D_2. The Simpson index corresponds to the probability that the same nucleotide sequence is obtained from two independent draws. It gives the expected number of shared sequences between two individuals, normalized by the product of their repertoire sizes, assuming that their receptor sequences were generated independently from the same source. Thus, it is deeply linked to the notion of "public" sequences found in several individuals, and making up the public repertoire [26,35,41]. This number, estimated to be $1/D_2 \sim 3 \cdot 10^{-10}$ for human TCR β chains from the model, is in fact very close to that measured in the data for out-of-frame sequences [34].

It is important to stress that, however large, these numbers are *not* the total number of possible receptor sequences, D_0, which is much larger. As we can see from the rank-frequency plot of generated TCR β chain sequences (Figure 11.3b, red), generation probabilities span over 20 orders of magnitude. The largest rank of $\sim 10^{30}$ is in fact a lower bound to D_0 limited by the finite sampling of sequences by the model. To better estimate D_0, one may count the total number of possible deletion profiles reported for each gene, and multiply that number by the total number of possible insertion profiles of at most L_{max} nucleotides, $(4^{L_{max}+1}-1)/3$, for each of the two junctions. Doing so with $L_{max} = 26$, the largest number of insertions reported in [34], yields an upper bound of $D_0 \sim 2 \cdot 10^{39}$ for the TCR β chain alone. However, because this estimate is very sensitive to the value of L_{max}, which is not precisely known and may depend on the sample size, it must be taken with some caution.

The above estimates only include heavy or β chains. Coupling this chain with the light or α chain adds further diversity. Since the shorter (α and light) chains have only one junctional region between the V and J genes, their diversity is much lower. For example, TCR α chains were estimated to have a generation Shannon entropy of $H_1 = 30$ bits, or $D_1 \sim 10^9$ [39]. The part of the entropy that is attributable to the gene choice is similar to that reported for the β chain, of the order of 10 bits. While that contribution was only a small fraction of the overall diversity for the β chain, it is comparable to that of insertions for the α chain. The number of possible α chain sequences can be estimated similarly to the β chain, yielding $D_0 \sim 5 \; 10^{21}$.

Assuming that the two chain rearrangements are independent, the overall diversity of the pool from which TCRs are generated is about $H_1 \sim 75$ bits, or $D_1 \sim 10^{23}$, and a total potential repertoire of size $D_0 \sim 10^{61}$. Note that this last estimate is much larger than the classically quoted number of 10^{15} from [42], which assumed a much more restricted junctional diversity. Analysis of recently published α-β sequence pairings should allow for more precise estimates of these diversity numbers for TCRs [17] and BCRs [15].

All these diversity numbers are very large. Clearly, a single individual is only able to sample a tiny fraction of the potential pool of receptor sequences, with a total T cells count of $\sim 3 \cdot 10^{11}$ in humans [1].

11.4 THYMIC SELECTION AND HYPERMUTATIONS

After sequences have been generated by V(D)J recombination, they undergo an initial selection process. For T cells, this takes place in the thymus and is called thymus selection. An analogous process occurs for B cells. Sequences that bind too strongly to the host's own self-proteins, as well as those that bind too weakly to them, are discarded. By analyzing the in-frame naive receptor repertoire, one can study how this initial selection process affects the diversity of the repertoire. While the recombination diversity, $P_{gen}(s)$, described the potential variability from the gene rearrangement process, this post-selection naive diversity, $P_{sel}(s)$, describes the statistics of sequences actually found in the naive repertoire. It is still a potential diversity, as it refers to a statistical ensemble of receptors, rather than a finite set of receptors found in a given individual.

One can define a sequence-dependent selection factor $Q(s) = P_{sel}(s)/P_{gen}(s)$ quantifying how the distribution of sequences is affected by thymic selection. As before, sampling from $P_{sel}(s)$ is impossible in practice because of the too large number of sequences, and models of the selection factor $Q(s)$ are needed. For example, it may take the factorized form

$$Q(s) = \prod_{i=1}^{L} q_{i;L(a_i)}, \qquad (11.6)$$

where $(a_1, a_2, ..., a_L)$ is the amino-acid sequence of the CDR3 region of length L, and the single-position factors $q_{i;L}(a)$ are inferred from the data using maximum likelihood. This model describes very well the statistics of naive and memory TCR β-chain sequences [43], α-chain sequences [44], and naive BCR heavy chain sequences [40]. The selection factors $Q(s)$ were shown to depend only on the amino-acid rather than nucleotide sequence, consistent with our hypothesis that selection acts on the protein product and its functional properties (folding, stability binding, etc.). Although selection factors may vary significantly from individual to individual in the statistical sense, these differences are relatively small. In addition, models inferred from the memory and naive sequence repertoires were found to be similar, suggesting that the selection factors $Q(s)$ capture universal functional properties of the receptor proteins.

Diversity numbers can be estimated from the model of Eq. 11.6. The entropy of the post-selection distributions of receptor sequences, $P_{sel}(s) = Q(s)P_{gen}(s)$ are shown in green in Figure 11.3a. The rank-frequency distribution and Hill diversities D_β of the post-selection ensemble of TCR β chain sequences are shown in green in Figures 11.3b and c.

Diversity is reduced by selection from 47 to 38 bits for TCR β chains, from 30 to 26 bits for α chains, and from 70 to 58 bits for BCR heavy chains, corresponding to $D_1 \sim 3 \cdot 10^{11}$ for β chains, $D_1 \sim 7 \cdot 10^7$ for α chains (or a combined TCR diversity of $2 \cdot 10^{19}$ assuming independence between the two chains), and $D_1 \sim 3 \cdot 10^{17}$ for heavy chains. About two bits of this reduction are due to the removal of visibly nonfunctional sequences (out-of-frame or having stop codons). However, most of the diversity loss is caused by negative selection against sequences that were unlikely to be produced in the first place. Frequent sequences are enriched by the selection process, while rare ones are more likely to be removed. This enhancement of inequalities between sequences is the main source of entropy reduction by selection.

It should be noted that these estimate rely on an effective model (11.6), which may miss many important aspects of the selection process. In particular, negative selection, which prunes the repertoire of specific sequences that bind to self-antigens, is likely not accounted for by the model. This further diversity loss would be specific to each individual and its set of self-antigens, which depends on its HLA types. To assess whether all the aspects of selection that are not individual specific are well captured by Eq. 11.6, one can ask whether the Simpson index calculated with the model, $1/D_2$, is consistent with the observed repertoire overlap between distinct individuals, as it should if the two repertoires were drawn independently from the same distribution $P_{sel}(s)$. Indeed the model and data showed good agreement [43], confirming that the model describes the statistics of sequences accurately.

Following their release into the periphery, cells undergo a somatic evolution process by which they divide, die, or proliferate depending on the signals they receive. In the case of T cells, it is not clear how this evolution affects the potential naive diversity, as TCR β-chain sequences expressed by memory cells are statistically indistinguishable from naive ones [43]. In contrast, BCRs experience somatic hypermutations as B cells proliferate upon antigen recognition, during the process of affinity maturation. These hypermutations are stochastic but do not occur uniformly across the receptor, favoring instead sequence context dependent "hotspots" [45,46]. High-throughput repertoire sequencing now makes it possible to build predictive statistical models of hypermutations by disentangling mutation from substitution rates using either synonymous mutants [47] or out-of-frame sequences [40,48]. Out-of-frame sequences have a raw mutation rate ranging from a 5% to 10%, implying an additional 0.4 bits per nucleotide. This additional diversity is a huge boost if this estimate holds for the whole length of the receptor sequence. However, the increase in diversity due to hypermutations should depend on how long cells have been allowed to evolve. As affinity maturation consists of alternating cycles of mutation and selection, the effects of hypermutations on diversity cannot entirely be decoupled from selective pressures. The inference of selection during affinity maturation using repertoire sequencing is currently a very active field of study [23,49–55].

11.5 REALIZED DIVERSITY

Thus far we have focused on the potential diversity of lymphocyte receptors. Its object is the probability that each receptor sequence has been generated, selected, and, in the case of BCR, hypermutated into its final form. One can also study the realized diversity of receptor clonotypes actually present in a given individual at a given time. The relative frequency of clonotypes in an individual can vary greatly depending on the history of cell divisions and deaths, and is in general distinct from the probabilities P_{gen} and P_{sel} discussed so far. Measuring accurate clonotype frequencies relies on trustworthy counts made possible by unique molecular barcodes associated to original mRNA molecule [19–21] (with the caveat that cells may express variable amounts of mRNA molecules). One can build the rank-frequency relation as before, by ranking clonotypes in a given individual from most common to rarest. This relation can be measured for different phenotypes (naive or memory, CD4 or CD8), in different tissues or organs, or at different ages, to study the organisation and evolution of diversity.

In Figure 11.4 we plot the rank-frequency relation for the unpartitioned TCR β-chain repertoires sampled from the blood of six individuals [44] and sequenced using unique molecular barcodes. A striking feature of these relations is that they seem to follow a power law, $f \propto 1/r^a$, where f and r denote the clonotype frequency and rank, with exponent a ranging from 0.65 to 1, with a mean of 0.78. This observation is consistent with previous reports on zebrafish BCR [6,25] or mouse TCR repertoires [5]. These power laws cannot be explained by a neutral model in which cells divide and die stochastically at a constant rate: calling μ and ν the division and death rates and assuming a constant input of new clones from the thymus, one can show that the distribution of clone sizes n takes the form $P(n) \propto (1/n) \, (\mu/\nu)^n$. Instead, power-laws are consistent with models where each clone evolves under a fluctuating fitness shaped by its changing antigenic environment [56].

Power-law frequency distributions make it challenging to estimate diversity measures D_β [32]. This difficulty can be understood by considering the geometric construction of diversities of Figure 11.2: examining the rank-frequency curve of Figure 11.4, no tangent of slope –1 can be easily defined. Mathematically, the normalization of the distribution strongly depends on the maximal rank, as $\Sigma_r 1/r^a$ is a diverging series, meaning that the distribution is dominated by a very large number of very small clonotypes. This is particularly problematic as these rare clonotypes are not well captured by incomplete sampling.

Most past studies of repertoire diversity have actually focused on the hardest diversity measure to estimate in the face of these sampling issues, namely the species richness index D_0. By sequencing a subset of the repertoire with low-throughput techniques and extrapolating to the entire repertoire, Arstila and collaborators found a lower bound to the total size of the TCR repertoire of 10^6 distinct β chains, each pairing to 25 distinct α chains, i.e. $2.5 \cdot 10^7$ distinct TCRs [27]. This bound has since been revisited using high-throughput sequencing data, yielding the same order of magnitude of a few millions [2,3].

In practice, most experiments are performed on samples of blood or tissues and do not sequence every single cell. Even experiments using a whole tissue are subject to losses. The problem of species richness estimation from incomplete samples is not specific to lymphocyte repertoires and has been extensively discussed in ecology. A number of estimators of D_0, such as Chao1 [57], the abundance-based coverage estimator [58], or more recently DivE proposed in the context of TCRs [29], have been developed to address this issue. Another estimator using multiple samples, Chao2 [59], has recently been used to yield a lower bound of 10^8 distinct TCR β chains in humans [28]. All these estimators implicitly assume that the distribution of frequencies is reasonably peaked, and may not be appropriate for broad distributions such as power laws.

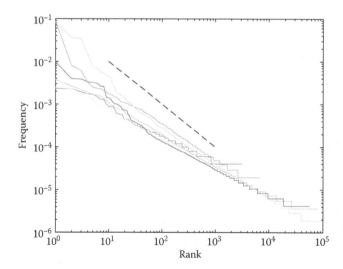

Figure 11.4 Clonotype frequency vs. rank in the sequenced un-partitioned repertoires of six individuals from Pogorelyy et al. (From Pogorelyy, M. V. et al., *PLoS Compute Biol*, 13(7), e10055722, 2017.) These relations are close to a power law with exponents ranging from –0.65 to –1. The dashed line shows a slope of –1.

To illustrate the inadequacy of most estimators to capture the true species richness of power-law distributed clone sizes, we numerically generated $D_0 = 10^7$ distinct clonotypes, and fixed their abundance to

$$C_r = (D_0/r)^\alpha, \tag{11.7}$$

where $r = 1,\ldots, D_0$ is the rank of the clonotype ordered by abundance, and $\alpha = 0.8$ to mimick the data of Figure 11.4. We simulated a sample comprising 1% of the entire dataset, by drawing S_r, the size of clonotype of rank r in the sample, from a Poisson distribution of mean $C_r/100$. We calculated Chao1,

$$D_0 \approx D_0^{\text{raw}} + \frac{n_1^2}{2n_2}, \tag{11.8}$$

where D_0^{raw} is the number of sampled clonotypes $(S_r > 0)$, n_1 is the number of singletons $(S_r = 1)$, and n_2 the number of doubletons $(S_2 = 2)$. This estimate gave $D_0 = 3 \cdot 10^6$ instead of the true value of 10^7. Dividing the dataset into five subsamples as in [28], and calculating Chao2 yields a similar estimate, $3.2 \cdot 10^6$. The reason for this underestimation is deep and does not depend much on the details of the estimator. When downsampling, one loses information about the rare clones, which dominate the species richness. Extrapolating their number from larger clones must rely on implicit or explicit assumptions about the clonal distribution, which are likely not satisfied by fat-tailed distributions such as power laws. It is therefore likely that most current estimates from high-throughput sequencing data are only lower bounds to the true species richness.

In fact, simple theoretical arguments based on thymic output estimates and neutral models of clonal evolution give upper bounds of 10^{10}-10^{11} [60,61]. However, since we have argued that the power-law in the rank-frequency curve did not support the hypothesis of neutrality, it is legitimate to ask what species richness would be predicted from a power-law distribution of clone sizes. Assuming that the rank-size relation is given by Eq. 11.7, the average clonotype size reads:

$$\langle C \rangle = \frac{1}{D_0} \sum_{r=1}^{D_0} \left(\frac{D_0}{r} \right)^\alpha \approx D_0^{1-\alpha} \int_1^{D_0} \frac{1}{r^\alpha} = \frac{1}{1-\alpha}, \tag{11.9}$$

where we have approximated the sum by an integral, which is valid for large D_0. Plugging $\alpha = 0.8$ gives an average clone size of five cells, and hence a species richness $D_0 = 3 \cdot 10^{11}/5 \sim 10^{11}$ of the same order of magnitude as total number of T cells. Note however that this estimate is very sensitive to the value of α, as the average clone size becomes $\sim \ln(D_0)$ for $\alpha = 1$, and $\sim \zeta(\alpha)D_0^{\alpha-1}$ for $\alpha > 1$, where $\zeta(\alpha)$ is the Riemann zeta function.

Although the validity of the power law across the entire spectrum of clone sizes is a matter of debate, this example emphasizes the need for models to extrapolate the size distribution to the very rare clonotypes, the knowledge of which is essential for evaluating species richness.

11.6 TOWARDS A FUNCTIONAL DIVERSITY

All the diversities discussed in this chapter apply to nucleotide sequences. These estimates demonstrate the potential of the adaptive immune system to generate a huge diversity of sequences, while identifying the biases of their generation and selection. However, they do not directly inform us about the functional diversity of the repertoire, defined as its capacity to recognize a wide variety of antigens. First, the binding properties of receptors are determined by their amino-acid sequences, the diversity of which is smaller due to the degeneracy of the genetic code. But more fundamentally, a given antigen can be recognized by many receptors—the flipside of cross-reactivity or polyspecificity. Mason [62] argued that if not for cross-reactivity, an individual would need a repertoire as large as the number of antigens it can encounter, or $\sim 10^{15}$ for TCRs, which is well beyond the number of lymphocytes a human or a mouse can afford. Simple models can help estimate the minimal size of the functional repertoire [5,63,64]. Theoretical arguments also suggests that cross-reactivity gives a certain freedom in the identity and binding properties of the receptors, implying that two individuals experiencing similar antigenic environments need not share common receptors through the convergent evolution of their repertoires [65].

Quantifying the functional diversity of the repertoire is arduous because it requires precise characterization of cross-reactivity by mapping the sequence of receptors to their binding properties. The identification of TCRs that bind to specific antigens using tetramer experiments in mice [66] shows that a single antigen is bound by 20-200 out of $4 \cdot 10^7$ CD4+ T cells, i.e., a fraction $5 \cdot 10^{-7}$–$5 \cdot 10^{-6}$ of the total population. Conversely, a single TCR can recognize many antigens. A lower bound of 10^6 has been reported for an autoimmune TCR from a human patient [67], but that number must be much larger ($> 5 \cdot 10^{-7} \times 10^{15} = 5 \cdot 10^8$) so that the TCR repertoire may cover the entire set of possible peptides.

Assessing cross-reactivity in a more quantitative and systematic way requires to massively measure the binding properties of a huge numbers of receptor-antigens pairs. High-throughput mutational scans combining binding assays with next-generation sequencing technologies now make it possible to measure the binding properties of a single receptor against many peptides [68], or of many mutagenized receptors against a single antigen [69]. Integrating these measurements into predictive models of receptor-antigen binding would provide powerful tools for analyzing lymphocyte repertoires. The diversity of receptor sequences could then be augmented by the more relevant diversity of antigens that can be recognized by them, with varying potencies and frequencies.

ACKNOWLEDGMENTS

This work was supported in part by grant ERCStG n. 306312, and by the National Science Foundation under Grant No. NSF PHY11-25915 through the KITP where part of the work was done.

REFERENCES

1. Jenkins, M.K., Chu, H.H., McLachlan, J.B., and Moon, J.J. (2009). On the composition of the pre-immune repertoire of T cells specific for Peptide-major histocompatibility complex ligands. *Annu Rev Immunol 28*, 275-294.

2. Robins, H.S. et al. (2009). Comprehensive assessment of T cell receptor beta-chain diversity in alpha-beta T cells. *Blood 114*, 4099-4107.

3. Warren, R.L. et al. (2011). Exhaustive T cell repertoire sequencing of human peripheral blood samples reveals signatures of antigen selection and a directly measured repertoire size of at least 1 million clonotypes. *Genome Res 21*, 790-797.

4. Hozumi, N., and Tonegawa, S. (1976). Evidence for somatic rearrangement of immunoglobulin genes coding for variable and constant regions. *Proc Natl Acad Sci 73*, 3628-3632.

5. Zarnitsyna, V.I., Evavold, B.D., Schoettle, L.N., Blattman, J.N., and Antia, R. (2013). Estimating the diversity, completeness, and cross-reactivity of the T cell repertoire. *Front Immunol 4*, 485.

6. Weinstein, J., Jiang, N., White, R., Fisher, D.S., and Quake, S.R. (2009). High-throughput sequencing of the zebrafish antibody repertoire. *Science 324*, 807-810.

7. Freeman, J.D., Warren, R.L., Webb, J.R., Nelson, B.H., Holt, R. (2009). Profiling the T cell receptor beta-chain repertoire by massively parallel sequencing. *Genome Res 19*, 1817-1824.

8. Robins, H.S. et al. (2010). Overlap and effective size of the human CD8+ T cell receptor repertoire. *Sci Transl Med 2*, 47ra64.

9. Benichou, J., Ben-Hamo, R., Louzoun, Y., and Efroni, S. (2012). Rep-Seq: Uncovering the immunological repertoire through next-generation sequencing. *Immunology 135*, 183-191.

10. Warren, E.H., Matsen, F., and Chou, J. (2013). High-throughput sequencing of B- and T-lymphocyte antigen receptors in hematology. *Blood 122*, 19-22.

11. Six A. et al. (2013). The past, present and future of immune repertoire biology - the rise of next-generation repertoire analysis. *Front Immunol 4*, 413.

12. Woodsworth, D.J., Castellarin, M., Holt, R. (2013). Sequence analysis of T cell repertoires in health and disease. *Genome Med 5*, 98.

13. Georgiou, G. et al. (2014). The promise and challenge of high-throughput sequencing of the antibody repertoire. *Nat Biotechnol 32*, 158-168.

14. Calis, J.J., and Rosenberg, B.R. (2014). Characterizing immune repertoires by high throughput sequencing: Strategies and applications. *Trends Immunol. 35(12)*, 581-590.

15. Dekosky, B.J. et al. (2014). In-depth determination and analysis of the human paired heavy- and light-chain antibody repertoire. *Nat Med 21*, 1-8.

16. Turchaninova M. et al. (2013). Pairing of T cell receptor chains via emulsion PCR. *Eur J Immunol 43*, 2507-2515.

17. Howie, B. et al. (2015). High-throughput pairing of T cell receptor a and b sequences. *Sci Trans Med 7*, 301ra131.

18. Shugay, M. et al. (2014). Towards error-free profiling of immune repertoires. *Nat Methods 11*, 653-655.

19. Vollmers, C., Sit, R.V., Weinstein, J.A., Dekker, C.L., and Quake, S.R. (2013). Genetic measurement of memory B cell recall using antibody repertoire sequencing. *Proc Natl Acad Sci 110*, 13463-13468.

20. Egorov, E.S. et al. (2015). Quantitative Profiling of Immune Repertoires for Minor Lymphocyte Counts Using Unique Molecular Identifiers. *J Immunol 194*, 6155-6163.

21. Best, K., Oakes, T., Heather, J.M., Shawe-Taylor, J., and Chain, B. (2015). Computational analysis of stochastic heterogeneity in PCR amplification efficiency revealed by single molecule barcoding. *Sci Rep 5*, 14629.

22. Greiff, V., Miho, E., Menzel, U., and Reddy, S.T. (2015). Bioinformatic and Statistical Analysis of Adaptive Immune Repertoires. *Trends Immunol 36*, 738-749.

23. Yaari, G., and Kleinstein, S.H. (2015). Practical guidelines for B cell receptor repertoire sequencing analysis. *Genome Med 7*, 121.

24. Greiff, V. et al. (2015). A bioinformatic framework for immune repertoire diversity profiling enables detection of immunological status. *Genome Med 7*, 49.

25. Mora, T., Walczak, A.M., Bialek, W., and Callan, C.G. (2010). Maximum entropy models for antibody diversity. *Proc Natl Acad Sci 107*, 5405-5410.

26. Venturi, V., Kedzierska, K., Turner, S.J., Doherty, P.C., and Davenport, M.P. (2007). Methods for comparing the diversity of samples of the T cell receptor repertoire. *J Immunol Methods 321*, 182-195.

27. Arstila, T.P. et al. (1999). A direct estimate of the human alphabeta T cell receptor diversity. *Science 286*, 958-961.

28. Qi, Q. et al. (2014). Diversity and clonal selection in the human T cell repertoire. *Proc. Natl. Acad. Sci 111(36)*, 13139-44.

29. Laydon, D.J. et al. (2014). Quantification of HTLV-1 Clon-ality and TCR Diversity. *PLoS Comput Biol 10*, 1-13.

30. Rényi, A. (1961). On measures of entropy and information. *Entropy 547*, 547-561.

31. Hill, A.M.O. (1973). Diversity and Evenness: A Unifying Notation and Its Consequences. *Ecology 54*, 427-432.

32. Mora, T., and Walczak, A.M. (2016). Renyi entropy, abundance distribution and the equivalence of ensembles. *Phys Rev E 93*, 052418.

33. Janeway, C., Murphy, K.P., Travers, P., and Walport, M. (2008). *Janeway's immunobiology*. Garland Science.

34. Murugan, A., Mora, T., Walczak, A.M., and Callan, C.G. (2012). Statistical inference of the generation probability of T cell receptors from sequence repertoires. *Proc Natl Acad Sci 109*, 16161-16166.

35. Venturi, V. et al. (2006). Sharing of T cell receptors in antigen-specific responses is driven by convergent recombination. *Proc Natl Acad Sci 103*, 18691-18696.

36. Volpe, J.M., Cowell, L.G., and Kepler, T.B. (2006). SoDA: Implementation of a 3D alignment algorithm for inference of antigen receptor recombinations. *Bioinformatics 22*, 438-444.

37. Gaëta, B.A. et al. (2007). iHMMune-align: Hidden Markov model-based alignment and identification of germline genes in rearranged immunoglobulin gene sequences. *Bioinformatics 23*, 1580-1587.

38. Munshaw, S., and Kepler, T.B. (2010). SoDA2: A Hidden Markov Model approach for identification of immunoglobulin rearrangements. *Bioinformatics 26*, 867-872.

39. Elhanati, Y., Marcou, Q., Mora, T., and Walczak, A.M. (2016). repgenHMM: A dynamic programming tool to infer the rules of immune receptor generation from sequence data. *Bioinformatics 32(13)*, 1943–1951.

40. Elhanati, Y. et al. (2015). Inferring processes underlying B cell repertoire diversity. *Philos Trans R Soc Lond, B, Biol Sci 370*, 20140243.

41. Venturi, V. et al. (2011). A mechanism for TCR sharing between T cell subsets and individuals revealed by pyrosequencing. *J Immunol 186*, 4285-4294.

42. Davis, M.M., and Bjorkman, P.J. (1988). T cell antigen receptor genes and T cell recognition. *Nature 334*, 395-402.

43. Elhanati, Y., Murugan, A., Callan, C.G., Mora, T., and Walczak, A.M. (2014). Quantifying selection in immune receptor repertoires. *Proc Natl Acad Sci 111*, 9875-9880.

44. Pogorelyy, M.V. et al. (2017). Persisting fetal clonotypes influence the structure and overlap of adult human T cell receptor repertoires. *PLoS Comput Biol 13(7)*, e1005572.

45. Shapiro, G.S., Aviszus, K., Ikle, D., and Wysocki, L.J. (1999). Predicting regional mutability in antibody V genes based solely on di- and trinucleotide sequence composition. *J Immunol 163*, 259-268.

46. Cowell, L.G., and Kepler, T.B. (2000). The Nucleotide-Replacement Spectrum Under Somatic Hypermutation Exhibits Microsequence Dependence That Is Strand-Symmetric and Distinct from That Under Germline Mutation. *J Immunol 164*, 1971-1976.

47. Yaari, G. et al. (2013). Models of somatic hypermutation targeting and substitution based on synonymous mutations from high-throughput immunoglobulin sequencing data. *Front Immunol 4*, 358.

48. Dunn-Walters, D.K., Dogan, A., Boursier, L., MacDonald, C.M., and Spencer, J. (1998). Base-Specific Sequences That Bias Somatic Hypermutation Deduced by Analysis of Out-of-Frame Human IgVH Genes. *J Immunol 160*, 2360-2364.

49. Uduman, M. et al. (2011). Detecting selection in immunoglobulin sequences. *Nucleic Acids Res 39*, W499-W504.

50. Yaari, G., Uduman, M., and Kleinstein, S.H. (2012). Quantifying selection in high-throughput Immunoglobulin sequencing data sets. *Nucleic Acids Res 40*, e134.

51. Kepler, T.B. et al. (2014). Reconstructing a B cell Clonal Lineage. II. Mutation, Selection, and Affinity Maturation. *Front Immunol 5*, 170.

52. Laserson, U. et al. (2014). High-resolution antibody dynamics of vaccine-induced immune responses. *Proc Natl Acad Sci 111*, 4928-4933.

53. Uduman, M., Shlomchik, M.J., Vigneault, F., Church, G.M., and Kleinstein, S.H. (2014). Integrating B cell lineage information into statistical tests for detecting selection in Ig sequences. *J Immunol 192*, 867-874.

54. Mccoy, C.O. et al. (2015). Quantifying evolutionary constraints on B cell affinity maturation. *Philos Trans R Soc Lond, B, Biol Sci 370*, 20140244.

55. Yaari, G., Benichou, J.I.C., Heiden, J.A.V., Kleinstein, S.H., and Louzoun, Y. (2015). The mutation patterns in B cell immunoglobulin receptors reflect the influence of selection acting at multiple time-scales. *Philos Trans R Soc Lond, B, Biol Sci 370*, 20140242.

56. Desponds, J., Mora, T., and Walczak, A.M. (2016). Fluctuating fitness shapes the clone-size distribution of immune repertoires. *Proc Natl Acad Sci 113*, 274-279.

57. Chao, A. (1984). Nonparametric estimation of the number of classes in a population. *Scand J Stat 11*, 265-270.

58. Chao, A., and Lee, S.M. (1992). Estimating the Number of Classes via Sanple Coverage. *J Am Stat Assoc 87*, 210-217.

59. Chao, A., and Bunge, J. (2002) Estimating the number of species in a stochastic abundance model. *Biometrics 58*, 531-539.

60. Kesmir, C., Borghans, J., and de Boer, R.J. (2000). Diversity of Human T Cell Receptors. *Science 288*, 1135.

61. Lythe, G., Callard, R.E., Hoare, R., and Molina-París, C. (2015). How many TCR clonotypes does a body maintain? *J Theor Biol 389*, 214-224.

62. Mason, D. (1998). A very high level of crossreactivity is an essential feature of the T- cell receptor. *Immunol Today 19*, 395-404.

63. Perelson, A.S., and Oster, G.F. (1979). Theoretical studies of clonal selection minimal antibody repertoire size and reliability of self non self discrimination. *J Theor Biol 81*, 645-670.

64. de Boer, R.J., and Perelson, A.S. (1993). How diverse should the immune system be? *Proc R Soc Lond, B, Biol Sci 252*, 171.

65. Mayer, A., Balasubramanian, V., Mora, T., and Walczak, A.M. (2015). How a well-adapted immune system is organized. *Proc Natl Acad Sci 112*, 5950-5955.

66. Moon, J.J. et al. (2007). Naive CD4+ T Cell Frequency Varies for Different Epitopes and Predicts Repertoire Diversity and Response Magnitude. *Immunity 27*, 203-213.

67. Wooldridge, L. et al. (2012). A single autoimmune T cell receptor recognizes more than a million different peptides. *J Biol Chem 287*, 1168-1177.

68. Birnbaum, M.E. et al. (2014). Deconstructing the peptide-MHC specificity of t cell recognition. *Cell 157*, 1073-1087.

69. Adams, R.M., Kinney, J.B., Mora, T., and Walczak, A.M. (2016). Measuring the sequence-affinity landscape of antibodies with massively parallel titration curves. *eLife 5*, e23156.

Antigen receptor diversification during immune responses

MIRI MICHAELI AND RAMIT MEHR

12.1 INTRODUCTION: IMMUNOGLOBULIN GENE DIVERSIFICATION DURING IMMUNE RESPONSES

Primary diversification of the TCR and BCR repertoire during T and B cell development is achieved via receptor variable region gene rearrangement. However, in contrast to T cells, B cells further diversify their receptors in germinal centers during immune responses (Victora and Mesin, 2014; Victora and Nussenzweig, 2012). Heavy chain constant regions are functionally diversified via class switch recombination (CSR) (Xu, Zan, Pone, Mai, and Casali, 2012). Heavy and light chain variable regions undergo affinity maturation—a term which refers to the combined result of diversification by somatic hypermutation (and in some species also gene conversion) and antigen-driven selection (Corcoran and Tarlinton, 2016). Somatic hypermutation (SHM) is about a million times faster than normal somatic mutation and affects only the rearranged variable region genes. Like CSR, SHM is initiated by the enzyme activation-induced cytidine deaminase (AID), but unlike CSR, SHM cannot occur in normal B cells *in vitro*, and affinity maturation requires T cell help at almost every stage and can only occur *in vivo*. Affinity maturation accounts for a large part of the diversity of memory B cell repertoires (Budeus et al., 2015).

The fact that most immunoglobulin variable region (IgV) genes sampled are heavily mutated poses, on one hand, a challenge that must be overcome when processing IgV gene sequencing data. On the other hand, many analysis methods based on identifying these mutations can yield very useful insights regarding B cell clonal dynamics and antigen-driven selection. This chapter reviews the problems and solutions posed by SHM, the SHM-based analysis methods and some insights gleaned from these analyses in our and some others' recent studies.

12.2 FIRST CHALLENGE: IgV GENE DATA PRE-PROCESSING AND ERROR CORRECTION

High throughput sequencing (HTS) enables the sequencing of genes from many samples simultaneously, yields more sequences per sample and is sensitive enough to identify different unique sequences, such as the mutated variants in the same B cell clone (Calis and Rosenberg, 2014; Robins, 2013). However, the software packages normally used for preprocessing of HTS data and mutation identification (reviewed in (Michaeli, Noga, Tabibian-Keissar, Barshack, and Mehr, 2012)) rely on being given a "reference" or "template" gene to which all sequences can be compared in order to identify sample molecular identification (MID) tags and primers and discard low-quality sequences. Such template genes do not exist for the somatically rearranged and mutated IgV genes. Thus, the computational immunology community has had to develop its own data cleaning and preprocessing tools for TCR and BCR repertoire sequencing, a.k.a. immune-sequencing or REP-seq (see, e.g., (Marquet et al., 2014; Michaeli, Barak, Hazanov, Noga, and Mehr, 2013; Michaeli et al., 2012; Moorhouse et al., 2014; Schaller et al., 2015; Vander Heiden et al., 2014)). We have developed Ig-HTS-Cleaner (Ig High Throughput Sequencing Cleaner), a program containing a simple cleaning procedure that successfully deals with pre-processing of Ig sequences derived from HTS, and Ig-Indel-Identifier (Ig Insertion–Deletion Identifier), a program for identifying legitimate and artifact insertions and/or deletions (indels). Our programs were designed for analyzing Ig gene sequences obtained by 454 sequencing, but they are applicable to all types of sequences and sequencing platforms. Ig-HTS-Cleaner and Ig-Indel-Identifier have been implemented in Java and saved as executable JAR files, supported on Linux and MS Windows (Michaeli et al., 2012).

The PCR reaction itself is a source of many errors. Best *et al.* (Best, Oakes, Heather, Shawe-Taylor, and Chain, 2015) have shown that gene amplification by PCR introduces substantial product heterogeneity, independent of primer sequence and bulk experimental conditions. This heterogeneity could be attributed both to inherited differences between different template DNA molecules, each of which may be randomly amplified to a different multiplicity, and to the inherent stochasticity of the PCR process. They concluded that PCR heterogeneity arises even when reaction and substrate conditions are kept as constant as possible and suggested that single molecule barcoding is essential in order to derive reproducible quantitative results from any protocol combining PCR with HTS. Single molecule barcoding is a method that uses unique molecular identifiers (UMIs; (Egorov et al., 2015; Kivioja et al., 2011; Turchaninova et al., 2016)), which are random strings of 10-15 nucleotides inserted into the primers during primer synthesis. Thus, if two or more identical sequences possess the same UMI, this multiplicity can be assigned to random PCR amplification, while identical sequences with different UMIs correspond to different molecules in the original DNA aliquot. The UMI method can also help correct sequencer errors, as each sequencing method has its own error profile (see, e.g., (Best et al., 2015; Loman et al., 2012)).

12.3 SECOND CHALLENGE: ANNOTATING SEQUENCES AND ASSIGNING THEM INTO CLONES

Sequence annotation, in the case of Ig genes, involves identification of the V and J segments (sometimes also D, though this is never very reliable) and of the part of the sequence each is derived from. There are many tools for this task, which differ in the databases they reply on and the method used for gene segment identification (Gaeta et al., 2007; Lefranc, 2003; Russ, Ho, and Longo, 2015; Volpe, Cowell, and Kepler, 2006). As explained in Section 12.2, assigning sequences into clonally-related groups is also not trivial. It is usually based on V and J gene segment identity and CDR3 region similarity. However, due to SHM, no fixed cutoff of similarity is appropriate for BCR genes. Instead, clustering-based algorithms are often used (Chen, Collins, Wang, and Gata, 2010).

12.4 THIRD CHALLENGE: ESTIMATING CLONAL SIZES AND OVERALL REPERTOIRE DIVERSITY

In basic IgV repertoire studies, the SHM problem was sometimes ignored by taking only one representative of each clone. However, this ignores the potential to extract information and insights from clone sizes and the mutations themselves. Thus, computational tools were developed for identifying the mutations and distinguishing them from PCR and sequencing errors (reviewed in (Pabst, Hazanov, and Mehr, 2015)). If the sequencing is based on genomic DNA, then the use of UMIs (Egorov et al., 2015; Kivioja et al., 2011; Turchaninova et al., 2016) can also supply the clone size information; however, if the original material was RNA, which enables the identification of the constant region and hence the isotype, then there is no way to know how many RNA molecules per cell were included in the sequences material. In the latter case, plasma cells would be over-represented relative to B cells in the resulting repertoire, unless the cells were pre-sorted according to subset.

12.5 B CELL RECEPTOR REPERTOIRE STUDIES IN HEALTH AND DISEASE

Several recent reviews have focused on the contribution of B cell repertoire studies to our understanding of the humoral immune system in general and its activity in certain diseases in particular (Boyd and Crowe, 2016; Calis and Rosenberg, 2014; Finn and Crowe, 2013; Mathonet and Ullman, 2013). Under certain conditions, one may find a general change in a property of the whole repertoire, such as CDR3 length distributions (Gibson et al., 2009; Pickman, Dunn-Walters, and Mehr, 2013). Assuming that clonal sizes are reliable, one may also address questions regarding overall repertoire diversity. Repertoire diversity, measured using tools borrowed from ecology (e.g., (Michaeli et al., 2014)), is a very interesting property to follow. It decreases during an immune response, as the repertoire becomes more clonal, and returns to pre-response levels thereafter (Ademokun et al., 2011). The latter return is sometimes impaired with aging (Tabibian-Keissar et al., 2016) where there is also a general repertoire diversity increase over time in peripheral blood (Dunn-Walters, 2016) and lymph nodes (Tabibian-Keissar et al., 2016), while surprisingly, the repertoires in the spleen show an opposite trend. Diversity may also decrease when a malignant clone takes over most of the space available for B cells, in which case it should return to higher levels after successful treatment (Warren, Matsen IV, and Chou, 2013). Finally, in certain immunodeficiencies, TCR and BCR repertoire diversity may also be reduced (Yu et al., 2014) or skewed (O'Connell et al., 2014).

More specific changes may occur in the frequencies of certain gene segments (Martin, Wu, Kipling, and Dunn-Walters, 2015) or even particular gene combinations (Michaeli et al., 2014). Over- or under-expression of particular gene segment combinations (relative to the expected based on the frequency of expression of each of the segments in the repertoire) may correspond to more than one clone using the same combination. Such cases are obviously common in responses to infections, e.g., with HIV (Hoehn et al., 2015), and in autoimmune or chronic inflammatory diseases (Hehle et al., 2015; Lomakin et al., 2014; Snir et al., 2015), as in both cases a limited number of antigenic epitopes may be driving the response. However, gene segment combinations over- or under-expressed in, e.g., autoimmune diseases were also found in B cell malignancies (Michaeli et al., 2014), possibly hinting at the connection between chronic inflammation and the eventual development of B cell malignancy.

12.6 SHM- AND LINEAGE TREE-BASED ANALYSIS METHODS: LINEAGE TREES

Despite the difficulties posed by SHM, many insights can be gleaned from analyzing the resulting mutations. Sometimes the mere existence of mutations is informative, as in the case of B cell chronic lymphocytic leukemia (B-CLL), where those patients with a mutated malignant clone have a better prognosis than those with a non-mutated malignant clone (Volkheimer et al., 2007). However, in most cases the identities, frequencies and locations of the mutations must be characterized. We have developed many methods of analysis of SHM, all of which rely on first creating the clonal lineage tree, for which we have written the program IgTree (Barak, Zuckerman, Edelman, Unger, and Mehr, 2008); sample trees are shown in Figure 12.1. The root of the tree is constructed from the germline segments from which the rearranged gene is composed, and a clonal consensus in the junction regions. Figure 12.2 shows the main steps in lineage tree generation, starting from the raw data.

Tree-based mutation identification is more precise than the common practice of merely counting mutations within groups of sequences, for the following reasons. First, there is no over-counting: if a mutation has occurred only once according to the deduced tree, it will only be counted once, even if it appears in many descendant sequences. Second, each mutation is identified relative to the nearest identifiable ancestor, and thus the nucleotide and amino acid changes are more precisely identified. Third, the IgTree algorithm can also identify reversion mutation, and fourth, it can deal with short gaps, assigning them to one mutational (insertion or deletion) event. Since the IgTree algorithm groups together identical sequences, but not if they came from different samples, it gives more precise information on clonal sizes. Thus, lineage tree analysis-based BCR/Ab repertoire analysis and diversity analyses are also more precise.

In some cases, merely drawing the lineage trees is highly informative. The tree structure can point at connections between sequences obtained from different tissues (Figure 12.3), isotypes or days of the response (Figure 12.4), different cell populations, and so on. Quantification of relationships between populations—as presented on the trees—is also possible (*manuscript in preparation*) and can be highly instructive.

Lineage trees also enable us to follow the history of the clone. One may express the receptors encoded by the sequences at each stage of diversification, thus directly following affinity maturation in antibodies of interest, as has been done for anti-HIV antibodies (e.g. Bonsignori et al., 2011). Alternatively, one may look at lineage trees from clones that were sampled more than once, and thus follow the dynamics—and even transformation—of malignant B cell clones, and glean information about disease ontogeny and course, as has been done for follicular lymphoma ((Carlotti et al., 2015) and *manuscript in preparation*) (Figure 12.5).

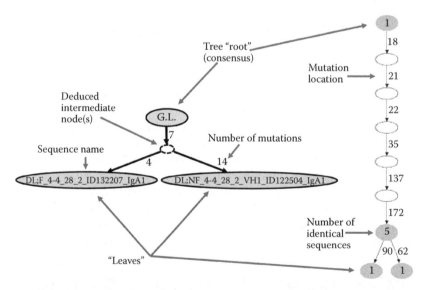

Figure 12.1 Sample lineage trees. In all trees, nodes correspond to sequences and edges to mutations. In the tree on the left, G.L. indicates the pre-mutation sequence, composed of germline-encoded segments and rearrangement junction nucleotides (tree "root"); the dashed ellipse indicates a sequence whose existence was deduced as a common ancestor to the sequences below it (tree "branching point"); and the two bottom ellipses (tree "leaves") indicate sequences found in the experiments, each showing the sequence name. The numbers next to the edges indicate the numbers of mutations separating the corresponding nodes. The tree on the right shows each mutation as a separate edge, with the mutation's location indicated next to it; since the order of mutations between tree root and the first branching point, or between two consecutive branching points, is always unknown, the mutations are ordered according to location on the sequence. The shaded nodes indicate sequences fund in the experiment, and the numbers within nodes indicate the numbers of separate sequences represented by the node.

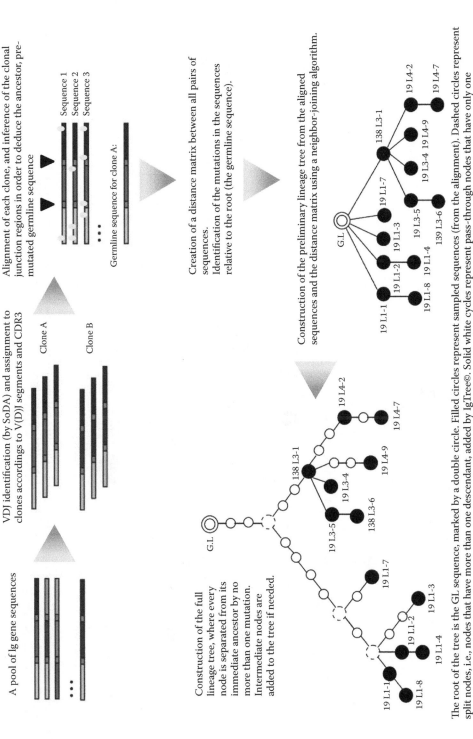

A pool of Ig gene sequences

VDJ identification (by SoDA) and assignment to clones accordings to V(D)J segments and CDR3

Clone A

Clone B

Alignment of each clone, and inference of the clonal junction regions in order to deduce the ancestor, premutated germline sequence

Sequence 1
Sequence 2
Sequence 3

Germline sequence for clone A:

Creation of a distance matrix between all pairs of sequences.
Identification of the mutations in the sequences relative to the root (the germline sequence).

Construction of the preliminary lineage tree from the aligned sequences and the distance matrix using a neighbor-joining algorithm.

Construction of the full lineage tree, where every node is separated from its immediate ancestor by no more than one mutation. Intermediate nodes are added to the tree if needed.

The root of the tree is the GL sequence, marked by a double circle. Filled circles represent sampled sequences (from the alignment). Dashed circles represent split nodes, i.e, nodes that have more than one descendant, added by IgTree©. Solid white cycles represent pass-through nodes that have only one descendant representing one mutation, added by IgTree©. The names of the sequences appears next to the sampled nodes [63].

Figure 12.2 The analysis steps leading from a pool of sequences to lineage trees.

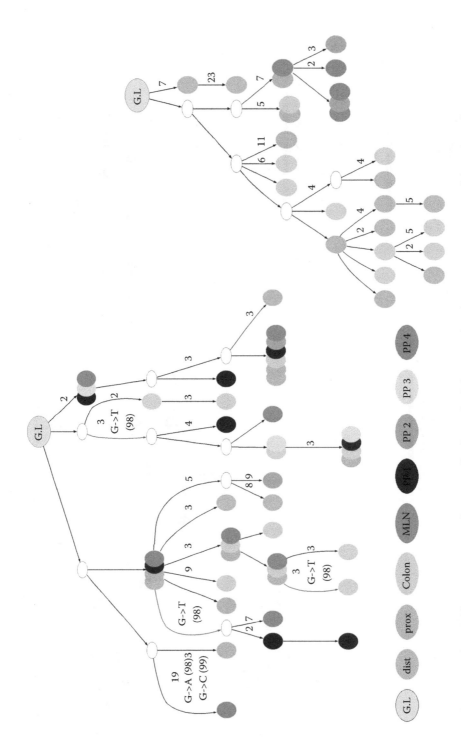

Figure 12.3 Clonal trees obtained from antigen-specific IgA B-cells after oral immunization show how responses are spread throughout the entire gut immune system. (From Bergqvist, P. et al., *Mucosal Immunology*, 6(1), 122-135, https://doi.org/10.1038/mi.2012.56, 2012.) (Bergqvist et al., 2012.) "G>T (98)" denotes a key mutation in position 98 that greatly increases the affinity to the antigen.

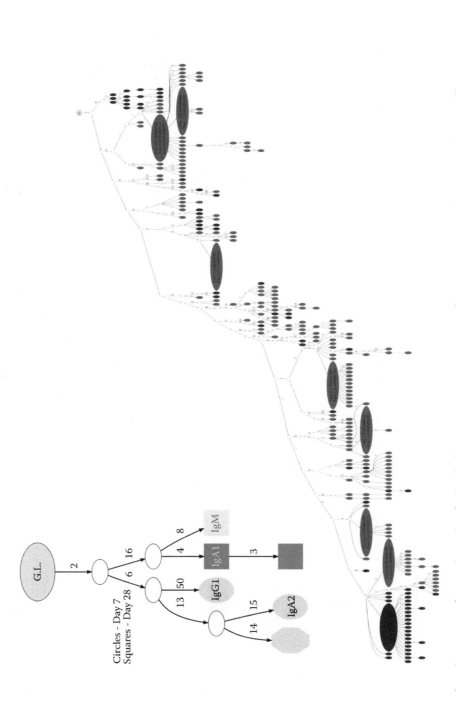

Figure 12.4 Left—a lineage tree from a clone identified in the human immune response to influenza vaccination showing switching to different isotypes in the same clone, while some of the B cells maintain the IgM isotype even 28 days post-immunization. (From Tabibian-Keissar, H. et al.,*European Journal of Immunology, 46(2),* 480–492, https://doi.org/10.1002/eji.201545586, 2016.) Right—a tree showing the mixing of IgA1 (dark gray) and IgA2 (gray) in one IgA clone in a human sample (O. Pabst's lab and ours, manuscript in preparation).

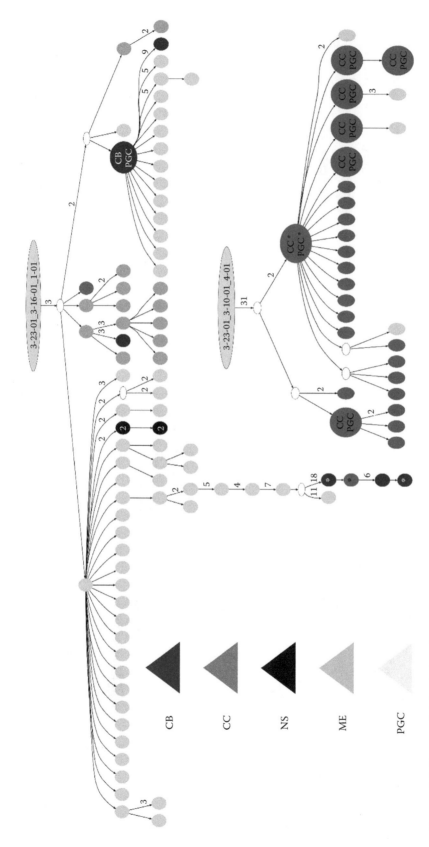

Figure 12.5 Two sample follicular lymphoma trees. (From Carlotti, E. et al., *PLoS ONE* 10(9), 1-20, https://doi.org/10.1371/journal.pone.0134833, 2015.) The root node in each tree contains a listing of the V, D, and J genes used in the corresponding Ig gene rearrangement. The different shades of gray correspond to different B cell phenotypes, as shown in the legend at left. The phenotypes are as follows: Pre-germinal center (PGC) (IgD+CD38+); germinal center centroblasts (CB) (IgD+CD38+CD10+CXCR4+); and centrocytes (CC) (IgD+CD38+CD10+CXCR4-); germinal center (PGC) (IgD+CD38+CD10+CXCR4+); and memory enriched (ME) (IgD-CD38-) B cells.

12.7 SHM- AND LINEAGE TREE-BASED ANALYSIS METHODS: LEARNING FROM THE MUTATIONS

Since lineage tree-based mutation identification is more precise, it is best to analyze the mutations introduced by SHM based on the list of mutations in each tree. The type of nucleotide substitution inserted by SHM depends on the particular DNA repair path used by the cell to resolve the initial U-G lesion created by AID (reviewed in (Hazanov and Michaeli, 2014)). Once all the mutations in all sequences are identified, various statistics—such as the fraction of mutations from/to each nucleotide, or the transition and transversion fractions—can be calculated and compared between samples (Zuckerman et al., 2010), sometimes leading to new insights regarding SHM.

SHM-introduced point mutations occur mostly in well-known "hotspot" motifs, such as RGYW/WRCY. Understanding SHM targeting may be aided by studying these AID targeting motifs. Our program PictoIg© (Zuckerman et al., 2010) identifies and enumerates sequence motifs up to 10 or more nucleotides upstream and downstream of the mutated location, based on previous studies limited to shorter sequence motifs (Spencer and Dunn-Walters, 2005). The program outputs sequence logos, where over- or under-represented nucleotides are drawn above or below the x axis, with the letter size proportional to the relative representation of the nucleotide in the given position, with indication of whether this relative representation is significantly different from that expected under a random process.

We also sometimes analyze the N-glycosylation motifs in the amino acid sequences. These motifs are defined as Asn-X-Ser/Thr, where X is any amino acid except proline; aspartate and glutamate are also disfavored in the X-position. Such motifs may be part of the rearranged pre-mutation sequence or be added to the sequence by SHM. N-glycosylation motifs have been identified in various B cell lymphomas (Forconi et al., 2004; Zhu et al., 2002a; Zhu et al., 2002b). We found (Hazanov, MSc thesis, Bar-Ilan University, 2010) that the number of existing glycosylation sites in the deduced pre-mutation heavy chain V gene sequences of the dominant clones of several lymphomas and in the deduced pre-mutation light chain V genes of Follicular Lymphoma were significantly higher than in normal controls. The number of new N-glycosylation motifs acquired through SHM was also significantly higher in lymphomas than in normal controls. The role of this increased N-glycosylation in lymphoma ontogeny and progression is so far unknown and would be interesting to elucidate.

The analysis of mutations, in particular when based on lineage tree structure, enables us also to address the question of which selection forces act on the diversifying B cell clones in a quantitative manner. Point mutations may be replacement (R) mutations, resulting in a change in the encoded amino acid or a silent (S) mutations, also called synonymous mutations as they do not lead to amino acid changes. Theoretically, a random mutation process in the absence of any selection would bring about an even distribution of R and S mutations throughout the diversifying gene. Out of 526 possible single base changes in the 61 codons of the 20 amino acids, ignoring stop codons, 392 produce R mutations and 134 are S mutations, leading to an expected ratio of R:S=2.925 (Jukes and King, 1979). This estimate is based on codon tables alone, ignoring the concept of "hot spots" and the fact that some codons are more "mutable", that is, susceptible to mutation, than others for the same amino acid. It has been taken to mean that a higher (lower) ratio than 2.925 indicates selection for (against) replacement mutations. An elaboration of this idea, using a binomial test to show where fractions of R mutations were significantly higher or lower than what is expected from random mutations under no selection, was presented in (Chang and Casali, 1994) and later improved by replacing the binomial by a multinomial model for the probability of excess or scarcity of R mutations in the complementarity determining regions (CDRs) or framework regions (FRs) of the variable region gene (Lossos, Tibshirani, Narasimhan, and Levy, 2000). All the above models, however, yield many false positives (Bose and Sinha, 2005; Dunn-Walters and Spencer, 1998). This and other issues were corrected by the "focused" binomial test (Hershberg, Uduman, Shlomchik, and Kleinstein, 2008; Uduman et al., 2011).

12.8 CURRENT LIMITATIONS AND FUTURE DIRECTIONS

While the study of Ig gene diversification and repertoires, as reviewed above, has been explosively accelerated in the last decade, much work is still needed in order to reach a fully standardized, automated analysis pipeline. It is still not easy to compare results of studies using the different analysis tools currently available in the BCR repertoire research community. The number of groups developing mutation analysis tools, in particular lineage-tree based ones, is even smaller. We are, however, confident that both experimental and computational method standards will emerge in the next few years. While efforts towards standardization are under way (see, e.g., http://airr.irmacs.sfu.ca/), the number of researchers and clinicians embarking on HTS studies of B cell repertoires is steadily growing. Deeper sequencing technologies may, in the future, enable the rapid reconstruction of any individual's genomic Ig gene segment library (Zehnder et al., 2010), thus paving the way to studies of the association between certain Ig gene segments of combinations and various diseases. Another application of deep REP-seq is the follow-up of T or B cell lymphoma clones during and after therapy, which—if standardized and made available for clinical use—would enable much earlier detection of relapses than the currently used standard blood tests. The number of studies of TCR and BCR repertoires and B cell lineages in infectious diseases, immunodeficiencies, chronic inflammatory and autoimmune diseases, and ageing is likely to continue growing rapidly in the foreseeable future, yielding unprecedented insights into the course of such diseases and suggesting avenues for therapy.

REFERENCES

Ademokun, A., Wu, Y.C., Martin, V., Mitra, R., Sack, U., Baxendale, H., … Dunn-Walters, D.K. (2011). Vaccination-induced changes in human B-cell repertoire and pneumococcal IgM and IgA antibody at different ages. *Aging Cell 10*(6), 922-930. https://doi.org/10.1111/j.1474-9726.2011.00732.x

Barak, M., Zuckerman, N.S., Edelman, H., Unger, R., and Mehr, R. (2008). IgTree (c): Creating immunoglobulin variable region gene lineage trees. *Journal of Immunological Methods, 338*(1-2), 67-74. JOUR. Retrieved from ISI:000259829600010

Bergqvist, P., Stensson, Hazanov, L., Holmberg, Mattsson, J., Mehr, R., … Lycke, N.Y. (2012). Re-utilization of germinal centers in multiple Peyer's patches results in highly synchronized, oligoclonal, and affinity-matured gut IgA responses. *Mucosal Immunology 6*(1), 122-135. https://doi.org/10.1038/mi.2012.56

Best, K., Oakes, T., Heather, J.M., Shawe-Taylor, J., and Chain, B. (2015). Computational analysis of stochastic heterogeneity in PCR amplification efficiency revealed by single molecule barcoding. *Scientific Reports 5*(November 2014), 14629. https://doi.org/10.1038/srep14629

Bonsignori, M., Hwang, K.-K., Chen, X., Tsao, C.-Y., Morris, L., Gray, E., … Haynes, B.F. (2011). Analysis of a clonal lineage of HIV-1 envelope V2/V3 conformational epitope-specific broadly neutralizing antibodies and their inferred unmutated common ancestors. *Journal of Virology 85*(19), 9998-10009. https://doi.org/10.1128/JVI.05045-11

Bose, B., and Sinha, S. (2005). Problems in using statistical analysis of replacement and silent mutations in antibody genes for determining antigen-driven affinity selection. *Immunology 116*(2), 172-183. https://doi.org/10.1111/j.1365-2567.2005.02208.x

Boyd, S.D., and Crowe, J.E. (2016). Deep sequencing and human antibody repertoire analysis. *Current Opinion in Immunology 40*, 103-109. https://doi.org/10.1016/j.coi.2016.03.008

Budeus, B., Schweigle de Reynoso, S., Przekopowitz, M., Hoffmann, D., Seifert, M., and Küppers, R. (2015). Complexity of the human memory B-cell compartment is determined by the versatility of clonal diversification in germinal centers. *Proceedings of the National Academy of Sciences 112*(38), E5281-E5289. https://doi.org/10.1073/pnas.1511270112

Calis, J.J.A., and Rosenberg, B.R. (2014). Characterizing immune repertoires by high throughput sequencing: Strategies and applications. *Trends in Immunology 35*(12), 581-590. https://doi.org/10.1016/j.it.2014.09.004

Carlotti, E., Wrench, D., Rosignoli, G., Marzec, J., Sangaralingam, A., Hazanov, L., … Gribben, J.G. (2015). High throughput sequencing analysis of the immunoglobulin heavy chain gene from flow-sorted B cell sub-populations define the dynamics of follicular lymphoma clonal evolution. *PLoS ONE 10*(9), 1-20. https://doi.org/10.1371/journal.pone.0134833

Chang, B., and Casali, P. (1994). The Cdr1 sequences of a major proportion of human germline Ig V-H genes are inherently susceptible to amino-acid replacement. *Immunology Today 15*(8), 367-373. JOUR. Retrieved from ISI:A1994NZ94100006

Chen, Z., Collins, A.M., Wang, Y., and Gata, B.A. (2010). Clustering-based identification of clonally-related immunoglobulin gene sequence sets. *Immunome Research 6*(SUPPL. 1), 1-7. https://doi .org/10.1186/1745-7580-6-S1-S4

Corcoran, L.M., and Tarlinton, D.M. (2016). Regulation of germinal center responses, memory B cells and plasma cell formation-an update. *Current Opinion in Immunology 39*, 59-67. https://doi.org/10.1016/j .coi.2015.12.008

Dunn-Walters, D.K. (2016). The ageing human B cell repertoire: A failure of selection? *Clinical and Experimental Immunology 183*(1), 50-56. https://doi.org/10.1111/cei.12700

Dunn-Walters, D.K., and Spencer, J. (1998). Strong intrinsic biases towards mutation and conservation of bases in human IgV(H) genes during somatic hypermutation prevent statistical analysis of antigen selection. *Immunology 95*(3), 339-345. JOUR. Retrieved from ISI:000076991800005

Egorov, E.S., Merzlyak, E.M., Shelenkov, A.A., Britanova, O.V., Sharonov, G.V., Staroverov, D.B., ... Chudakov, D.M. (2015). Quantitative profiling of immune repertoires for minor lymphocyte counts using unique molecular identifiers. *Journal of Immunology 194*(12), 6155-6163. https://doi.org/10.4049 /jimmunol.1500215

Finn, J.A., and Crowe, J.E. (2013). Impact of new sequencing technologies on studies of the human B cell repertoire. *Current Opinion in Immunology 25*(5), 613-618. https://doi.org/10.1016/j.coi.2013.09.010

Forconi, F., Capello, D., Berra, E., Rossi, D., Gloghini, A., Cerri, M., ... Gaidano, G. (2004). Incidence of novel N-glycosylation sites in the B-cell receptor of lymphomas associated with immunodeficiency. *British Journal of Haematology 124*(5), 604-609. JOUR. Retrieved from ISI:000189304300004

Gaeta, B.A., Malming, H.R., Jackson, K.J.L., Bain, M.E., Wilson, P., and Collins, A.M. (2007). iHMMune-align: hidden Markov model-based alignment and identification of germline genes in rearranged immuno-globulin gene sequences. *Bioinformatics 23*(13), 1580-1587. JOUR. Retrieved from ISI:000248620400002

Gibson, K.L., Wu, Y.C., Barnett, Y., Duggan, O., Vaughan, R., Kondeatis, E., ... Dunn-Walters, D.K. (2009). B-cell diversity decreases in old age and is correlated with poor health status. *Aging Cell 8*(1), 18-25. JOUR. Retrieved from ISI:000262877900002

Hazanov H., Michaeli M., Lavy-Shahaf, G. and Mehr, R. (2014). Informatic tools for immunoglobulin gene sequence analysis. In A.K. Kaushik and Y. Pasman (Ed.), *Comparative immunoglobulin Genetics* (pp. 223-240). Waretown, NJ: Apple Academic Press, Inc.

Hehle, V., Fraser, L.D., Tahir, R., Kipling, D., Wu, Y.-C., Lutalo, P.M.K., ... Spencer, J. (2015). Immunoglobulin kappa variable region gene selection during early human B cell development in health and systemic lupus erythematosus. *Molecular Immunology 65*(2), 215-223. https://doi.org/10.1016/j.molimm.2015.01.017

Hershberg, U., Uduman, M., Shlomchik, M.J., and Kleinstein, S.H. (2008). Improved methods for detecting selection by mutation analysis of Ig V region sequences. *International Immunology 20*(5), 683-694. JOUR. Retrieved from ISI:000255325200005

Hoehn, K.B., Gall, A., Bashford-Rogers, R., Fidler, S.J., Kaye, S., Weber, J.N., ... Pybus, O.G. (2015). Dynamics of immunoglobulin sequence diversity in HIV-1 infected individuals. *Philosophical Transactions of the Royal Society of London. Series B, Biological Sciences 370*(1676), 20140241-. https://doi.org/10.1098/rstb .2014.0241

Jukes, T.H., and King, J.L. (1979). Evolutionary nucleotide replacements in Dna. *Nature 281*(5732), 605-606. JOUR. Retrieved from ISI:A1979HQ78400072

Kivioja, T., Vähärautio, A., Karlsson, K., Bonke, M., Enge, M., Linnarsson, S., and Taipale, J. (2011). Counting absolute numbers of molecules using unique molecular identifiers. *Nature Methods 9*(1), 72-74. https:// doi.org/10.1038/nmeth.1778

Lefranc, M.P. (2003). IMGT databases, web resources and tools for immunoglobulin and T cell receptor sequence analysis, http://imgt.cines.fr. *Leukemia 17*(1), 260-266. https://doi.org/10.1038/sj.leu.2402637 \r2402637 [pii]

Lomakin, Y.A., Zakharova, M.Y., Stepanov, A.V., Dronina, M.A., Smirnov, I.V., Bobik, T.V., ... Gabibov, A.G. (2014). Heavy-light chain interrelations of MS-associated immunoglobulins probed by deep sequencing and rational variation. *Molecular Immunology 62*(2), 305-314. https://doi.org/10.1016/j .molimm.2014.01.013

Loman, N.J., Misra, R.V., Dallman, T.J., Constantinidou, C., Gharbia, S.E., Wain, J., and Pallen, M.J. (2012). Performance comparison of benchtop high-throughput sequencing platforms. *Nature Biotechnology 30*(5), 434-439. https://doi.org/10.1038/nbt.2198

Lossos, I.S., Tibshirani, R., Narasimhan, B., and Levy, R. (2000). The inference of antigen selection on Ig genes. *Journal of Immunology 165*(9), 5122-5126. JOUR. Retrieved from ISI:000090076000047

Marquet, M., Garot, A., Bender, S., Carrion, C., Rouaud, P., Lecardeur, S., ... Pinaud, E. (2014). The Eµ enhancer region influences H chain expression and B cell fate without impacting IgVH repertoire and immune response in vivo. *Journal of Immunology 193*(3), 1171-1183. https://doi.org/10.4049/jimmunol.1302868

Martin, V., Wu, Y.C., Kipling, D., and Dunn-Walters, D.K. (2015). Age-related aspects of human IgM+ B cell heterogeneity. *Annals of the New York Academy of Sciences 1362*(1), 153-163. https://doi.org/10.1111 /nyas.12823

Mathonet, P., and Ullman, C.G. (2013). The application of next generation sequencing to the understanding of antibody repertoires. *Frontiers in Immunology 4*(SEP), 1-5. https://doi.org/10.3389/fimmu.2013.00265

Michaeli, M., Barak, M., Hazanov, L., Noga, H., and Mehr, R. (2013). Automated analysis of immunoglobulin genes from high-throughput sequencing: Life without a template. *Journal of Clinical Bioinformatics 3*(1), 15. https://doi.org/10.1186/2043-9113-3-15

Michaeli, M., Noga, H., Tabibian-Keissar, H., Barshack, I., and Mehr, R. (2012). Automated cleaning and pre-processing of immunoglobulin gene sequences from high-throughput sequencing. *Frontiers in Immunology 3*(DEC), 1-16. https://doi.org/10.3389/fimmu.2012.00386

Michaeli, M., Tabibian-Keissar, H., Schiby, G., Shahaf, G., Pickman, Y., Hazanov, L., ... Mehr, R. (2014). Immunoglobulin gene repertoire diversification and selection in the stomach - from gastritis to gastric lymphomas. *Frontiers in Immunology 5*(JUN), 1-14. https://doi.org/10.3389/fimmu.2014.00264

Moorhouse, M.J., van Zessen, D., IJspeert, H., Hiltemann, S., Horsman, S., van der Spek, P.J., ... Stubbs, A.P. (2014). ImmunoGlobulin galaxy (IGGalaxy) for simple determination and quantitation of immunoglobulin heavy chain rearrangements from NGS. *BMC Immunology 15*(1), 59. https://doi.org/10.1186/s12865-014-0059-7

O'Connell, A.E., Volpi, S., Dobbs, K., Fiorini, C., Tsitsikov, E., de Boer, H., ... Notarangelo, L.D. (2014). Next generation sequencing reveals skewing of the T and B cell receptor repertoires in patients with Wiskott-Aldrich syndrome. *Frontiers in Immunology 5*(JUL). https://doi.org/10.3389/fimmu.2014.00340

Pabst, O., Hazanov, H., and Mehr, R. (2015). Old questions, new tools: Does next-generation sequencing hold the key to unraveling intestinal B-cell responses? *Mucosal Immunology 8*(1), 29-37. https://doi .org/10.1038/mi.2014.103

Pickman, Y., Dunn-Walters, D., and Mehr, R. (2013). BCR CDR3 length distributions differ between blood and spleen and between old and young patients, and TCR distributions can be used to detect myelodys-plastic syndrome. *Phys Biol 10*(5), 56001. https://doi.org/10.1088/1478-3975/10/5/056001

Robins, H. (2013). Immunosequencing: applications of immune repertoire deep sequencing. *Current Opinion in Immunology 25*(5), 646-652. https://doi.org/10.1016/j.coi.2013.09.017

Russ, D.E., Ho, K.-Y., and Longo, N.S. (2015). HTJoinSolver: Human immunoglobulin VDJ partitioning using approximate dynamic programming constrained by conserved motifs. *BMC Bioinformatics 16*(1), 1-11. https://doi.org/10.1186/s12859-015-0589-x

Schaller, S., Weinberger, J., Jimenez-Heredia, R., Danzer, M., Oberbauer, R., Gabriel, C., and Winkler, S.M. (2015). ImmunExplorer (IMEX): a software framework for diversity and clonality analyses of immu-noglobulins and T cell receptors on the basis of IMGT/HighV-QUEST preprocessed NGS data. *BMC Bioinformatics 16*(1), 252. https://doi.org/10.1186/s12859-015-0687-9

Snir, O., Mesin, L., Gidoni, M., Lundin, K.E.A., Yaari, G., and Sollid, L.M. (2015). Analysis of celiac dis-ease autoreactive gut plasma cells and their corresponding memory compartment in peripheral blood using high-throughput sequencing. *Journal of Immunology 194*(12), 5703-5712. https://doi.org/10.4049 /jimmunol.1402611

Spencer, J., and Dunn-Walters, D.K. (2005). Hypermutation at A-T base pairs: the A nucleotide replacement spectrum is affected by adjacent nucleotides and there is no reverse complementarity of sequences flanking mutated A and T nucleotides. *Journal of Immunology 175*(8), 5170-5177. https://doi.org/10.4049/jimmunol.175.8.5170

Tabibian-Keissar, H., Hazanov, L., Schiby, G., Rosenthal, N., Rakovsky, A., Michaeli, M., ... Barshack, I. (2016). Aging affects B-cell antigen receptor repertoire diversity in primary and secondary lymphoid tissues. *European Journal of Immunology 46*(2), 480-492. https://doi.org/10.1002/eji.201545586

Turchaninova, M.A., Davydov, A., Britanova, O.V., Shugay, M., Bikos, V., Egorov, E.S., ... Chudakov, D.M. (2016). High-quality full-length immunoglobulin profiling with unique molecular barcoding. *Nat Protocols 11*(9), 1599-1616. https://doi.org/10.1038/nprot.2016.093

Uduman, M., Yaari, G., Hershberg, U., Stern, J.A., Shlomchik, M.J., and Kleinstein, S.H. (2011). Detecting selection in immunoglobulin sequences. *Nucleic Acids Research 39*(SUPPL. 2), 1-6. https://doi.org/10.1093/nar/gkr413

Vander Heiden, J.A., Yaari, G., Uduman, M., Stern, J.N.H., O'Connor, K.C., Hafler, D.A., ... Kleinstein, S.H. (2014). PRESTO: A toolkit for processing high-throughput sequencing raw reads of lymphocyte receptor repertoires. *Bioinformatics 30*(13), 1930-1932. https://doi.org/10.1093/bioinformatics/btu138

Victora, G.D., and Mesin, L. (2014). Clonal and cellular dynamics in germinal centers. *Current Opinion in Immunology 28*(1), 90-96. https://doi.org/10.1016/j.coi.2014.02.010

Victora, G.D., and Nussenzweig, M.C. (2012). Germinal centers. *Annu Rev Immunol 30*, 429-457. https://doi.org/10.1146/annurev-immunol-020711-075032

Volkheimer, A.D., Weinberg, J.B., Beasley, B.E., Whitesides, J.F., Gockerman, J.P., Moore, J.O., ... Levesque, M.C. (2007). Progressive immunoglobulin gene mutations in chronic lymphocytic leukemia: Evidence for antigen-driven intraclonal diversification. *Blood 109*(0006–4971 (Print)), 1559-1567. JOUR.

Volpe, J.M., Cowell, L.G., and Kepler, T.B. (2006). SoDA: implementation of a 3D alignment algorithm for inference of antigen receptor recombinations. *Bioinformatics 22*(4), 438-444. JOUR. Retrieved from ISI:000235277300008

Warren, E.H., Matsen IV, F.A., and Chou, J. (2013). High-throughput sequencing of B- And T-lymphocyte antigen receptors in hematology. *Blood 122*(1), 19-22. https://doi.org/10.1182/blood-2013-03-453142

Xu, Z., Zan, H., Pone, E.J., Mai, T., and Casali, P. (2012). Immunoglobulin class-switch DNA recombination: Induction, targeting and beyond. *Nature Reviews. Immunology 12*(7), 517-531. https://doi.org/10.1038/nri3216

Yu, X., Almeida, J.R., Darko, S., Van Der Burg, M., Deravin, S.S., Malech, H., ... Milner, J.D. (2014). Human syndromes of immunodeficiency and dysregulation are characterized by distinct defects in T-cell receptor repertoire development. *Journal of Allergy and Clinical Immunology 133*(4), 1109-1115.e14. https://doi.org/10.1016/j.jaci.2013.11.018

Zehnder, L., Collins, A.M., Nadeau, K.C., Egholm, M., Miklos, D.B., Birgitte, J., ... Zehnder, J.L. (2010). Individual variation in the germline Ig gene repertoire inferred from variable region gene rearrangements. *Journal of Immunology 184*, 6986-6992. https://doi.org/10.4049/jimmunol.1000445

Zhu, D.L., McCarthy, H., Ottensmeier, C.H., Johnson, P., Hamblin, T.J., and Stevenson, F.K. (2002a). Acquisition of potential N-glycosylation sites in the immunoglobulin variable region by somatic mutation is a distinctive feature of follicular lymphoma. *Blood 99*(7), 2562-2568. JOUR. Retrieved from ISI:000174559300040

Zhu, D.L., McCarthy, H., Ottensmeier, C.H., Johnson, P., Hamblin, T.J., and Stevenson, F.K. (2002b). High incidence of novel N-glycosylation sites in the immunoglobulin variable region genes of follicular lymphoma. *Blood 100*(6), 2270-2271. JOUR. Retrieved from ISI:000177884800053

Zuckerman, N.S., Hazanov, H., Barak, M., Edelman, H., Hess, S., Shcolnik, H., ... Mehr, R. (2010). Somatic hypermutation and antigen-driven selection of B cells are altered in autoimmune diseases. *Journal of Autoimmunity 35*(4), 325-335. https://doi.org/10.1016/j.jaut.2010.07.004

Quantitative modeling of mast cell signaling

LILY A. CHYLEK, DAVID A. HOLOWKA, BARBARA A. BAIRD, AND WILLIAM S. HLAVACEK

13.1 INTRODUCTION

Cells exist in environments that necessitate responses. Growth, death, movement, and other fundamental acts are all influenced by decisions made on the basis of environmental cues. Decision-making is mediated by cell signaling systems, which translate inputs into outputs through networks of interacting proteins, lipids, and other biomolecules.

A signaling process begins when a cell surface receptor interacts with an extracellular ligand and undergoes a change detectable within the cell. Two common examples of such changes are oligomerization and conformational alterations. From the receptor, multitudinous biochemical events can emanate. These events, which include catalysis of post-translation modifications and formation of multi-protein complexes, can culminate in consequences such as migration, secretion, and changes in gene expression.

To understand how cells make decisions, and to potentially predict and manipulate these decisions, we need to understand the process by which a signaling system translates inputs to outputs. We can uncover the pieces of this puzzle through experimental measurements, such as western blots revealing dynamics of protein phosphorylation or a microscopy image revealing locations of biomolecules. To integrate these puzzle pieces into a picture of the cell's inner workings, we need to assemble a model: a representation summarizing how we think the system works.

13.2 MODELS IN CELL BIOLOGY

Models are ubiquitous in biology. They often take the form of maps that show proteins connected by arrows that represent various types of influences or interactions. The value of these diagrams is that they provide a visual overview that can be comprehended more readily than a textual description of the system's components and connections. However, our ability to enumerate and illustrate such connections tends to outstrip our ability to predict the outcomes that those interactions lead to, especially when trying to account for the quantitative factors that are inherent to signaling systems, such as the number of copies of a protein, the affinity of an interaction, or relative competition among binding partners. Another compounding factor is the intricacy of the "wiring" itself: cell signaling systems are rife with feedback and feed-forward loops (Alon, 2007), cross-talk (Guo and Wang, 2009), and redundancies (Sun and Bernards, 2014). These factors contribute to a variety of behaviors that seem at first perplexing: hysteresis (Das et al., 2009), oscillations (Wollman and Meyer, 2012), and desensitization (Weetall et al., 1993). It can be difficult to develop an intuition about these phenomena. A strategy to extend our reasoning capabilities about these complex and quantitative systems is to make our maps executable: to represent biomolecular interactions in a way that enables a computer to simulate them.

A spectrum of approaches has been used to model aspects of cell signaling, from molecular dynamics simulations of molecular movements on the sub-nanosecond timescale (Karplus and McCammon, 2002) to Boolean networks representing a coarse-grained view of the overall network (Albert and Thakar, 2014). Here, we will focus on models based on chemical kinetics (Aldridge et al., 2006) because they combine features that are especially relevant for studying cell signaling in a combined modeling-experimental framework: 1) these models take into account laws of physics and chemistry that govern molecular interactions, 2) they have the potential to encompass a large set of proteins, and 3) they can be used to simulate timescales from seconds to minutes to hours, which are timescales on which experimental measurements are commonly performed. We will focus on IgE receptor signaling, which is of special interest because it has been modeled from ligand-receptor binding up to second messenger generation and because the role of aggregation in initiation of signaling is relatively well-understood.

13.3 QUANTITATIVE ANALYSIS OF IgE RECEPTOR SIGNALING

One of the earliest signaling systems to be investigated through mathematical modeling and quantitative experiments is signaling via the high-affinity receptor for IgE, also known as FcεRI (Dembo and Goldstein, 1978). This multi-subunit receptor is found on the surface of mast cells and basophils. Stimulation of this receptor can lead to release of histamine and other mediators that are involved in the allergic immune response (Kraft and Kinet, 2007). Additionally, IgE receptor signaling is similar to signaling by other antigen recognition receptors, so studying this system has relevance for general understanding of immunity beyond allergies.

FcεRI forms a stable, one-to-one complex with an IgE antibody (McDonnell et al., 2001), which is specific to a particular antigen. IgE is bivalent for antigen binding, meaning that its two Fab arms can each bind to a separate antigen site. Antigens that are multivalent are capable of cross-linking multiple receptors and forming receptor aggregates. These aggregates can initiate signaling by allowing kinases co-localized with clustered receptors to phosphorylate neighboring receptors. The resulting signaling cascade, including influx of extracellular Ca^{2+}, leads to release of pre-formed inflammatory mediators in a process called degranulation (Figure 13.1). Aggregation is the mode of signal initiation used by other immunoreceptors, as well as a process found at various stages of diverse signaling systems. For example, aggregation of the adaptor protein LAT, for which mathematical models have been developed (Chylek et al., 2014d), is an aspect of T-cell receptor (TCR) signaling (Balagopalan et al., 2015). The parallels between FcεRI and other signaling systems make it a useful model system.

The mast cell system offers an unusual level of experimental tractability. One reason is that the antigen the cells will respond to is determined by the specificity of the IgE antibodies that are bound to cell-surface FcεRI. Exposing cells to different IgEs, separately or in combination, results in cells that are responsive to different (combinations of) stimuli.

Additionally, a variety of synthetic antigens can be constructed by attaching small molecules recognized by antibodies, called haptens, to polymer scaffolds; these ligands can then bind to hapten-specific IgE. This feature has been leveraged to study a wide range of structurally distinct ligands, which give rise to a variety

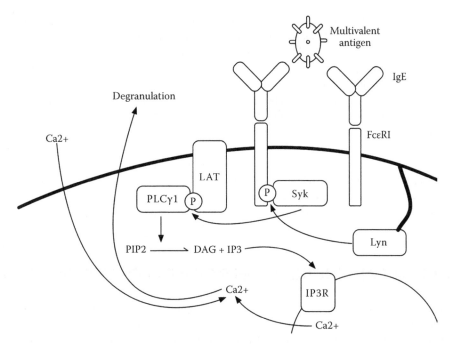

Figure 13.1 An illustration of molecules involved in initiation of IgE receptor signaling. A one-to-one complex is formed between FcεRI and an IgE antibody. Each of the IgE's two Fab arms is capable of interacting with an antigen. A multivalent antigen is able to cross-link (aggregate) two or more IgE-receptor complexes. These receptor aggregates can then undergo phosphorylation by the kinase Lyn, which is tethered to the membrane via palmitoylation and myristolation. Lyn associates with receptors via its intrinsically disordered unique domain and/or through colocalization in lipid rafts (Holowka et al., 2005, Young et al., 2003). Lyn phosphorylates the receptor at several residues in its cytoplasmic subunits, each of which contains an immunoreceptor tyrosine-based activation motif (ITAM). An ITAM contains two tyrosine residues that can be phosphorylated. The beta subunit ITAM contains an atypical third tyrosine. The N-terminal tyrosine in the beta ITAM, when phosphory-lated, can associate with the SH2 domain of Lyn. The pair of disulfide-linked gamma subunits each contain one ITAM that, when doubly phosphorylated, can associate with the tandem Src homology 2 (SH2) domains of the kinase Syk. Syk can then proceed to phosphorylate an array of downstream targets, including the adaptor Lat, which can then bind to phospholipase Cγ1 (Plcg1). Plcg1 cleaves the phospholipid PIP2, yielding diacylglycerol (DAG) and inositol trisphosphate (IP3). Interactions of IP3 with the IP3 receptor on the endoplasmic reticulum leads to calcium mobilization. Store-operated calcium entry (SOCE) enables influx of extracellular calcium into the cytoplasm. These events enable release of inflammatory mediators through degranulation.

of responses. One of the most commonly used ligands is DNP-BSA, which is a bovine serum albumin (BSA) molecule conjugated to multiple 2,4-dinitrophenyl (DNP) haptens. This ligand stimulates robust signaling and degranulation, but a drawback is that it is chemically heterogeneous; different DNP-BSA molecules may bear different numbers of DNP groups, and two molecules with the same number of DNP groups may have them conjugated to different lysine residues of the protein. Thus, the mechanisms of ligand-receptor interactions are difficult to deconvolute. More controlled ligands have been constructed and used to shed light on what qualities of a ligand influence the signaling response.

Valency has been found to be an important factor. Monovalent ligands, such as DNP-lysine and DNP-aminocaproyl-L-tyrosine (DCT) fail to stimulate signaling because they do not enable formation of receptor aggregates. Nevertheless, monovalent ligands are a useful tool for studying inhibition of signals triggered by multivalent ligands, because an excess of monovalent ligand is capable of breaking up aggregates (Subramanian et al., 1996), leading to downregulation of signaling.

Most bivalent ligands generate minimal degranulation (Paar et al., 2002), suggesting that the kind of aggregates that they form do not stimulate sufficient signaling within the cell. However, it is worth noting that some bivalent antibodies that bind to FcεRI directly do stimulate signaling (Ortega et al., 1988), suggesting that the steric constraints and/or binding properties of different ligands may have a deciding effect.

Trivalent ligands tend to stimulate a more robust range of cellular responses. A set of trivalent ligands built on a rigid double-stranded DNA scaffold revealed that the longer the length of the scaffold, the weaker the resulting degranulation and phosphorylation of most, but not all, signaling proteins, including the receptor itself and the adaptor protein Lat (Sil et al., 2007). Degranulation decreased with ligand length, as did stimulated Ca^{2+} mobilization, but in a less drastic manner. These results support the concept of transphosphorylation by receptor-associated kinases being important to early signaling, with larger distances between receptors reducing the efficiency of transphosphorylation. These results also point to the existence of diverging pathways that enable some signaling components to be more independent of receptor phosphorylation than others.

Other trivalent DNP ligands include one built on a polyethylene glycol scaffold (Posner et al., 2007) and one consisting of a trimeric fibritin foldon domain bound to DNP (Mahajan et al., 2014). The range of ligands available for manipulating clustering of IgE-FcεRI complexes has enabled a controlled analysis of the intracellular information-processing system that connects inputs to outputs, and many of these analyses have included modeling.

13.4 CHEMICAL KINETIC MODELS OF IgE RECEPTOR SIGNALING

Most early modeling studies of this system focused on a prerequisite for receptor-mediated signaling: ligand-receptor binding. Models for the kinetics of the system took the form of ordinary differential equations (ODEs) that represented the changing concentrations of chemical species in the model, which were controlled by the processes of ligand capture, receptor crosslinking, and cyclization to form rings (Posner et al., 1991, Posner et al., 1995, Subramanian et al., 1996, Xu et al., 1998, Das et al., 2008). Equilibrium models in the form of algebraic expressions were also developed. Some of these models were fit to binding data, which often took the form of fluorescence measurements (Erickson et al., 1986). The fluorescence of IgE labeled with fluorescein isothiocyanate (FITC) is reduced in the presence of the hapten DNP. Thus, measurements of FITC fluorescence quenching can be translated to a quantity of IgE sites bound. Additionally, in some studies ligands were also fluorescently labeled and the amount of ligand bound to IgE was quantified, providing additional data for parameter estimation (Xu et al., 1998, Hlavacek et al., 1999). These combined modeling and experimental studies were used to postulate mechanisms and estimate rate constants involved in ligand-receptor binding.

These studies of events on the cell surface provided a starting point for investigations into what occurs inside the cell. In 1997, IgE receptor signaling became the subject of an early modeling study of intracellular signaling in a mammalian system (Wofsy et al., 1997) (Figure 13.2). Going beyond ligand-receptor interactions, this model was used to investigate the relationship between receptor aggregation, receptor phosphorylation, and association of aggregates with the kinase Lyn. The ligand considered in this model and the associated experiments was a covalently cross-linked dimer of IgE that can bind to a pair of receptors. Phosphorylation sites in the receptor were simplified to a single site. Such simplifications may or may not be appropriate and in general should be carefully evaluated (Chylek, 2013). Parameters for the model were obtained through a combination of published estimates and values obtained through fitting to experimental data. The model was used to make predictions about how Lyn is redistributed as receptor aggregates form. A conclusion of this study was that late-forming aggregates are less likely to contain Lyn than early-forming aggregates. However, the model also predicted that under some conditions, late-forming aggregates can recruit Lyn away from aggregates formed earlier. This prediction was confirmed experimentally, an example of how a model can help make a prediction that would be difficult to arrive at otherwise (Wofsy et al., 1997).

The next step in model development was addition of another kinase, Syk. However, this step required a rethinking of methodology. Recall that kinetic models for cell signaling systems tend to be built by writing ODEs, as in the seminal study of Kholodenko et al. (1999) of signaling by the epidermal growth factor receptor (EGFR). With this approach, an ODE must be written for every chemical species that is potentially populated in the system being modeled. As the number of interactions grows, the number of potentially populated species can explode. A model that included recruitment and activation of Syk entailed 354 distinct

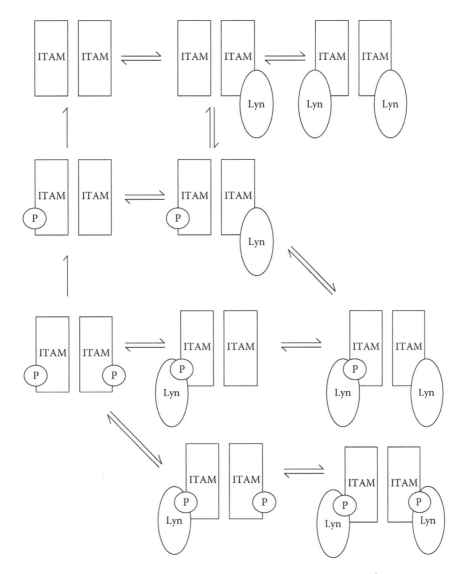

Figure 13.2 A subset of the reactions included in the model of Wofsy et al. (1997). These reactions represent interactions between a receptor dimer, crosslinked by a covalently-linked dimer of IgE, and Lyn kinase. Lyn can interact with an unphosphorylated receptor via its unique domain. Lyn can interact with a phosphorylated receptor via its SH2 domain. In this model, receptor phosphorylation sites are lumped together as one single phosphorylation site. This model does not explicitly include phosphatases. Phosphatase activity is implied in the rapid dephosphorylation of receptors that are not bound to Lyn. In addition to the reactions shown here, the model also contains reactions for binding between receptor and ligand (the IgE dimer).

species (Faeder et al., 2003). Despite its large size from the perspective of equations, from the perspective of molecules the model only contained four signaling molecules (a ligand, the receptor, Lyn, and Syk) out of the many that are known to be involved in mast cell signaling. It was apparent that continued progress in model development would necessitate a new approach to how we think about models.

13.5 THE ADVENT OF RULE-BASED MODELING

So far, models have been built on the notion of reactions, where each reaction describes the behavior of a very specific set of chemical species. The number of reactions can be reduced by making them less specific (more general), and thus less numerous. A way to do this is to describe a generalized reaction, called a rule, and to task a computer with enumerating the specific reactions (Chylek et al., 2014b; Chylek et al., 2015). A rule describes the necessary and sufficient conditions required for an interaction to occur. For example, a rule may state that for Lyn to bind a phosphorylated site in the receptor, Lyn must have an unbound SH2 domain and the phosphorylated site in the receptor must also be unbound. Any other molecular details that are assumed or known to not influence the interaction, such as phosphorylation and occupancy of other receptor sites, are omitted from the rule. A rule is a generalized representation of a reaction that could occur in many different instances that vary in their nonessential molecular details.

The specific, potentially numerous reactions implied by a set of rules can be enumerated by a program that processes the rules. From this point, ODEs can be derived from the list of reactions for numerical integration, or the reactions can be used as event generators in a stochastic simulation based on Gillespie's method (Gillespie, 2007). In this way, a signaling network can be represented, by the human modeler, using a relatively compact set of rules and the drudgery of translating those rules into reactions is performed by a computer program (Faeder et al., 2009).

Several languages and software packages have been developed to aid rule-based modeling. One of the most commonly used is BioNetGen. We will focus on BioNetGen, which enables both stochastic and deterministic simulations. In BioNetGen's modeling language, called BNGL, the connectivity of molecules of interest are represented essentially as graphs, along with their relevant internal components, which can include domains, motifs, and amino acid residues. If desired, components can have multiple possible states representing component properties such as location, post-translational modification status, conformation, or other variables.

For example, the text "Syk(tSH2,Y519~0~P)" is a string-based encoding of a graphical representation of the kinase Syk, which is taken here to contain a tandem pair of SH2 domains called tSH2 and a tyrosine called Y519. The text indicates that this tyrosine can either be unphosphorylated (0) or phosphorylated (P). An example of a rule is:

```
Syk(tSH2) + FcR(gITAM~PP) -> Syk(tSH2!1).FcR(gITAM~PP!1) k1
```

This rule states that the tSH2 domain in Syk can bind to a (doubly) phosphorylated ITAM in the gamma subunit of the IgE receptor. The bonded components are labeled with "!1". We are assuming that the phosphorylation state of the tyrosine in Syk, Y519, has no bearing on this interaction, and thus it is omitted from the rule. Reactions enumerated from this rule would include a reaction where Y519 in Syk is phosphorylated, and one where it is not phosphorylated. Both reactions would proceed with the same rate constant, k1. If we had reason to expect that the phosphorylation status of Y519 in Syk would affect binding of its tSH2 domain, which is true of some tyrosine residues in this kinase (Grädler et al., 2013), the rule could be modified to include its phosphorylation state.

The 2003 model for IgE receptor signaling that was developed using rule-based methods revealed the effects of kinase copy numbers, dephosphorylation kinetics, and how the beta subunit of the receptor can act as either an amplifier or inhibitor (Faeder et al., 2003).

13.6 REPRESENTING A SIMPLE REACTION NETWORK WITH RULES, REACTIONS, AND EQUATIONS

To illustrate how ODE-based and rule-based models represent the same chemical kinetics, we will go over a simple example toy model for IgE receptor signaling. We will assume that the IgE receptor has two binding sites, located in its beta and gamma subunits, for associating with the kinases Lyn and Syk, respectively, and that interactions with each kinase occurs independently of the other. We will consider the process by which the receptor becomes associated with both kinases.

The receptor (R) may first bind to Lyn (L), forming complex C_L, or it may first bind to Syk (S) forming complex C_S. From there, a final complex is formed when C_L binds to Syk or when C_S binds to Lyn. These complexes are illustrated in Figure 13.3a. This set of interactions implies four reactions, illustrated in Figure 13.3b.

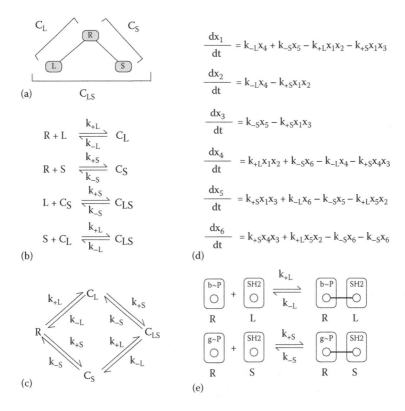

Figure 13.3 A comparison of representations of a chemical reaction network. **(a)** The receptor (R) can bind to Lyn (L) and to Syk (S). A complex of the receptor with Lyn only, the receptor with Syk only, and the receptor with both Lyn and Syk are named R_L, R_S, and R_{LS} respectively. **(b)** The list of reactions describing the binding processes of panel a. C_L is a complex of the receptor and Lyn only. C_S is a complex of the receptor and Syk only. C_{LS} is a complex of the receptor, Lyn, and Syk. **(c)** The reactions in this system form a reaction network. In the reaction scheme shown, vertices are receptor complexes, and the arrows between them represent the chemical reactions that account for formation or destruction of each species. Each reaction is associated with a rate constant. **(d)** The ordinary differential equations (ODEs) derived from the chemical reaction network. The variables x_1, x_2, x_3, x_4, x_5, and x_6 represent the concentrations of the species R, L, S, C_L, C_S, and C_{LS} respectively. These equations describe the changes of each species' concentration, as determined by reaction rates, over time. **(e)** The rules representing an equivalent set of reactions. These rules can be processed by rule-based modeling software to yield the reactions and equations shown in other panels of this figure, or used directly to advance the state of a system if one is using network-free simulation techniques (described later).

Each reaction is associated with a forward and reverse rate constant. We assume that the rate constant of Lyn or Syk binding is identical for when the other kinase is already bound to the receptor. Figure 13.3c organizes these reactions into a network that illustrates the receptor transitioning from fully unbound to fully bound.

From the reactions of Figure 13.3c, we can obtain the ODEs presented in Figure 13.3d. The variables x_1, x_2, x_3, x_4, x_5, and x_6 represent the concentrations of the species R, L, S, C_L, C_R, and C_{LS}, respectively. The equations describe the change in concentration of each of these species over time. The equations are found by considering which reactions either contribute to the formation or consumption of the species in question. For example, C_L is formed by binding of Lyn to the receptor, and consumed by dissociation of Lyn from the receptor (leaving L and R), as well as by binding of Syk (forming the next species, C_{LS}). We obtain terms in the equation by multiplying the rate constant by the concentration(s) of species involved in the reaction. The sum of these terms makes up the complete ODE. There are six ODEs in total.

In Figure 13.3e, we show the same process represented by rules. In each rule, we list the reaction centers in each molecule, that is, the part of the molecule that is involved in the interaction. For binding of Lyn to the receptor, the reaction centers are the phosphorylated beta subunit of the receptor (b~P) and the Lyn SH2 domain. For binding of Syk to the receptor, the reaction centers are the phosphorylated gamma subunit of

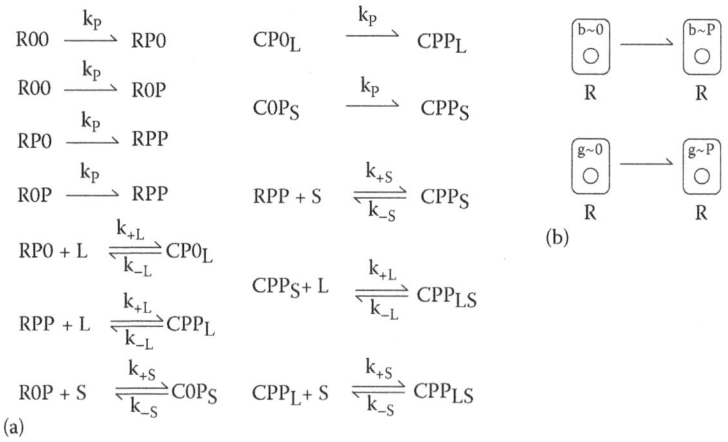

$$R00 \xrightarrow{k_p} RP0 \qquad CP0_L \xrightarrow{k_p} CPP_L$$

$$R00 \xrightarrow{k_p} R0P \qquad C0P_S \xrightarrow{k_p} CPP_S$$

$$RP0 \xrightarrow{k_p} RPP$$

$$R0P \xrightarrow{k_p} RPP \qquad RPP + S \underset{k_{-S}}{\overset{k_{+S}}{\rightleftharpoons}} CPP_S$$

$$RP0 + L \underset{k_{-L}}{\overset{k_{+L}}{\rightleftharpoons}} CP0_L$$

$$RPP + L \underset{k_{-L}}{\overset{k_{+L}}{\rightleftharpoons}} CPP_L \qquad CPP_S + L \underset{k_{-L}}{\overset{k_{+L}}{\rightleftharpoons}} CPP_{LS}$$

$$R0P + S \underset{k_{-S}}{\overset{k_{+S}}{\rightleftharpoons}} C0P_S \qquad CPP_L + S \underset{k_{-S}}{\overset{k_{+S}}{\rightleftharpoons}} CPP_{LS}$$

(a)

(b)

Figure 13.4 An extension to the model of Figure 13.3. **(a)** This panel shows the chemical reactions that would need to be written if one were to add a simple mechanism whereby receptors are phosphorylated via a first-order reaction. The species R00, RP0, R0P, and RPP represent, respectively, the receptor in an unphosphorylated form, phosphorylated at beta only, phosphorylated at gamma only, and phosphorylated at both sites. The same nomenclature extends to the complex species (C0P, CP0, and CPP). To turn these reactions into a system of ODEs, the equations of Figure 13.3d would have to be modified, and new equations would need to be written to account for the new species. **(b)** In contrast, only two additional rules would need to be added to the rules of Figure 13.3e for the model to be expanded. The original rules would not need to be modified.

the receptor (g~P) and the Syk SH2 domain. Because we assume that the other kinase does not affect the rate of the interaction, it is omitted from the rule. The first rule encompasses reactions 1 and 3 in Figure 13.3b, whereas the second rule encompasses reactions 2 and 4 in Figure 13.3b.

It is important to emphasize that this toy model is simplistic in multiple respects. One simplification is that the receptor is taken to be permanently in a phosphorylated state. To illustrate how the two modeling approaches fare when model extension is pursued, we will consider what happens when we include the receptor switching from an unphosphorylated to phosphorylated state.

In the reaction network, we would need to introduce an entirely new set of species to account for a receptor that is completely unphosphorylated, phosphorylated only at the beta chain, phosphorylated only at the gamma chain, and phosphorylated at both. (Each chain contains multiple tyrosine residues, but as a simplification we are lumping all of the sites in a given chain as a single site of phosphorylation.) We would then have to consider two versions of each of the receptor-kinase complexes, differing based on receptor phosphorylation state. We would also have to account for phosphorylation of a receptor site when the other site is phosphorylated and bound. The 12 reactions are shown in Figure 13.4a. There are a total of 10 distinct chemical species, and an equation would need to be written for each one.

In contrast, in the rule-based model we would only need to add two more rules, each describing the independent phosphorylation of one receptor site (Figure 13.4b). These rules can be combined with the rules of Figure 13.3e, without having to edit the original rules. From this example it can be seen that expanding the rule-based model to account for more details will be a faster (and less error-prone) task than writing the reactions and equations by hand.

13.7 TOWARDS COMPREHENSIVENESS AND MODULARITY

As our knowledge of signaling proteins grows, we want to develop models that encompass more molecular players, especially when we have ever-increasing ways to probe and quantify cellular behaviors. For example, mass spectrometry (MS) has made it possible to track phosphorylation states of hundreds to thousands of specific protein sites simultaneously (Cox and Mann, 2011). Super-resolution microscopy has revealed detailed pictures of how molecules spatially organize themselves within the cell (Shelby et al., 2013).

Microfludic evices make it possible to implement complex time-varying inputs and to monitor what cells do in response (Cheong et al., 2009). To remain relevant, modeling techniques have needed to advance to keep up with the array of directions in which experimental data are expanding.

One of these advances has been the development of new simulation techniques. Although generating reactions from a rule set is feasible for many models, for some models the number of possible reactions is too large for even this process to be manageable. In some cases, it is the result of the model including many different proteins in the signaling network. In other cases, there may be only a few different types of proteins that can, however, combine with each other in seemingly endless configurations. An example of such a situation is the problem of a bivalent receptor (e.g., the FcεRI-IgE complex) and a trivalent ligand (e.g., one of the several trivalent ligands described above). The branching aggregates that may arise in this scenario are too numerous to be enumerated (Yang et al., 2008, Monine et al., 2010), but as described above, it is a biologically relevant process and thus something that we would like to be able to simulate.

A solution to this problem came in the mid 2000's with the development of network-free simulation methods (Danos et al., 2007, Yang et al., 2008). As the name suggests, this method bypasses the step of generating a chemical reaction network by using the rules themselves as event generators in a stochastic simulation protocol based on kinetic Monte Carlo (Voter, 2007). Roughly, the rates of rules are calculated based on the properties of individually tracked sites in a model, and a waiting time is determined. A rule is selected for execution, reactive sites are selected, the system state is updated (through site state changes consistent with the selected rule), and time is incremented. Several variants of this algorithm exist and are encoded in the general-purpose software tools DYNSTOC (Colvin et al., 2009), RuleMonkey (Colvin et al., 2010), NFsim (Sneddon et al., 2011), and KaSim (http://www.kappalanguage.org/).

Taking advantage of network-free simulation, large models have been built and analyzed. An example is a large model for TCR signaling that, like FcεRI, is a multi-subunit immunoreceptor. The model was fit to MS-based time-resolved measurements of phosphorylation at specific protein sites that characterize signaling during the first 60 s of TCR stimulation, yielding an unprecedented number of matched simulation and experimental time courses, and the model was also found to be predictive (Chylek et al., 2014a). Another example of a large model is one for early events in EGFR signaling (Stites et al., 2015), which was also used to analyze proteomic datasets characterizing protein copy numbers in particular cell lines and affinities of protein-protein interactions. Recently developed fitting software (Thomas et al., 2016) will facilitate further efforts to optimize parameter values of large models so that these models are consistent with high-throughput experimental measurements.

In parallel with construction of these models, rigorous methods for model visualization and annotation were developed to handle the issue of how we can represent what a model contains and where the information comes from (Chylek et al., 2011). These methods include visualization of models as extended contact maps and their annotation with model guides. Model guides may take the form of a wiki (Creamer et al., 2012), pointing the way towards community-driven modeling efforts where new models can be built upon the old.

Recently, we used these visualization, simulation, and annotation techniques to develop a large model for IgE receptor signaling that also serves as a library from which more specialized models can be obtained (Chylek et al., 2014c). This model incorporates many features of IgE receptor signaling that had previously been part of separate signaling models. It also includes proteins and interactions that had not been considered in models before. A subset of components from this library was used to develop a model addressing a question raised in one of the differential ligand response studies discussed above (Sil et al., 2007): namely, why do some responses depend heavily on upstream phosphorylation whereas others do not? The model predicted that bistability in lipid synthesis, resulting from positive feedback loops, may be a factor. A model lacking positive feedback predicted that when phosphorylation of the adaptor Lat was reduced, all downstream outputs would be reduced to an equal or greater extent. In contrast, a model including a positive feedback loop involving the adaptor protein Gab2 and the lipid kinase phosphoinositide-3 kinase (PI3K) predicted that under some conditions, a subset of downstream outputs would be buffered from reductions in upstream phosphorylation. These results provide a possible explanation for why ligands that induce different levels of receptor phosphorylation can induce similar levels of some downstream phosphorylation targets: as long as upstream phosphorylation exceeds a minimum level, positive feedback can sustain robust activation of certain downstream pathways. These predictions are experimentally testable by, for example, disrupting the feedback loop through a knockdown or knockout of one of its components.

13.8 CONSIDERATIONS ON HOW A MODEL IS BUILT

A rule essentially states three pieces of information: (1) which molecules are interacting, (2) which sites are directly affected by the interaction (by becoming bound, unbound, or otherwise modified), and (3) which sites are not directly affected by the interaction but exert an influence on the interaction.

To explore what is meant by each piece of information, let us return to the example of Syk interacting with FcεRI, and model it in more detail by considering the two SH2 domains separately. We can write a rule stating that the N-terminal SH2 domain of Syk binds to the C-terminal tyrosine in the gamma ITAM of FcεRI, and that this interaction proceeds with a forward rate constant, k:

```
Syk(nSH2) + Rec(g_Y2) -> Syk(nSH2!1).Rec(g_Y2!1) k
```

We can also specify that the kinetics of the interaction are affected by whether the other SH2 domain of Syk is already bound to the receptor:

```
Syk(nSH2,cSH2) + Rec(g_Y2) -> Syk(nSH2!1,cSH2).Rec(g_Y2!1) k1
Syk(nSH2,cSH2!1) + Rec(g_Y1!1,g_Y2) -> Syk(nSH2!2,cSH2!1).Rec(g_Y1!1,g_Y2!2) k2
```

The first rule states that the C-terminal SH2 domain of Syk is unbound. The second rule states that this C-terminal SH2 domain is already bound to the receptor. The forward rate constant for this second rule, k2, will be larger than k1 because Syk is already tethered to the receptor, increasing the likelihood that the N-terminal SH2 domain will encounter its binding partner.

The primary literature is rich in information about biomolecular interactions. Many models are based on rules gleaned from potentially hundreds of individual studies of investigators who characterized signaling systems, one interaction at a time. These types of studies have been carried out using biochemical techniques such as immunoprecipitation (Markham et al., 2007) or more biophysical techniques like Förster resonance energy transfer (FRET) (Piston and Kremers, 2007). Other studies have used more high-throughput techniques, such as MS-based proteomics or protein microarrays, to identify a large number of interaction partners simultaneously (Hause et al., 2012). One consideration to keep in mind is to what extent different studies were performed under different conditions and whether this affects the compatibility of different data sets.

The specific sites involved in interactions have been uncovered by implementing mutations (e.g., mutating a particular tyrosine to a phenylalanine and determining whether a certain interaction is affected by the change). Some experiments have also shed light on what protein components, beyond the ones that are directly interacting, can influence the interaction. When this type of contextual information is available, it is usually a good idea to make a rule more specific by including it.

Once a rule is formulated, parameters, which can come from many different sources, must be supplied. The parameters for some specific interactions have been quantified through experimental studies. Sometimes these studies identify both forward and reverse rate constants, whereas others only identify the ratio of the two (in the form of an affinity or dissociation constant); this latter type of measurement is still useful because it constrains our estimates of rate constants.

Other interactions have not been studied at the level of affinities and rate constants, but measurements for analogous interactions can sometimes suggest a typical value. In cases where a specific value has not been determined, fitting (i.e., the optimization of parameter values to achieve simulated behavior matching experimental data) is useful. A general-purpose fitting tool compatible with software for rule-based modeling has recently been developed (Thomas et al., 2016). This tool implements a genetic algorithm that makes it possible to optimize multiple parameters simultaneously while also leveraging parallel computing resources.

As a modeler learns more about protein interactions and writes more rules, the model grows, and the eventual scope of a model must be defined. By scope, we mean how much of a network's proteins, protein components, and interactions should be included in a model. The answer is determined by the question that the model is being formulated to address. For example, if the goal is to develop a model that reproduces a defined set of experimental time courses of phosphorylation, the proteins containing phosphosites that were measured should be the focus of the model, along with any players needed to fill out the connections between them. In other cases, the scope might not be so clearly defined at first. For example, one might need to develop a model with the goal of reproducing a certain overall cellular behavior (e.g., desensitization) that could result from the confluence of multiple biochemical pathways (e.g., various positive and negative signals). There is no clear-cut procedure for deciding what to include in such a model, but the trial-and-error process of discovering which components of a network are needed to produce a specific behavior can be an informative and surprising undertaking in itself.

Although the literature contains a great deal of information about interaction networks, it doesn't spell out the answer to every question. Sometimes, possibilities that are not emphasized or even explored in individual studies can actually be significant when the system is regarded as a whole. The modeler's starting point is to take information that is already known, to turn it into an executable form, and to determine whether it forms a coherent picture or whether there are gaps that need to be filled.

How do we know when gaps exist? We begin by trying to ground a model in reality by comparing it to relevant experimental data and working towards agreement between the two (by including various known network components and exploring reasonable parameter values). The presence of gaps is suggested when a model seems like it should be able to match an experimental data set, but it cannot. Discrepancies between model and data are often the start of something interesting, because they indicate that some factor (in the model, experiments, or both) has not been considered.

Sometimes, to fill these gaps we need to propose new interactions that have not been reported before. At other times, we need to look at available information in a different way; it is possible that the necessary factors have already been found, but that their combined effect hasn't been appreciated. In either case, the model should then be used to make experimentally testable predictions that could be used to support or disprove the model.

For example, in the TCR modeling study discussed above, the authors found that the conventionally accepted pathway for recruitment of the protein WAS (WASP) to the T-cell receptor was insufficient to account for observed rapid dynamics of WAS phosphorylation. An alternative, shortcut pathway was needed. The shortcut's individual components had been described before, but had not been regarded as forming a pathway for fast recruitment of WAS. The model also pointed to previously uncharacterized roles for the tyrosine phosphatase PTPN6 (SHP1). Both aspects of the model were supported by experiments prompted for the purpose of testing the model (Chylek et al., 2014a) as well as in later studies (Paensuwan et al., 2015).

Model visualization is almost always helpful, especially if a model is large. In addition to making a model more understandable, visualisation can also serve as a basis for identification of network motifs, such as feedback loops (Chylek et al., 2014c).

The parameter values of a model can be explored in several ways. If there is reason to think that the model could exhibit bistability (the existence of two steady states, which can result from, for example, positive feedback), bifurcation analysis is a possibility. This type of analysis can be performed by incrementing a parameter from a low value to a high value and plotting the steady-state value of the resulting outputs for each value of that parameter. Then, the parameter is incremented from high to low, and outputs are plotted again. If there is a range of parameter values where a given output has a different value in the two cases (the low-to-high case and the high-to-low case), then that is a region of bistability. Bifurcation analysis has been employed in recent studies of B-cell antigen receptor signaling (Barua et al., 2012) and FcεRI signaling (Chylek et al., 2014c).

Another common type of analysis that can be applied to any model is sensitivity analysis, whereby a parameter is altered by a certain percentage, and then the difference in output values is quantified. The ratio of the two is a sensitivity coefficient that informs us about which parameters in the model have the greatest bearing on specific model behaviors (Barua et al., 2012).

In a similar vein, one can explore what a model does under the conditions of various "virtual experiments." Knockdowns, overexpressions, mutations, and the like can all be achieved by (usually straightforward) modifications of the model. For example, a knockdown is achieved by lowering the copy number of a protein, an overexpression by increasing copy number, and a mutation by modifying the functionality of a component in a protein. This type of exploration may reveal interesting directions for future studies.

At each step in the history of quantitative investigation of FcεRI signaling, the content of models has been determined by multiple factors, including the state of knowledge in the field, the type of experimental data available for comparison, and the status of modeling software itself. The models of FcεRI signaling form an example of how different considerations influence the content of a cell signaling model, and how the very concept of what a model is has grown over time, from a picture of interactions, to a system of equations, to an executable program of rules.

ACKNOWLEDGMENT

Funding from NIGMS/NIH (grant P50GM085273) is gratefully acknowledged.

REFERENCES

Albert, R. and Thakar, J. (2014). Boolean modeling: A logic-based dynamic approach for understanding signaling and regulatory networks and for making useful predictions. *Wiley Interdiscip Rev Syst Biol Med* 6, 353-369.

Aldridge, B.B., Burke, J.M., Lauffenburger, D.A., and Sorger, P.K. (2006). Physicochemical modelling of cell signalling pathways. *Nat Cell Biol 8*, 1195-1203.

Alon, U. (2007). Network motifs: Theory and experimental approaches. *Nat Rev Genet 8*, 450-456.

Balagopalan, L., Kortum, R.L., Coussens, N.P., Barr, V.A., and Samelson, L.E. (2015). The linker for activation of T cells (LAT) signaling hub: From signaling complexes to microclusters. *J Biol Chem 290*, 26422-26429.

Barua, D., Hlavacek, W.S., and Lipniacki, T. (2012). A computational model for early events in B cell antigen receptor signaling: Analysis of the roles of Lyn and Fyn. *J Immunol 189*, 646-658.

Cheong, R., Wang, C.J., and Levchenko, A. (2009). Using a microfluidic device for high-content analysis of cell signaling. *Sci Signal 2*, l2.

Chylek, L.A. (2013). Decoding the language of phosphorylation site dynamics. *Sci Signal 6*, jc2.

Chylek, L.A., Akimov, V., Dengjel, J., Rigbolt, K.T., Hu, B., Hlavacek, W.S., and Blagoev, B. (2014a). Phosphorylation site dynamics of early T-cell receptor signaling. *PLoS One 9*, e104240.

Chylek, L.A., Harris, L.A., Tung, C.S., Faeder, J.R., Lopez, C.F., and Hlavacek, W.S. (2014b). Rule-based modeling: A computational approach for studying biomolecular site dynamics in cell signaling systems. *Wiley Interdiscip Rev Syst Biol Med 6*, 13-36.

Chylek, L.A., Holowka, D.A., Baird, B.A., and Hlavacek, W.S. (2014c). An interaction library for the FcεRI signaling network. *Front Immunol 5*, 172.

Chylek, L.A., Hu, B., Blinov, M.L., Emonet, T., Faeder, J.R., Goldstein, B., Gutenkunst, R.N., Haugh, J.M., Lipniacki, T., Posner, R.G., Yang, J., and Hlavacek W.S. (2011). Guidelines for visualizing and annotating rule-based models. *Mol BioSyst 7*, 2779–2795.

Chylek, L.A., Wilson, B.S., and Hlavacek, W.S. (2014d). Modeling biomolecular site dynamics in immunoreceptor signaling systems. *Adv Exp Med Biol 844*, 245-262.

Chylek, L.A., Harris, L.A., Faeder, J.R., and Hlavacek, W.S. (2015). Modeling for (physical) biologists: An introduction to the rule-based approach. *Phys Biol 12*, 045007.

Colvin, J., Monine, M.I., Faeder, J.R., Hlavacek, W.S., Von Hoff, D.D., and Posner, R.G. (2009). Simulation of large-scale rule-based models. *Bioinformatics 25*, 910-917.

Colvin, J., Monine, M.I., Gutenkunst, R.N., Hlavacek, W.S., Von Hoff, D.D., and Posner, R.G. (2010). RuleMonkey: Software for stochastic simulation of rule-based models. *BMC Bioinformatics 11*, 404.

Cox, J. and Mann, M. (2011). Quantitative, high-resolution proteomics for data-driven systems biology. *Annu Rev Biochem 80*, 273-299.

Creamer, M.S., Stites, E.C., Aziz, M., Cahill, J.A., Tan, C.W., Berens, M.E., Han, H., Bussey, K.J., Von Hoff, D.D., Hlavacek, W.S., and Posner, R.G. (2012). Specification, annotation, visualization and simulation of a large rule-based model for ERBB receptor signaling. *BMC Syst Biol 6*, 107.

Danos, V., Feret, J., Fontana, W., Harmer, R., and Krivine, J. (2007). Rule-based modeling of cellular signaling. *Lect Notes Comput Sci 4703*, 17-41.

Das, J., Ho, M., Zikherman, J., Govern, C., Yang, M., Weiss, A., Chakraborty, A.K., and Roose, J.P. (2009). Digital signaling and hysteresis characterize Ras activation in lymphoid cells. *Cell 136*, 337-351.

Das, R., Baird, E., Allen, S., Baird, B., Holowka, D., and Goldstein, B. (2008). Binding mechanisms of PEGylated ligands reveal multiple effects of the PEG scaffold. *Biochemistry 47*, 1017-1030.

Dembo, M. and Goldstein, B. (1978). Theory of equilibrium binding of symmetric bivalent haptens to cell surface antibody: Application to histamine release from basophils. *J Immunol 121*, 345-353.

Erickson, J., Kane, P., Goldstein, B., Holowka, D., and Baird, B. (1986). Cross-linking of IgE-receptor complexes at the cell surface: A fluorescence method for studying the binding of monovalent and bivalent haptens to IgE. *Mol Immunol 23*, 769-781.

Faeder, J.R., Hlavacek, W.S., Reischl, I., Blinov, M.L., Metzger, H., Redondo, A., Wofsy, C., and Goldstein, B. (2003). Investigation of early events in FcεRI-mediated signaling using a detailed mathematical model. *J Immunol 170*, 3769-3781.

Faeder, J.R., Blinov, M.L., and Hlavacek, W.S. (2009). Rule-based modeling of biochemical systems with BioNetGen. *Methods Mol Biol 500*, 113-167.

Gillespie, D.T. (2007). Stochastic simulation of chemical kinetics. *Annu Rev Phys Chem 58*, 35-55.

Grädler, U., Schwarz, D., Dresing, V., Musil, D., Bomke, J., Frech, M., Greiner, H., Jäkel, S., Rysiok, T., Müller-Pompalla, D., and Wegener, A. (2013). Structural and biophysical characterization of the Syk activation switch. *J Mol Biol 425*, 309-333.

Guo, X. and Wang, X.F. (2009). Signaling cross-talk between TGF-β/BMP and other pathways. *Cell Res 19*, 71-88.

Hause, R.J. Jr, Leung, K.K., Barkinge, J.L., Ciaccio, M.F., Chuu, C.P., and Jones, R.B. (2012). Comprehensive binary interaction mapping of SH2 domains via fluorescence polarization reveals novel functional diversification of ErbB receptors. *PLoS One 7*, e44471.

Hlavacek, W.S., Perelson, A.S., Sulzer, B., Bold, J., Paar, J., Gorman, W., and Posner, R.G. (1999). Quantifying aggregation of IgE-FcεRI by multivalent antigen. *Biophys J 76*, 2421-2431.

Holowka, D., Gosse, J.A., Hammond, A.T., Han, X., Sengupta, P., Smith, N.L., Wagenknecht-Wiesner, A., Wu, M., Young, R.M., and Baird, B. (2005). Lipid segregation and IgE receptor signaling: A decade of progress. *Biochim Biophys Acta 1746*, 252-259.

Karplus, M. and McCammon, J.A. (2002). Molecular dynamics simulations of biomolecules. *Nat Struct Biol 9*, 646-652.

Kholodenko, B.N., Demin, O.V., Moehren, G., and Hoek, J.B. (1999). Quantification of short term signaling by the epidermal growth factor receptor. *J Biol Chem 274*, 30169-30181.

Kraft, S. and Kinet, J.P. (2007). New developments in FcεRI regulation, function and inhibition. *Nat Rev Immunol 7*, 365-378.

Mahajan, A., Barua, D., Cutler, P., Lidke, D.S., Espinoza, F.A., Pehlke, C., Grattan, R., Kawakami, Y., Tung, C.S., Bradbury, A.R., Hlavacek, W.S., and Wilson, B.S. (2014). Optimal aggregation of FcεRI with a structurally defined trivalent ligand overrides negative regulation driven by phosphatases. *ACS Chem Biol 9*, 1508-1519.

Markham, K., Bai, Y., and Schmitt-Ulms, G. (2007). Co-immunoprecipitations revisited: An update on experimental concepts and their implementation for sensitive interactome investigations of endogenous proteins. *Anal Bioanal Chem 389*, 461-473.

McDonnell, J.M., Calvert, R., Beavil, R.L., Beavil, A.J., Henry, A.J., Sutton, B.J., Gould, H.J., and Cowburn, D. (2001). The structure of the IgE Cε2 domain and its role in stabilizing the complex with its high-affinity receptor FcεRIα. *Nat Struct Biol 8*, 437-441.

Monine, M.I., Posner, R.G., Savage, P.B., Faeder, J.R., and Hlavacek, W.S. (2010). Modeling multivalent ligand-receptor interactions with steric constraints on configurations of cell-surface receptor aggregates. *Biophys J 98*, 48-56.

Ortega, E., Schweitzer-Stenner, R., and Pecht, I. (1988). Possible orientational constraints determine secretory signals induced by aggregation of IgE receptors on mast cells. *EMBO J 7*, 4101-4109.

Paar, J.M., Harris, N.T., Holowka, D., and Baird, B. (2002). Bivalent ligands with rigid double-stranded DNA spacers reveal structural constraints on signaling by FcεRI. *J Immunol 169*, 856-864.

Paensuwan, P., Ngoenkam, J., Khamsri, B., Preechanukul, K., Sanguansermsri, D., and Pongcharoen, S. (2015). Evidence for inducible recruitment of Wiskott-Aldrich syndrome protein to T cell receptor-CD3 complex in Jurkat T cells. *Asian Pac J Allergy Immunol 33*, 189-195.

Piston, D.W. and Kremers, G.J. (2007). Fluorescent protein FRET: The good, the bad and the ugly. *Trends Biochem Sci 32*, 407-414.

Posner, R.G., Erickson, J.W., Holowka, D., Baird, B., and Goldstein, B. (1991). Dissociation kinetics of bivalent ligand-immunoglobulin E aggregates in solution. *Biochemistry 30*, 2348-2356.

Posner, R.G., Geng, D., Haymore, S., Bogert, J., Pecht, I., Licht, A., and Savage, P.B. (2007). Trivalent antigens for degranulation of mast cells. *Org Lett 9*, 3551-3554.

Posner, R.G., Wofsy, C., and Goldstein, B. (1995). The kinetics of bivalent ligand-bivalent receptor aggregation: Ring formation and the breakdown of the equivalent site approximation. *Math Biosci 126*, 171-190.

Shelby, S.A., Holowka, D., Baird, B., and Veatch, S.L. (2013). Distinct stages of stimulated FcεRI receptor clustering and immobilization are identified through superresolution imaging. *Biophys J 105*, 2343-2354.

Sil, D., Lee, J.B., Luo, D., Holowka, D., and Baird, B. (2007). Trivalent ligands with rigid DNA spacers reveal structural requirements for IgE receptor signaling in RBL mast cells. *ACS Chem Biol 2*, 674-684.

Sneddon, M.W., Faeder, J.R., and Emonet, T. (2011). Efficient modeling, simulation and coarse-graining of biological complexity with NFsim. *Nat Methods 8*, 177-183.

Stites, E.C., Aziz, M., Creamer, M.S., Von Hoff, D.D., Posner, R.G., and Hlavacek, W.S. (2015). Use of mechanistic models to integrate and analyze multiple proteomic datasets. *Biophys J 108*, 1819-1829.

Subramanian, K., Holowka, D., Baird, B., and Goldstein, B. (1996). The Fc segment of IgE influences the kinetics of dissociation of a symmetrical bivalent ligand from cyclic dimeric complexes. *Biochemistry 35*, 5518-5527.

Sun, C. and Bernards, R. (2014). Feedback and redundancy in receptor tyrosine kinase signaling: Relevance to cancer therapies. *Trends Biochem Sci 39*, 465-474.

Thomas, B.R., Chylek, L.A., Colvin, J., Sirimulla, S., Clayton, A.H., Hlavacek, W.S., and Posner, R.G. (2016). BioNetFit: A fitting tool compatible with BioNetGen, NFsim, and distributed computing environments. *Bioinformatics 32*, 798-800.

Voter, A.F. (2007). Introduction to the kinetic Monte Carlo method. In K.E. Sickafus, E.A. Kotomin, and B.P. Uberuaga (Eds.), *Radiation Effects in Solids* (pp. 1-21). Dordrecht: Springer.

Weetall, M., Holowka, D., and Baird, B. (1993). Heterologous desensitization of the high affinity receptor for IgE (FcεR1) on RBL cells. *J Immunol 150*, 4072-4083.

Wofsy, C., Torigoe, C., Kent, U.M., Metzger, H., and Goldstein, B. (1997). Exploiting the difference between intrinsic and extrinsic kinases: Implications for regulation of signaling by immunoreceptors. *J Immunol 159*, 5984-5992.

Wollman, R. and Meyer, T. (2012). Coordinated oscillations in cortical actin and Ca2+ correlate with cycles of vesicle secretion. *Nat Cell Biol 14*, 1261-1269.

Xu, K., Goldstein, B., Holowka, D., and Baird, B. (1998). Kinetics of multivalent antigen DNP-BSA binding to IgE-FcεRI in relationship to the stimulated tyrosine phosphorylation of FcεRI. *J Immunol 160*, 3225-3235.

Yang, J., Monine, M.I., Faeder, J.R., and Hlavacek, W.S. (2008). Kinetic Monte Carlo method for rule-based modeling of biochemical networks. *Phys Rev E 78*, 031910.

Young, R.M., Holowka, D., and Baird, B. (2003). A lipid raft environment enhances Lyn kinase activity by protecting the active site tyrosine from dephosphorylation. *J Biol Chem 278*, 20746-20752.

Physical models in immune signaling

JAYAJIT DAS

Physical models are created to explain select behaviors of a system of interest. The goal of a physical model is to elucidate a small number of mechanisms to explain not only a specific system, but also a class of systems that might show similar behaviors. In physical models, the pursuit of finding "the sameness" across different systems takes precedence over describing every minute detail in a particular system (Phillips, 2017). In the words of Jeremy Gunawardena (Gunawardena, 2014), "The model that explains everything, explains nothing." The inspiration for creating such models comes from physical sciences, in particular physics and chemistry where these models provided "foundational insights" (Phillips, 2017) into the real system. Broadly, the development process of physical models can be described in the following steps: (i) Choose a small set of features in the biological system of interest. The model should be able to explain these features or behaviors. The choice of the features is a crucial component in determining the usefulness and generality of the model. The modeler's intuition plays a key role in this endeavor. (ii) Make approximations and hypothesize mechanism(s). Physical models approximate detailed biological systems by few reduced variables and then hypothesize mechanism(s) using the reduced or coarse-grained variables to explain the chosen features. In some cases it might be possible to execute an exhaustive scan of all possible hypotheses (Lever et al., 2016b; Ma et al., 2009). (iii) Create a mathematical description for the model. This step creates a quantitative description of the hypothesized mechanism(s). (iv) Evaluate the consequences of the mathematical description. Depending on the complexity of the model this step is carried out by pen-and-paper calculations and/or numerical simulations. The results of the calculations and simulations are then compared against available experimental data. (v) Test predictions. Once the model is able to explain the available data, it is then used to predict new features/behaviors that were not considered in building or validating the model. In this chapter we will restrict our discussion to comparing qualitative features between the model predictions and the experiments. There is an extensive literature where parameters in reduced models are estimated carefully by fitting model results with experimental data (Nelson et al., 2015). The interested reader can find more details on this topic in Chapter 15.

Now we will analyze two physical models: both were developed to explain specific features of T cell signaling.

14.1 KINETIC PROOF READING (KPR)

Immune cells of the adaptive immunity such as T cells are able to discriminate (e.g., become activated or remain tolerant) between closely related ligands with high precision. The kinetic proofreading (KPR) model was proposed by McKeithan to explain this behavior (McKeithan, 1995). The KPR mechanism was originally proposed by Hopfield to explain low rate of error in protein synthesis, and DNA replication (Hopfield, 1974). McKeithan adapted this mechanism to explain the ability of T cells to distinguish ligands with nearby affinities with high precision. We will briefly describe how the development of the KPR mechanism can be cast in the steps mentioned in the introduction.

Step (i). Antigen discrimination is one of the primary functions of T cells. However, T cells carry out other tasks as well, e.g., help mediate cell-cell communication by participating in cytokine signaling (Huse et al., 2006). McKeithan chose to focus on a specific property of T cell antigen discrimination, namely, how do different antigens, characterized by the half-life of the TCR-antigen complex, produce different degrees of T cell activation?

T cell receptors (TCRs) on T cells interact with short peptide fragments (8 to 11 mers) bound to MHC molecules (or pMHC) residing on antigen presenting cells. The peptide fragments are derived from naturally occurring host proteins (or self-peptides) or proteins associated with pathogens (or foreign peptides) (Murphy and Weaver, 2016). Self-peptide bound MHC molecules form complexes with TCRs lasting for fractions of seconds, whereas foreign peptides gives rise to TCR-pMHC complexes with lifetimes that range from tens of seconds to minutes. Typically out of the 70,000 to 300,000 MHC molecules on an antigen presenting cell, only a small fraction (20 to 100 molecules) is occupied by foreign peptides, and the rest of the MHC population is bound to self-peptides (Murphy and Weaver, 2016). The puzzle McKeithan attempted to solve was how T cells become activated by a small number of high affinity foreign peptides but not by a large number of weak affinity self-peptides.

Before we start discussing McKeithan's model it will be helpful to introduce a few properties of the ligand discrimination program.

1. *Sensitivity.* This property refers to the amount of change in T cell activation with the increase in the number or dose of a particular ligand (pMHC). We expect the T cell activation in the model to be sensitive, i.e., a large increase in activation when the number of high affinity ligands increases from zero 0 to few molecules (~10). However, the same T cells should remain inactivated when the number of weak affinity self-peptide-MHC complexes increase by a large number. This behavior is quantified by the next property.

2. *Specificity.* This term indicates how specific the T cell activation is to the ligand (pMHC) affinity given by the half-life of the TCR-pMHC complex. For example, when T cells are stimulated by a small (~10 molecules) number of ligands of low (half-life ~ 10 sec) or high (half-life ~ 1 sec) affinity, only the high affinity ligands are able to produce T cell activation. Thus the antigen discrimination program in T cells is simultaneously both highly sensitive and specific.

3. *Speed.* This term refers to the time scale of key signaling events that occur upon TCR-peptide-MHC interaction. The early key signaling events (e.g., Ca++ release, full phosphorylation of the protein Erk) that are tightly correlated with T cell activation occur within seconds to minutes of TCR engagement (Huse et al., 2007). The model is expected to generate such time scales (or speed) for the T cell signaling kinetics.

Step (ii). The number of molecular events that are initiated upon TCR-pMHC binding is enormous. The events are composed of a wide range of chemical modifications including phosphorylation, dephosphorylation, complex formation, and hydrolysis of membrane lipids. In addition, physical changes such as clustering of selective receptors and actin remodeling come into play. The culmination of these signaling events leads to specific gene expressions that produce T cell activation marked by a several effector functions, such as cytokine secretion, cell proliferation, and the release of cytotoxins for target cell lysis (Murphy and Weaver, 2016). McKeithan's ingenuity was to coarse grain the above details by a series of simple chemical modifications (Figure 14.1). The reduction of these details made it possible to clearly connect the TCR-pMHC half-life to the amount of active complexes produced during the signaling kinetics. The simplifications also posed the danger of ignoring details that could play important roles in regulating activation. We will discuss implications of these simplifications later in the section.

McKeithan invoked the kinetic proof reading mechanism by hypothesizing a step where once the TCR unbinds from an intermediate complex, all the chemical modifications are reversed and the complex returns to the starting inactive state. A similar kinetic proofreading step proposed by Hopfield and Ninio recycled intermediate complexes to generate high fidelity in protein synthesis or DNA replication (Hopfield, 1974; Ninio, 1975). A key feature of the KPR step is the recycling of the erroneous intermediate complexes to the native state with a finite rate before they are taken up for further processing. This step breaks detailed balance in the kinetics and thus the execution of the biochemical reactions requires a continuous supply of energy (see Appendices II-V for further details).

Step (iii). McKeithan described the kinetics in the model (Figure 14.1) using first and second order mass action kinetics. The mass action kinetics represents an approximate and reduced description of the actual kinetics (Gunawardena, 2014). For example, the binding interaction between the TCR and pMHC involves electrostatic interactions between many protein residues and solvent molecules. Moreover, interactions between multiple TCR and pMHC molecules are further influenced by the quasi two-dimensional confinement of these molecules between the opposing APC and T cell membranes (Huang et al., 2010; Qi et al., 2006). Therefore, the mass-action rate, $d[TM]/dt = k_{on}[T][M] - k_{off}[TM]$, provides an approximate description of the kinetics with the benefit of clearly relating the time dependence of the concentrations on the kinetic rates and the total concentrations of the reacting species. The off rate, k_{off}, determines the half-life ($\sim 1/k_{off}$) of the complex and has been used to characterize the affinity of a peptide-MHC toward a TCR. However, the

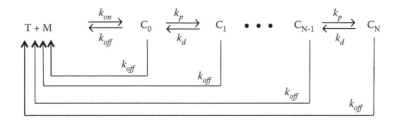

Figure 14.1 Schematic representation of McKeithan's model. The free TCR (T) and free pMHC (M) molecules interact to generate a complex (C_0) that undergoes multiple chemical modifications to via a series of intermediate partially activated complexes C_1, ..., C_{N-1} to generate the active complex C_N. The KPR step in the model is the complete deactivation of the any of the activated complex where the ligand (pMHC) unbinding takes the complex to the starting inactive state (T + M).

relation between potency of a ligand to activate T cells and $t_{1/2}$ is more nuanced and is better characterized by an aggregate dwell time for the ligand. The aggregate dwell time is a function of both k_{off} and k_{off}/k_{on} (Govern et al., 2010). The mass action kinetics in the KPR model (Figure 14.1) are described by the following ordinary differential equations.

$$\frac{d[T]}{dt} = -k_{on}[T][M] + k_{off}([C_0] + [C_1] + \cdots + [C_N])$$

$$\frac{d[M]}{dt} = -k_{on}[T][M] + k_{off}([C_0] + [C_1] + \cdots + [C_N])$$

$$\frac{d[C_0]}{dt} = k_{on}[T][M] - (k_{off} + k_p)[C_0] + k_d[C_1]$$

$$\frac{d[C_1]}{dt} = k_p[C_0] - (k_{off} + k_p + k_d)[C_1] + k_d[C_2]$$

$$\frac{d[C_2]}{dt} = k_p[C_1] - (k_{off} + k_p + k_d)[C_2] + k_d[C_3]$$

$$\cdots$$

$$\frac{d[C_N]}{dt} = k_p[C_{N-1}] - (k_{off} + k_p + k_d)[C_N]$$

The first three equations contain second order binding reactions; however, the rest of the reactions are of first order and therefore it is possible to analyze the kinetics easily in the steady state.

Step (iv). For insight into the effect of the KPR step, we first solve the kinetics for a three-state system when there are only two complexes, C_0 and C_1, and the unbound state with T_0 number of TCR and M_0 number of pMHC molecules. Here the steady state is given by,

$$[C_1] = \frac{k_p[C_0]}{(k_{off} + k_p + k_d)} = \alpha'[C_0] \tag{14.1}$$

where, $\alpha' = k_p/(k_{off} + k_p + k_d)$, and,

$$[C_0] = \frac{k_{on}}{k_{off}}(T_0 - (1 + \alpha')[C_0])(M_0 - (1 + \alpha')[C_0])$$

The above equation is a quadratic equation in $[C_0]$ which can be easily solved to obtain $[C_1]$ using Eq. (14.1),

$$[C_1] = \alpha' f(T_0, M_0, k_{on}, k_{off})$$

For the parameter values, $k_{off} > k_p > k_d$, and, $K_D (= k_{off}/k_{on}) \gg T_0 > M_0$, we can show (see Appendix I),

$$[C_1] = 1/(k_{off})^2 \cdot T_0 M_0 k_{on} + O((T_0/K_D)^2, (M_0/K_D)^2) \tag{14.2a}$$

At this point, it will be instructive to analyze the steady state of the above system without the KPR step where the relation between $[C_0]$ and $[C_1]$ is given by,

$$[C_1] = \frac{k_p[C_0]}{k_d}$$

The relation corresponding to that in Eq. (14.2a) in this case is given by,

$$[C_1] = 1/k_{off} \cdot T_0 M_0 k_{on} + O((T_0/K_D)^2, (M_0/K_D)^2) \qquad (14.2b)$$

Comparing Eq. (14.2a) and (14.2b) we find that the presence of the KPR step gives rise to a larger change $(1/k_{off}^2$ vs $1/k_{off})$ in $[C_1]$ with the ligand half-life or k_{off} and thus produces a better ligand discrimination property.

The cost of executing the KPR step is a continuous dissipation of energy, which must be supplied to the system. Dissipation is a common feature of signaling kinetics that arises due to the breakdown of detailed balance in the kinetics. The detailed balance condition is tied to the presence of microscopic reversibility in the kinetics. There is a relation between network topology and microscopic reversibility which can be utilized in building models that are required to break the detailed balance condition. See Appendices II-V for details.

McKeithan carried out the analysis for N number of intermediate species in the limit $k_d = 0$ which further simplifies the calculations. At the steady state the intermediate complex concentrations are recursively related:

$$[C_1] = \frac{k_p [C_0]}{(k_{off} + k_p)} = \alpha [C_0]$$
$$[C_2] = \alpha [C_1]$$
$$\dots$$
$$[C_N] = \alpha [C_{N-1}]$$

where,

$$\alpha = k_p/(k_p + k_{off}) < 1$$

Therefore,

$$[C_N] = \alpha^N [C_0]$$

where, $[C_0]$ satisfies the quadratic equation,

$$[C_0] = \frac{k_{on}}{k_{off}} \left(T_0 - \frac{1-\alpha^{N+1}}{1-\alpha}[C_0] \right) \left(M_0 - \frac{1-\alpha^{N+1}}{1-\alpha}[C_0] \right)$$

As before, one can show,

$$[C_N] = (k_p/k_{off})^{N+1} \cdot T_0 M_0 k_{on} + O((T_0/K_D)^2, (M_0/K_D)^2) \qquad (14.3)$$

The factor $1/(k_{off})^{N+1}$ in Eq. (14.3) increases the specificity of the response dramatically. For example, if k_{off} values for a weak and strong affinity ligands are $(k_{off})_{weak} = 1.0 k_p$ and $(k_{off})_{strong} = 0.1 k_p$, then the ratio of the activated complex formed for these two ligands will be $[C_N]_{weak}/[C_N]_{strong} = (0.1/1)^{N+1} = 10^{-(N+1)}$; therefore, a 10 fold difference in the affinity has been amplified into a difference of 10^{N+1} fold (1000 fold when N = 2). However, this occurs at a cost of decreased sensitivity to the ligands and larger activation times τ. The sensitivity decreases as the value of $[C_N]$ decreases exponentially (as $\alpha^N[C_0]$) with increasing N. The time scale to for an activation step is about $1/k_p$ the in mass action kinetics, thus the activation time increases with increasing N as $\tau \sim N/k_p$. The above model ignored stochastic fluctuations in the copy numbers of the molecular species. Chemical reactions are inherently stochastic in nature due to thermal fluctuations and including the such fluctuations can quantitatively and even qualitatively change the kinetics. The stochastic modeling of the KPR model is described in Appendices II-V.

Step (v). The KPR model developed here should be used to make qualitative instead of quantitative comparisons with experiments. This is because the model makes many simplifying assumptions, and the details not considered in the model could affect the numerical values of the species concentrations (say, C_N) that are compared with experiments. It is difficult to determine the precise number (N) of intermediate complexes during T cell signaling because the kinases (e.g., ZAP70) and phosphatases involved in the modifying the TCR complex can also possess multiple activation states. Within these limitations the KPR model is able to explain the high specificity of T cell activation. Predictions from a modified version of McKeithan's model agreed well with experiments done for activation of Mast cells by triggering FcεRI receptors (Faeder et al., 2003).

However, an important limitation of the above model is the linear increase of the abundance of the activated species with ligand concentration (Eq. (14.3)) (François et al., 2013). This implies that self-peptides if present in large numbers can still activate the T cells. This is not consistent with the measurements. Furthermore, recent experiments with well defined antigens show a bell-curve shaped dose response (lower activation both at low and very high antigen doses) for high affinity ligands (Lever et al., 2016a). The KPR model is qualitatively inconsistent with these results, and coupling of the KPR model with feed-forward chemical reactions can restore such features in the kinetics (Lever et al., 2016a).

14.2 OPEN QUESTIONS

The KPR model was developed to explain the highly sensitive ligand discrimination property of T cells. However, in the recent years mechanical interactions between T cells and antigen presenting cells and reorganization of actin polymers beneath the T cell plasma membrane have been found to play an important role in generating ligand sensitive responses (Feng et al., 2017). Furthermore, complex biochemical modifications involving feedback interactions at very early stages of TCR triggering important for initiation of T cell signaling (Chakraborty and Weiss, 2014). Thus it is an interesting question to investigate the precise contribution of the KPR mechanism in giving rise to the ligand discrimination program in T cells in the presence of the above effects. This question is also related to a broader question of "retroactivity" in signal transduction networks where one is interested in how the input/output relation in a small signaling module changes when the module is embedded in a larger signaling network (Del Vecchio et al., 2008).

14.3 FEEDBACKS

Feedbacks are common motifs in signaling networks. A positive (or negative) feedback augments (or inhibits) production of a molecular species. Positive feedbacks have been found to generate sharp changes and memory in activation of specific molecular species during signaling (Das et al. 2009a). Negative feedbacks can give rise to oscillations (Hoffmann et al., 2002) in the kinetics, and combinations of positive and negative feedbacks can generate transient activation in signaling species (Mukherjee et al., 2013a). Physical models have been quite successful in elucidating mechanisms by which feedbacks affect signaling responses (Ferrell Jr and Xiong, 2001; Murray, 1989; Nelson et al., 2015). We will discuss an example of a positive feedback in regulating T cell activation here (Das et al., 2009a). We will not explicitly outline the steps as in the KPR model here and hope the reader will be able to identify those from the description below.

Ras-SOS positive feedback during early time T cell activation. T cells produce binary responses (activation or tolerance) when the dose of a high affinity peptide-MHC molecule crosses a threshold value. However, when the antigen dose is increased, many experiments showed that the increase in the numbers of the very upstream signaling markers such as phosphorylated ITAMs associated with TCRs are gradual or analogue in nature. Therefore, a question of interest is how this analogue input signal is converted into a digital output or a binary response. The kinetic proofreading mechanism proposed by McKeithan attempts to explain such behavior; however, there are issues regarding the low sensitivity of the response with increasing antigen dose in the model. An alternate or even a complementary mechanism to KPR that can generate such a behavior is a positive feedback. There are several examples of positive feedback (Altan-Bonnet and Germain, 2005; Mukherjee et al., 2013b) in the membrane proximal lymphocyte signaling events that can potentially produce sharp increase in abundances in downstream activation markers, such as phosphorylated Erk. One such positive feedback involves the activation of a protein Ras. Ras is a membrane bound protein that plays an important role in cell growth and proliferation (Mor and Philips, 2006). Ras becomes active when it binds GTP but is inactive when bound to GDP (Margarit et al., 2003). The transition between the active and inactive forms of Ras occurs at a much slower time scale (~hours) than that of the signaling time scales (~mins). Lymphocytes possess enzymes that make these transitions occur at faster time scales. SOS (Son of Sevenless) and Rasgrp1 are two enzymes in T and B cells that make the activation of Ras (RasGDP→ RasGTP) occur in minutes. The enzyme RasGAP, on the other hand, regulates the de-activation process, RasGTP→ RasGDP.

The reactions RasGDP↔RasGTP represent exchange of GDP/GTP molecules within Ras (Mor and Philips, 2006). Ras activation is an important event in lymphocyte signal transduction, as RasGTP initiates activation of MAP kinase cascades that control cell functions such as proliferation, cytokine secretion, cell survival, and apoptosis. The positive feedback in Ras activation arises via SOS (Jun et al., 2013; Mor and Philips, 2006). A SOS molecule contains an allosteric site that can bind to either RasGTP or RasGDP, and when the allosteric site is occupied with RasGTP, the rate of Ras activation increases over 75 fold (Das et al., 2009a; Iversen et al., 2014). Thus, once few molecules of RasGTP are present, they can increase the rate of RasGTP production by binding to the allosteric site of SOS. This creates a positive feedback in Ras activation. The enzyme Rasgrp1 also mediates Ras activation; however, unlike SOS, it does not possess any allosteric site to further regulate its catalytic rate. A role of Rasgrp1 could be to produce enough numbers of RasGTP initially to ignite the positive feedback in Ras activation via SOS. The goal of a physical model in this case could be to determine the mechanisms underlying the interplay between the two enzymes SOS and Rasgrp1 in producing Ras activation and how that activation can be used to explain digital T cell responses against a gradual change in antigen dose.

In order to develop a physical model, we need to make several simplifying approximations akin to those in the KPR model. The interactions involving Ras, SOS, Rasgrp1, and RasGAP include several other molecular species such as GTP and GDP, Grb2 (a protein that binds SOS to the TCR-pMHC complex), DAG (a lipid component in the plasma membrane), the protein PKC (activates Rasgrp1) (Jun et al., 2013), Ca++ ions (molecules that regulate RasGAP activation) (Mor and Philips, 2006), and membrane lipids (molecules that regulate access of RasGTP to SOS allosteric site) (Iversen et al., 2014; Jun et al., 2013). We will coarse-grain these interactions in creating a simple model in which SOS and Rasgrp1 produce RasGTP from RasGDP following enzymatic reactions and RasGAP carries out the reverse reaction RasGTP→ RasGTP as an enzyme. The positive feedback induced by SOS in RasGTP production was first found in *in vitro* experiments, and the existence of the allosteric and the catalytic pockets in the SOS molecule was supported by crystallographic studies. Thus, the inclusion of the positive feedback via SOS in the model aiming to describe the Ras activation in T cells is a hypothesis, which needs to be further tested against experiments. This was confirmed in a set of experiments combined with *in silico* modeling in T and B cells. We will describe the model developed in (Das et al., 2009a) using a simple model involving the kinetics of RasGTP abundances alone.

Deterministic model: The simple model we describe here captures the basic features of the kinetics, such as bistability and hysteresis, produced by the detailed biochemical model in Das et al. (2009a). The deterministic kinetics of the abundance of RasGTP ($[R_T]$) in a volume V in the simple model is given by the ODE below:

$$\frac{d[R_T]}{dt} = \frac{k_E[E][R_D]}{K_{ME} + [R_D]} + \frac{k_F[R_D][R_T]}{K_{MF} + [R_D]} - \frac{k_d[R_T]}{K_{MD} + [R_T]} = g(R_T) - d(R_T) \tag{14.4}$$

where $[R_D] \equiv$ RasGDP abundance in a volume V, $[R_T] \equiv$ RasGTP abundance in V, and, $[R_D] + [R_T] = R_0 \equiv$ the total Ras abundance in V. This simple model ignores the role of SOS with an allosteric site that is empty or occupied with RasGDP in producing Ras activation for the sake of simplicity. In Eq. (14.4), [E] denotes the abundance of the enzyme RasGRP1 in V. We used a Michaelis-Menten form (Murray, 1989) to simplify the rates for enzymatic activation/deactivation of RasGDP/RasGTP. The Michaelis-Menten approximation holds when the abundance of the substrate ($[R_D]$ or $[R_T]$) is larger than that of the enzyme (RasGRP1/SOS/ SOS$_{allo}$-RasGTP or RasGAP). The enzymes in this situation are rendered activated by the incoming signal, e.g., SOS in the cytosol is recruited to the plasma membrane by binding to the protein Grb2 associated with the TCR signaling complex that is formed upon TCR, pMHC binding. Thus, the abundances of the enzymes at low signal intensities are likely to be much smaller than the substrates. The first term in Eq. (14.4) describes the enzymatic activation of Ras-GDP by the enzymes RasGRP1 and SOS without the positive feedback. The second term describes Ras activation by the enzyme complex SOS$_{allo}$-RasGTP, when the allosteric pocket of SOS is occupied by RasGTP. Since the copy number of SOS$_{allo}$-RasGTP is dependent on the copy number of RasGTP, one can approximately describe the dependence of [SOS$_{allo}$-RasGTP] as proportional to the number of free RasGTP. Thus, the Ras activation rate in the above equation becomes linearly dependent on [RasGTP]. [SOS$_{allo}$-RasGTP] also depends on the number of SOS molecules. We have assumed an implicit dependence of [SOS] on the rate k_F as $k_F \propto$ [SOS]. The last term describes the enzymatic de-activation of RasGTP by RasGAP. In order to understand the steady state behavior of the above kinetics, we graphically analyzed the dependence of terms $g([R_T])$ and $d([R_T])$ on $[R_T]$ (Figure 14.2). The curves for $g([R_T])$ and $d([R_T])$ will intersect at the fixed point(s) ($[R_T^*]$) of Eq. (14.4). The stability (stable or unstable) of the fixed points is determined by the derivatives, $g'([R_T])$ and $d'([R_T])$ or the slopes of the curves at the point(s) of intersection. If $[R_T]$ is changed by a small amount δR_T from its value $[R_T^*]$ at a fixed point, then the kinetics of δR_T, to the first order of δR_T, is given by,

$$\frac{d(\delta R_T)}{dt} = \left[g'\left(R_T^* \right) - d'\left(R_T^* \right) \right] \delta R_T$$

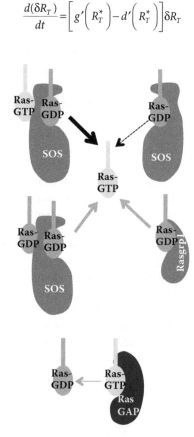

Figure 14.2 Schematic diagram showing Ras activation and de-activation. This figure shows Ras activation by the enzymes SOS and Rasgrp1. The complexes in which the alloestric site in SOS is occupied by RasGTP or RasGDP are indicated. The enzyme RasGAP catalyzes Ras deactivation.

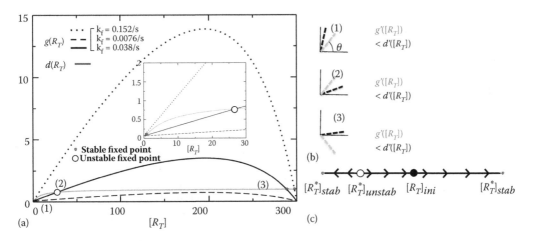

Figure 14.3 Steady state analysis of Ras activation in the simple model. **(a)** Shows the variation of $g([R_T])$ and $d([R_T])$ with $[R_T]$ for three different values of $k_F = 0.038/5$ s^{-1} (low), 0.038 s^{-1} (intermediate), and, 0.038×4 s^{-1} (high). $[R_T]$ was given by the number of Ras-GTP molecules in a volume $V = 4$ μm$^2 \times 0.02$ μm. The values of the other parameters are the following: $k_E = 0.01$ s^{-1}, $kd = 0.1$ s^{-1}, $K_{ME} = 144$ molecules, $K_{MF} = 120$ molecules, $[E] = 10$ molecules, and, $K_{MD} = 7.7$ molecules. The fixed points are given by the intersection points of the curves corresponding to $g([R_T])$ and $d([R_T])$. The inset shows the close up of the curves in range $0 \leq [R_T] \leq 30$ molecules. **(b)** Schematic diagrams show the tangents to the curves for $g([R_T])$ and $d([R_T])$ at the intersection points corresponding to $k_f = 0.038$ s^{-1}. The derivatives, $g'([R_T])$ and $d'([R_T])$, are given by the slopes equal to $\tan(\theta)$ where θ is the angle between the tangent vector and the x-axis. This relation allows one to easily check the stability of the fixed points by visually inspecting the points of intersections of the curves. **(c)** Shows the flow of the initial condition to the fixed points for the case $k_F = 0.038$ s^{-1}.

Thus, when $g'([R_T^*]) - d'([R_T^*]) < 0$ (or >0), the fixed point $[R_T] = [R_T^*]$ is a stable (or an unstable) fixed point. We can now analyze the graphs for $g([R_T])$ and $d([R_T])$ at low, intermediate, and, high values of k_F and $[E]$. Increasing the values of k_F and $[E]$ represent increasing the SOS and the Rasgrp1 abundances in V, respectively. We first consider the variation of k_F at $[E]$ fixed at a small value ($[E] = 10$ molecules) (Figure 14.3a). Under this condition, the $g([R_T])$ and $d([R_T])$ curves intersect at a single point at low and high values of k_F; and at intermediate values of k_F, the curves intersect at three points (Figure 14.3a). By analyzing the slopes of the curves at the points of intersection (Figure 14.3b), we can easily check that the fixed point at the lowest and the highest value of $[R_T^*]$ are stable fixed points. The fixed point at the intermediate value of $[R_T^*]$ is an unstable fixed point. The unstable fixed point arises at intermediate values of k_F (Figure 14.3a). This phase diagram fixed points (Figure 14.3c) provides the following interpretation of the Ras activation kinetics. At low k_F values or SOS abundances, regardless of the initial value of $[R_T]$, the system sustains a low value of $[R_T]$ because of the dominance of the reactions mediating Ras de-activation over Ras activation. At high k_F values, the situation is reversed, for any initial value of $[R_T]$ the kinetics sustains a large value of $[R_T]$ at the steady state. At intermediate values of k_F, there is an unstable fixed point at an intermediate value of $[R_T] = [R_T^*]_{unstab}$. Therefore, if the initial $[R_T] = [R_T]_{ini}$ is less than $[R_T^*]_{unstab}$, the system settles to a lower $[R_T^*]$ value at the steady state as there is not enough RasGRP molecules to ignite the positive feedback. In contrast, if $[R_T]_{ini} > [R_T^*]_{unstab}$, the available RasGTP molecules use the positive feedback to produce a higher value of $[R_T^*]$ (Figure 14.3c).

The dependence of the steady state behavior on the initial state is the manifestation of the presence of multiple stable fixed points in the kinetics. This behavior can also give rise to a memory in Ras activation is also known as hysteresis, where the Ras activation at particular signal input is dependent on whether the current input value was attained from a higher or a lower signal input (Figure 14.4a). Next we considered the variation of Ras activation with $[E]$ when k_F was held fixed at an intermediate value (Figure 14.4b). As $[E]$ was increased from $[E] = 0$, the unstable fixed point and the stable fixed point at the smallest $[R_T^*]$ value moved closer to each other and eventually these two fixed points "annihilated" each other to be survived by the stable fixed point at the largest $[R_T^*]$ value. The behavior can be interpreted as follows. Increasing the Rasgrp1 abundance (or $[E]$) produced RasGTP molecules that helped ignite the positive feedback in SOS to generate a high Ras activation.

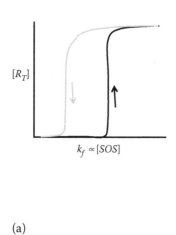

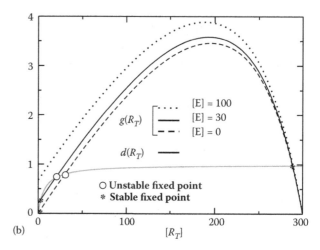

(a)

(b)

Figure 14.4 Hysteresis and dependence of Ras activation on [Rasgrp1]. **(a)** Schematic diagram showing the increase of steady state Ras activation (black line) as [SOS] was increased for initial [R_T] fixed at a small value. The steady state [R_T] decreases (grey line) following a different trajectory when [SOS] is decreased for a state containing large values of initial [R_T]. **(b)** Shows the fixed points as [E] is varied in the simple model. $k_F = 0.038$ s^{-1} and the other parameter values are the same as in Figure 14.3b.

Therefore, as the Rasgrp1 abundance (or [E]) increased the starting RasGTP (or [R_T]$_{ini}$) amount required to sustain the largest [R_T*] decreased, and beyond a threshold value the larger Rasgrp1 abundances were sufficient to generate enough RasGTP molecules to produce the largest Ras activation via the SOS feedback.

Stochastic model: The effect of the intrinsic noise fluctuations can be analyzed by solving the Master equation corresponding to Eq. (14.4). If we denote the number of RasGTP molecules in a single cell by n, then the distribution of RasGTP abundance in a cell population at a time t is given by the probability distribution function $P(n,t)$. The time evolution of $P(n,t)$ is given by the Master Equation,

$$\frac{\partial P(n,t)}{\partial t} = d(n+1)P(n+1,t) + g(n-1)P(n-1,t) - (d(n)+g(n))P(n,t) = \sum_{\substack{n'=0 \\ n' \neq n}}^{N} L_{nn'}P(n',t) \qquad (14.5)$$

where,

$$L_{nn'} = d(n')\delta_{n',n+1} + g(n')\delta_{n',n-1} - (d(n)+g(n))\delta_{n',n}$$

The time dependent Master equation in Eq. (14.5) can be solved exactly by calculating the eigenvalues and eigenvectors of L. This approach is described in Appendix III. This is a powerful method which allows one not only to exactly calculate probability distribution functions for copy numbers but also to calculate probability distributions of other relevant variables, such as the first passage time distributions or maximal value distributions (Das, 2013). A Mathematica code for solving Eq. (14.5) is provided at the link http://planetx .nationwidechildrens.org/~jayajit/das_chapter/Mathematica_codes. We also discuss a graphical method for calculation of the steady state solutions analytically in Appendix IV. The advantages of using these approaches are discussed in Appendices III–V.

The solutions reveal that stochastic fluctuations have a profound effect on Ras activation, in particular in the bistable region, in Ras activation single cells. The results show that Ras activation in a cell population can show a bimodal behavior, i.e., a subgroup of cells will contain large Ras activation vs the rest at low Ras activation at a time t, even when all the cells started at time t=0 with identical initial conditions (Das et al., 2009a). Therefore, the stochastic fluctuations in Ras activation create large enough numbers of RasGTP molecules in a subgroup of cells where it is able to engage the positive feedback and produce higher RasGRP concentrations. This behavior was confirmed in experiments with SOScat.

14.4 OPEN QUESTIONS

The above analysis ignores several features that could be important in regulating Ras activation in lymphocytes. The well-mixed assumption breaks down when reactants diffuse at a slower rate compared to the reaction time scales. This situation is particularly relevant for proteins (e.g., Ras) residing in the plasma membrane where the proteins diffuse at a much smaller rate compared to the cytosol. The presence of positive feedback in reactions can give rise to spatial spreading of activated species (e.g., RasGTP) in travelling waves (Das et al., 2009b). A recent experiment using lipid anchored Ras molecule on lipid bilayers and modeling demonstrated the presence of many states in SOS activation giving rise to a broad distribution of turnover rates for SOS-induced Ras activation (Iversen et al., 2014). Iversen et al. suggested an extension of the model by introducing a distribution of k_{cat} values.

Another relevant issue is the question of retroactivity. The Ras activation module discussed here is connected with other signaling modules. The participant signaling molecules in these modules can interact via positive and negative feedbacks. In addition, there is active intercellular transport of Ras between endo-membranes of organelles (e.g., Golgi bodies). It is important to know how the bistability and hysteresis in Ras activation is influenced by the above spatial effects, retroactivity, and active transport. Some of these issues were studied recently in *in silico* modeling in the context of EGFR signaling (Kochanczyk et al., 2017).

14.5 APPENDIX I: DERIVATIONS OF EQ. (14.2) AND EQ. (14.3)

Derivation of Eq. (14.2)

$$[C_0] = \frac{k_{on}[T][M]}{k_{off}} = \frac{k_{on}}{k_{off}}(T_0 - [C_0] - [C_1])(M_0 - [C_0] - [C_1])$$

$$\Rightarrow [C_0] = \frac{k_{on}}{k_{off}}(T_0 - (1+\alpha')[C_0])(M_0 - (1+\alpha')[C_0])$$

Define, $x = [C_0]$. The above equation is given by

$$x^2 - \left[\frac{K_D}{1+\alpha'} + T_0 + M_0\right]x + \frac{T_0 M_0}{(1+\alpha')} = 0$$

$$\Rightarrow x = \frac{1}{2}\left(\frac{K_D}{1+\alpha'} + T_0 + M_0\right)\left[1 \pm \sqrt{1 - \frac{4T_0 M_0}{(1+\alpha')\left(\frac{K_D}{1+\alpha'} + T_0 + M_0\right)^2}}\right]$$

$$= \frac{1}{2}\left(\frac{K_D}{1+\alpha'} + T_0 + M_0\right)\left[1 \pm \left(1 - \frac{2T_0 M_0}{(1+\alpha')\left(\frac{K_D}{1+\alpha'} + T_0 + M_0\right)^2}\right) + h.o.\right]$$

Choosing the stable (-ve sign) solution,

$$x \approx \frac{T_0 M_0}{K_D + (1+\alpha')(T_0 + M_0)}$$

Replacing the above form for $[C_0]$ in Eq. (14.1) we get Eq. (14.2a).
Eq. (14.3) can be derived by summing the geometric series,

$$[C_0] = \frac{k_{on}}{k_{off}}(T_0 - (1 + \alpha + \alpha^2 + \cdots + \alpha^N)[C_0])(M_0 - (1 + \alpha + \alpha^2 + \cdots + \alpha^N)[C_0])$$

$$= \frac{k_{on}}{k_{off}}\left(T_0 - \frac{1 - \alpha^{N+1}}{1 - \alpha}[C_0]\right)\left(M_0 - \frac{1 - \alpha^{N+1}}{1 - \alpha}[C_0]\right)$$

14.6 APPENDIX II: MODELING STOCHASTIC KINETICS

The copy numbers of molecular species in chemical reactions can change randomly with time. These stochastic fluctuations in the copy numbers, known as the intrinsic noise fluctuations, arise naturally due to thermal fluctuations in the system (Kampen, 1992). Therefore, two isolated identical chemical reaction systems that start reacting at the same initial condition (e.g., the same copy numbers of reactants species) will contain different copy numbers of the reacting species at any later time as the chemical reactions progress in the systems. There can be additional sources of variations in the copy numbers of molecular species resulting from the differences in cellular environments between individual cells, that often manifest as cell-cell differences in total abundances of a protein species or reaction rate constants (Swain et al., 2002). Such cell-cell variations are usually known as extrinsic noise fluctuations. In the presence of these fluctuations, a state represented by a specific set of copy numbers of molecular species in a single cell occurs at any time with a certain probability. The time evolution for the probability distribution function of the states is described by the Master equation (Goel and Dyn, 1974; Kampen, 1992). We derive the Master equation for a simple set of chemical reactions (Figure 14.5) pertaining to the kinetic proofreading model described here (Das, 2016).

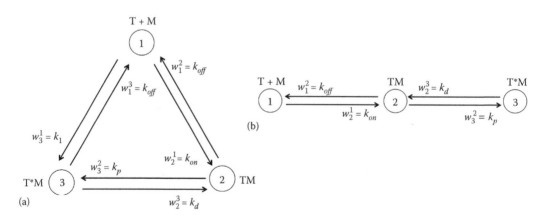

Figure 14.5 A three state model for KPR. **(a)** A single TCR (T) binds to a single pMHC (M) to create the complex TCR-pMHC (TM). The TM complex undergoes a chemical modification (e.g., tyrosine phosphorylation) to produce the active complex, T*M. The active complex dissociates to the initial inactive state containing free TCR and pMHC molecules. This is the KPR step. A very small rate k_1 is assumed to directly convert the free TCR and pMHC molecules to the active T*M state to keep some of the calculations finite. k_1 can be taken to be of very small value such that it does not realistically affect the kinetics in the time scales of interest. The chemical reactions move the system between three states, (1) T+M: free TCR and pMHC, (2) TM: the bound complex, and, (3) T*M: the active complex. **(b)** The model in **(a)** without the KPR step.

14.6.1 DERIVATION OF THE MASTER EQUATION

Consider the chemical modifications in Figure 14.5a. There are three states: the unbound single molecules of T and M (state #1), the bound complex (state #2), TM, and, the active complex T*M (state #3). The system starts from an initial state i_0 (e.g., state#1 or $i_0 = 1$) at $t = 0$ and transitions to the other states due to the chemical modifications (Figure 14.5). We will derive an equation that describes the time evolution of the states in terms of the conditional probability $P(i,t|i_0,0)$. $P(i,t|i_0,0)$ denotes the probability that the system is in the state i at time t (>0) given that the system was in the state i_0 at t = 0. We denote this conditional probability as $p_i(t)$ for brevity. In the next few steps we will determine the change in $p_i(t)$ for a small increment of time from t to $t + \Delta t$. Δt is small enough to not allow more than one reaction to occur in Δt. $p_i(t + \Delta t)$ can be expressed in terms of $p_i(t)$ as,

$$p_i(t+\Delta t) = \sum_{\substack{j=1 \\ j\neq i}}^{3} T(i,t+\Delta t|j,t)p_j(t) + Q(i;t+\Delta t,t)p_i(t) \tag{14.6}$$

where $T(i,t + \Delta t|j,t)$ is the probability for the transition $j \rightarrow i$ to occur between $t + \Delta t$ and t, and $Q(i;t + \Delta t,t)$ is the probability that no reaction occurred and the system remained in the state i in the same time interval.

The above equation is derived using the basic addition rule of probability for mutually exclusive events (Rényi, 2007). For example, three mutually exclusive events can occur in the time interval t to $t + \Delta t$ to produce the state $i = 1$ at $t = t + \Delta t$: (1) The system was in the state $i = 1$ at time t and it remained in the same state throughout the interval. (2) The system was in the state $i = 2$ at time t and the reaction $2 \rightarrow 1$ changed the state to $i = 1$. (3) The system was in the state $i = 3$ at time t and it transitioned to the state $i = 1$ due to the reaction $3 \rightarrow 1$. In relating $p_1(t + \Delta t)$ to $p_1(t)$, Eq. (14.6) sums up the probabilities for the each of the above mentioned mutually exclusive events (1) to (3). The same calculations can be done for any other $p_i(t + \Delta t)$ as well. Note the usefulness of the assumption regarding the size of Δt (i.e., no more than one reaction can occur) in determining the number the mutually exclusive events.

Now we need to calculate the transition probability $T(i,t + \Delta t|j,t)$ using the reaction propensities. This can be done using a frequentist approach (Rényi, 2007). For example, for the reaction $2 \rightarrow 1$, $T(1,t + \Delta t|2,t) = k_{off}\Delta t = w^2_1\Delta t$ where the transition rate is w^j_i and $w^j_i \Delta t$ is the probability for the transition $j \rightarrow i$. The probability that no reaction occurs in the time interval t to $t+\Delta t$ is calculated using the conservation of the total probability, i.e., the probability for the system to stay in the state i in the interval + the probability for the system to leave the state i in the interval = 1. Thus, the probability for leaving the state i in the interval is $\Sigma_j T(j,t+ \Delta t|i,t)$, where, the sum is over all the possible reactions $i \rightarrow j$ ($j \neq i$). For example, when $i = 1$, both the reactions $1 \rightarrow 2$ and $1 \rightarrow 3$ can displace the system from the state $i = 1$, thus $Q(1; t + \Delta t, t) = 1-k_{on}\Delta t - k_1\Delta t = 1-w^1_2\Delta t-w^1_3\Delta t$. Eq. (14.6) now can be rewritten as:

$$p_i(t+\Delta t) = \sum_{\substack{j=1 \\ j\neq i}}^{3} w_i^j p_j(t)\Delta t + p_i(t)\left[1 - \sum_{\substack{j=1 \\ j\neq i}}^{3} w_j^i\Delta t\right]$$

Rearranging the terms:

$$[p_i(t+\Delta t) - p_i(t)]/\Delta t = \sum_{\substack{j=1 \\ j\neq i}}^{3} w_i^j p_j(t) - \sum_{\substack{j=1 \\ j\neq i}}^{3} w_j^i p_i(t)$$

In the limit $\Delta t \rightarrow 0$:

$$\frac{\partial p_i(t)}{\partial t} = \sum_{\substack{j=1 \\ j \neq i}}^{3} \left[w_i^j p_j(t) - w_j^i p_i(t) \right] = \sum_{j=1}^{3} L_{ij} p_j(t) \tag{14.7}$$

where $L_{ij} = w_i^j (1 - \delta_{ij}) - \left[\sum_{j=1}^{3} w_i^j (1 - \delta_{ij}) \right] \delta_{ij}$. δ_{ij} is the Kronecker delta function, $\delta_{ij} = 1$ when $i = j$ and $\delta_{ij} = 0$ when $i \neq j$. This is the Master equation. Note the above equation also satisfies a conservation law:

$$\frac{\partial \sum_{i=1}^{3} p_i(t)}{\partial t} = \sum_{i=1}^{3} \sum_{j=1}^{3} L_{ij} p_j(t) = 0$$

The conserved quantity, i.e., the sum of all the probabilities is chosen to be $\Sigma_i p_i(t) = 1$. We will now describe a method for solving the Master equation.

14.7 APPENDIX III: SOLUTION OF THE MASTER EQUATION USING EIGEN-DECOMPOSITION OF L

The Master equation in Eq. (14.7) can be viewed as a set of coupled first order ordinary differential equations represented by a matrix equation:

$$\frac{d\mathbf{p}(t)}{dt} = \mathbf{L}\mathbf{p}(t) \tag{14.8}$$

where p_i in Eq. (14.7) is the ith element of the column matrix $\mathbf{p}(t)$, and L_{ij} in Eq. (14.7) is the ij^{th} element of the 3×3 matrix $\mathbf{L}$. The initial condition is given by:

$$\mathbf{p}(0) = \mathbf{f}. \tag{14.9}$$

Eqs. (14.8) and (14.9) can be easily generalized to higher dimensions. The elements of $\mathbf{p}(t)$ are non-negative and the elements of $\mathbf{L}$ are real numbers. Eq. (14.8) can be solved exactly by calculating the eigenvectors and eigenvalues for the matrix $\mathbf{L}$. The execution of this method can become challenging as the dimension of $\mathbf{L}$ becomes large. This is common for signaling networks where the dimension of $\mathbf{L}$ quickly becomes enormous for realistic numbers of reacting biochemical species and their copy numbers. There are several approximation techniques to deal with such situations (Munsky and Khammash, 2006). We will derive the solution for a general case with n number of states ($n=3$ represents Eq. (14.8)) using the Dirac-notation (Dirac, 1935). This notation is widely used in Quantum Physics and allows us to describe the matrix operations in a compact but clear manner. We briefly introduce the notation here. $|p\rangle$ and $\langle q|$ denote the column and the row matrices, respectively, and $\langle q|p \rangle$ denotes the scalar product between the vectors, i.e., $\langle q|p \rangle = \sum_{i=1}^{n} q_i p_i$. $\{q_1,...,q_n\}$ and

$\{p_1,...,p_n\}$ denote the elements of the **q** row and the **p** column matrices, respectively. The element p_i in Eq. (14.7) is $p_i \equiv \langle i|p \rangle$ and the ij^{th} element of **L** is, $L_{ij} \equiv \langle i|L|j \rangle \cdot |i \rangle$ (or $\langle i| $) represents a $1 \times n$ (or $n \times 1$) column (or row) vector where the ith element is 1 and the rest of the elements are zero. In this notation, $p_i \equiv \langle i|p \rangle$ and Eq. (14.8) takes the form $\dfrac{d|p(t) \rangle}{dt} = \mathbf{L}|p(t) \rangle$ and Eq. (14.7) is represented by:

$$\frac{\partial \langle i|p \rangle}{\partial t} = \sum_{j=1}^{n} \langle i|L|j \rangle \langle j|p \rangle \qquad (14.10)$$

Where $\left| e_R^{(\lambda_i)} \right\rangle$, and $\left\langle e_L^{(\lambda_i)} \right|$ denote the right and left eigenvectors of **L** corresponding to the eigenvalue λ_i, i.e., $\mathbf{L}\left| e_R^{(\lambda_i)} \right\rangle = \lambda_i \left| e_R^{(\lambda_i)} \right\rangle$ and $\left\langle e_L^{(\lambda_i)} \right| \mathbf{L} = \lambda_i \left\langle e_L^{(\lambda_i)} \right|$. The eigenvectors, $\left\{ \left| e_R^{(\lambda_1)} \right\rangle,..,\left| e_R^{(\lambda_n)} \right\rangle \right\}$, and $\left\{ \left\langle e_L^{(\lambda_1)} \right|,..,\left\langle e_L^{(\lambda_n)} \right| \right\}$ form an orthonormal basis set for any $1 \times n$ matrix or vector (e.g., $|p \rangle$ in Eq. (14.10)), i.e., $\left\langle e_L^{(\lambda_j)} \middle| e_R^{(\lambda_i)} \right\rangle = \delta_{ij}$.

Now $|p \rangle$ can be written as a linear superposition of the vectors $\left| e_R^{(\lambda_i)} \right\rangle$ as:

$$|p(t) \rangle = \sum_{i=1}^{n} a_i(t) \left| e_R^{(\lambda_i)} \right\rangle \qquad (14.11)$$

Thus, the time evolution in $|p(t) \rangle$ can be described as a time evolution in $\{a_i(t)\}$. We will use the resolution of the identity (or the completeness) relation (Mathews and Walker, 1970),

$$\sum_{j=1}^{n} |j \rangle \langle j| = \mathbf{I} \qquad (14.12)$$

where, I is the $n \times n$ identity matrix, and the left hand side of Eq. (14.12) denotes the outer product of the row and the column vectors, $\langle j|$, and, $|j \rangle$, respectively.

Substituting Eq. (14.11) in Eq. (14.10), and using Eq. (14.12) gives us,

$$\sum_{i=1}^{n} \left| e_R^{(\lambda_i)} \right\rangle \frac{\partial a_i(t)}{\partial t} = \sum_{i=1}^{n} a_i(t) L \left| e_R^{(\lambda_i)} \right\rangle = \sum_{i=1}^{n} \lambda_i a_i(t) \left| e_R^{(\lambda_i)} \right\rangle \qquad (14.13)$$

Equating the coefficients for the individual eigenvectors form both sides of Eq. (14.13),

$$\frac{\partial a_i(t)}{\partial t} = \lambda_i a_i(t)$$
$$\Rightarrow a_i(t) = e^{\lambda_i t} a_i(0)$$

Thus, the solution is given by,

$$|p(t) \rangle = \sum_{i=1}^{n} a_i(t) \left| e_R^{(\lambda_i)} \right\rangle = \sum_{i=1}^{n} e^{\lambda_i t} a_i(0) \left| e_R^{(\lambda_i)} \right\rangle \qquad (14.14)$$

The $\{a_i(0)\}$ is calculated from the initial state $\left|p(0)\right\rangle$ as

$$\left|p(0)\right\rangle = \sum_{i=1}^{n} a_i(0)\left|e_R^{(\lambda_i)}\right\rangle$$

$$\Rightarrow \left\langle e_L^{(\lambda_j)}\middle|p(0)\right\rangle = \sum_{i=1}^{n} a_i(0)\left\langle e_L^{(\lambda_j)}\middle|e_R^{(\lambda_i)}\right\rangle = \sum_{i=1}^{n} a_i(0)\delta_{ij} = a_j(0).$$

We can express $a_j(0)$ in terms of f_i (Eq. (14.9)) as,

$$a_j(0) = \left\langle e_L^{(\lambda_j)}\middle|p(0)\right\rangle = \sum_{i=1}^{n} \left\langle e_L^{(\lambda_j)}\middle|i\right\rangle\left\langle i\middle|p(0)\right\rangle = \sum_{i=1}^{n} \left\langle e_L^{(\lambda_j)}\middle|i\right\rangle f_i$$

Therefore, the solution for $p_i(t)$ is given by,

$$p_i(t) = \left\langle i\middle|p(t)\right\rangle = \sum_{j=1}^{n} e^{\lambda_j t} a_j(0)\left\langle i\middle|e_R^{(\lambda_j)}\right\rangle = \sum_{j=1}^{n}\sum_{k=1}^{n} e^{\lambda_j t} f_k \left\langle e_L^{\lambda_j}\middle|k\right\rangle\left\langle i\middle|e_R^{\lambda_j}\right\rangle \tag{14.15}$$

A program written in Mathematica is available at the link http://planetx.nationwidechildrens.org/~jayajit /das_chapter/Mathematica_codes that solves the kinetics in Figure 14.5 using Eq. (14.8)-(14.15).

14.8 APPENDIX IV: SOLUTION OF THE MASTER EQUATION AT THE STEADY STATE USING A GRAPHICAL METHOD

Here we introduce a graphical method for solving the Master equation at the steady state (or $dp_i/dt = 0$). The method serves two purposes. (i) It provides a straightforward technique to express the solution in a closed form for simple networks. (ii) It provides a deeper understanding into the kinetics. The method is based on Kirchhoff's method that solves a set of coupled linear algebraic equations for finding currents in electrical

networks. The Master equation (Eq. 14.7) at the steady state, i.e., $\sum_{i=1}^{3} L_{ij}p_j = 0$ poses a similar problem for

evaluating $\{p_j\}$. We apply the method on the example with three states for the sake of pedagogy. We will closely follow the notations and the steps developed in (Zia and Schmittmann, 2007) for this part. Generalization of this approach to a larger network is straightforward. The method is executed in three steps.

Step(0): Create a graph for the reaction network. Each vertex in the graph represents a unique state that can occur in the network. The vertices in Figure 14.5 show the three possible states that arise in the system. A directed edge (or a line with an arrowhead) from vertex i to vertex j is drawn if transition probability (or $w^j_i \Delta t \neq 0$) for the transition is non-vanishing.

Step(1): Construct all possible distinct spanning tree graphs from the graph created in *Step*(0). A spanning tree graph is a graph that connects all the vertices in a graph with the minimum number of undirected edges (Trudeau, 2013). Thus, a spanning tree does not contain any loop. For a graph with N number of vertices it is possible to construct N^{N-2} number of spanning trees, therefore, for N = 3 there will be $3^1 = 3$ different spanning trees (Figure 14.6). We index the spanning trees by $\{t_\alpha\} = \{t_1, t_2, t_3\}$.

Step(2): Construct directed graphs out of the spanning trees created in the previous step by replacing the undirected edges by directed edges when there is a non-zero transition probability associated with it. To solve for p_1 we need to consider the directed graphs where every arrow in the spanning trees points to a

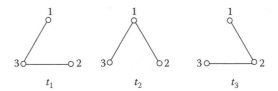

Figure 14.6 Spanning trees for the three state model. Shows the three spanning trees indexed by $\{t_\alpha\}$ = $\{t_1, t_2, t_3\}$.

flow toward vertex #1 (Figure 14.7). In the same way, for evaluating p_2 and p_3, we will consider directed graphs where the edges point to vertex #2 and #3, respectively (Figure 14.6). Once the graphs contributing towards the calculation of p_i are identified, we can start calculating the terms in the p_i's that arise from these graphs.

Step(3): Calculate contributions of the spanning trees, t_1, t_2, and t_3 to $\{p_i\}$. The contribution of the spanning tree t_α to p_i is denoted by $U(t_{\alpha(i)})$. $U(t_{\alpha(i)})$ is calculated by multiplying the transitions rates (or w^j_i's) for the transitions associated with the directed edges in the spanning tree (Figure 14.7).

Thus, $U(t_{1(1)})$, $U(t_{2(1)})$, and, $U(t_{3(1)})$, are given by,

$$U(t_{1(1)}) = w_3^2 w_1^3 = k_p k_{off}, U(t_{1(2)}) = w_1^3 w_1^2 = k_{off}^2, U(t_{1(3)}) = w_1^2 w_2^3 = k_{off} k_d$$

The other $\{U(t_{\alpha(i)})\}$ are calculated in the same manner. p_i is given by

$$p_i = \frac{1}{Z} \sum_{\alpha=1}^{3} U(t_{\alpha(i)}) \tag{14.16}$$

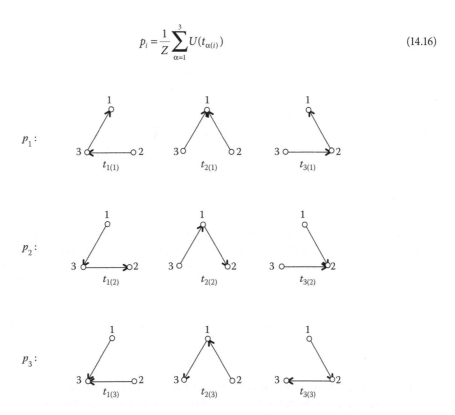

Figure 14.7 Directed graphs contributing to the calculations of $\{p_i\}$ following Eq. (14.16). The spanning trees (t_1, t_2, and t_3) corresponding to p_i are denoted by $t_{1(i)}$, $t_{2(i)}$, and $t_{3(i)}$.

where the partition function Z is defined as:

$$Z = \sum_{i=1}^{3} \sum_{\alpha=1}^{3} U(t_{\alpha(i)}).$$

In Appendices V-VI we use the graphical formulation developed here to gain deeper understanding into the kinetics, e.g., probe the presence of microscopic reversibility in the kinetics.

14.9 APPENDIX V: NETWORK ARCHITECTURE AND THE DETAILED BALANCE CONDITION

The energy utilized by a chemical reaction network is intimately tied with the presence or absence of the detailed balance condition. The presence of the detailed balance condition in turn is tied to the existence of microscopic reversibility in the kinetics. The presence of microscopic reversibility in stochastic kinetics is evaluated by the Kolmogorov criterion (Zia and Schmittmann, 2007). We introduce the concept of the Kolmogorov criterion and the detailed balance condition using our simple example in Figure 14.5. Generalization of these concepts to more complicated reaction networks is straightforward. The Kolmogorov criterion in a stochastic kinetics checks for the equality of probabilities for a series of transitions for two cases where the transitions begin and end at the same state but the changes occur in opposite ("forward" and "reverse") directions (Figure 14.5). Consider, the forward and reverse transitions occurring in the closed loop, namely, $1 \rightarrow 2 \rightarrow 3 \rightarrow 1$ (forward), and, $1 \leftarrow 2 \leftarrow 3 \leftarrow 1$ (reverse). The respective probabilities for the transitions are given by,

$$\Pi_1^1 = \pi^{forward}(1 \rightarrow 2 \rightarrow 3 \rightarrow 1) = w_2^1 w_3^2 w_1^3$$
$$\Pi_1^2 = \pi^{reverse}(1 \leftarrow 2 \leftarrow 3 \leftarrow 1) = w_1^2 w_2^3 w_3^1$$

The Kolmogorov criterion states that in the presence of microscopic reversibility, the two probabilities should be equal, i.e.,

$$\pi^{forward}(1 \rightarrow 2 \rightarrow 3 \rightarrow 1) = \pi^{reverse}(1 \leftarrow 2 \leftarrow 3 \leftarrow 1)$$
$$\Rightarrow w_1^2 w_2^3 w_3^1 = w_2^1 w_3^2 w_1^3 \tag{14.17}$$

The above condition (Eq. (14.17)) imposes constraints on the values of rate constants in the KPR network. Note, in the absence of the KPR step (Figure 14.5b), the probability of the transition in the forward ($1 \rightarrow 2 \rightarrow 3 \rightarrow 2 \rightarrow 1$) direction is equal to that in the reverse ($1 \leftarrow 2 \leftarrow 3 \leftarrow 2 \leftarrow 1$) direction regardless of the values of the rate constants. In this case,

$$\pi^{forward}(1 \rightarrow 2 \rightarrow 3 \rightarrow 2 \rightarrow 1) = w_2^1 w_3^2 w_2^3 w_1^2$$
$$\pi^{reverse}(1 \leftarrow 2 \leftarrow 3 \leftarrow 2 \leftarrow 1) = w_1^2 w_2^3 w_3^2 w_2^1$$

Thus, the possibility of the breakdown of the detailed balance condition is tied to the presence of loop structures in the graphs representing the chemical reaction kinetics. The presence of microscopic reversibility implies the presence of the detailed balance condition in the kinetics, which gives rise to Boltzmann distributions in the steady state, i.e., $p_i \propto \exp(\Phi_i)$, where, Φ_i is a potential function. Below we derive an important equality, which we will use to derive the Boltzmann distribution for the probabilities $\{p_i\}$ in the next section. The presence of microscopic reversibility in the closed loop 1-2-3-1 (Figure 14.5a) demands,

$$\Pi_1^1 = \pi(1 \to 2 \to 3 \to 1) = \pi(1 \to 2)\pi(2 \to 3 \to 1)$$
$$\Pi_1^1 = \pi(1 \leftarrow 2 \leftarrow 3 \leftarrow 1) = \pi(2 \leftarrow 3 \leftarrow 1)\pi(1 \leftarrow 2)$$

Therefore,

$$\frac{\Pi_2^1}{\Pi_1^2} = \frac{\pi(1 \to 2)}{\pi(1 \leftarrow 2)} = \frac{\pi(2 \leftarrow 3 \leftarrow 1)}{\pi(2 \to 3 \to 1)} = e^{\Phi_2 - \Phi_1} \tag{14.18}$$

The last equality in Eq. (14.18) shows that in the presence of microscopic reversibility or the detailed balance condition the ratio of the probabilities for transitioning from $1 \to 2$ and the reverse $(2 \to 1)$ does not depend on the specific path taken to execute the operation, i.e., path independence of the ratio. This simple result has a profound implication. The path independence implies that the ratio can only depend on the start and the end states and not on the states in between which allows us to write the ratio as using functions (or "potential energies") that depend on the start and the end states alone.

14.9.1 BOLTZMANN DISTRIBUTION AS A RESULT OF THE DETAILED BALANCE CONDITION IN THE KINETICS

It is now easy to derive that when the detailed balance condition in Eq. (14.18) is obeyed $\{p_i\}$ would always follow a Boltzmann distribution, i.e., $p_i \propto \exp(\Phi_i)$ or $p_i/p_j = \exp(\Phi_i - \Phi_j)$ $(i \neq j)$. For our simple example (Figure 14.5) we can show p_1/p_3 is given by a Boltzmann distribution by calculating p_1 and p_3 at the steady state using the solution obtained by the graphical method (Eq. 14.16). Consider the terms contributing to p_1 and p_3 in Eq. (14.16) (Figure 14.8).

$$U(t_{1(1)}) = U(t_{1(3)}) \times \frac{\Pi_3^1}{\Pi_1^3} = U(t_{1(3)}) \times e^{\Phi_1 - \Phi_3}$$

$$U(t_{2(1)}) = U(t_{2(3)}) \times \frac{\Pi_3^1}{\Pi_1^3} = U(t_{2(3)}) \times e^{\Phi_1 - \Phi_3} \tag{14.19}$$

$$U(t_{3(1)}) = U(t_{3(3)}) \times \frac{\Pi_3^1}{\Pi_1^3} = U(t_{3(3)}) \times e^{\Phi_1 - \Phi_3}$$

The path independence of Π_j^i, which is only valid when the detailed balance condition holds, is used for writing down the third equality in the above equations.

Therefore, $p_1 = 1/Z \sum_{\alpha=1}^{3} U(t_{\alpha(1)}) = \frac{e^{\Phi_1 - \Phi_3}}{Z} \sum_{\alpha=1}^{3} U(t_{\alpha(3)}) = e^{\Phi_1 - \Phi_3} p_3$. Similarly one can also show, $p_2 = e^{\Phi_2 - \Phi_3} p_3$.

The equalities in Eq. (14.19) can be generalized to any complex stochastic networks.

14.9.2 ENTROPY PRODUCTION AND QUANTIFICATION OF DISSIPATION

The chemical reaction networks, e.g., the KPR network, interact with the local environment. The interaction can arise due to reactions associated with the KPR consuming the energy generated by ATP hydrolysis. Some of this energy is irreversibly lost or dissipated as the reactions proceed. The breakdown of the detailed balance condition leads to a continuous dissipation of energy even in the steady state where the probability distributions of the copy numbers of molecules in different states do not change with time (Das, 2016). The dissipation

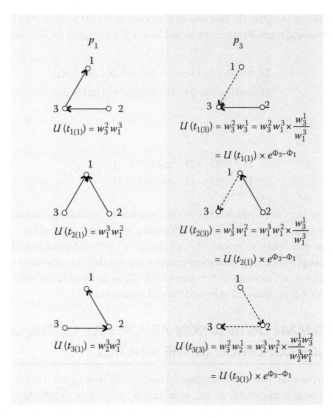

Figure 14.8 Relation between the directed graphs contributing to p_1 and p_3. The edges pointing in the opposite directions in the sub graphs for p_3 in comparison to that p_1 are shown with dashed lines with arrowheads. The $U(t_{\alpha(i)})$ terms for the graphs are shown below the respective graphs.

can be quantified by the entropy production. The precise relationship between energy dissipation and entropy production has been a subject of intense research in the recent years (Ge and Qian, 2010; Jarzynski, 2011).

The entropy of the system or the system entropy is defined as, $S_{sys} = -\sum_i p_i(t) \ln[p_i(t)]$ (Imparato and Peliti, 2007; Schnakenberg, 1976; Seifert, 2012; Zia and Schmittmann, 2007), where the sum over i can also represent a sum over single cells in a cell population (or an ensemble of stochastic trajectories). S_{sys} follows the kinetics (Imparato and Peliti, 2007; Schnakenberg, 1976; Seifert, 2012; Zia and Schmittmann, 2007),

$$\frac{dS_{sys}(t)}{dt} = -\underbrace{\sum_{\substack{i,j \\ j \neq i}} w_j^i p_j \ln\left(\frac{w_j^i p_i}{w_i^j p_j}\right)}_{\frac{dS_{total}}{dt}} - \underbrace{\sum_{\substack{i,j \\ j \neq i}} w_i^j p_j \ln\left(\frac{w_j^i}{w_i^j}\right)}_{\frac{dS_{med}}{dt}} = \frac{dS_{total}}{dt} - \frac{dS_{med}}{dt} \tag{14.20}$$

According to Eq. (14.20), the entropy S_{total} never decreases (Imparato and Peliti, 2007; Seifert, 2012), i.e., $dS_{total}/dt \geq 0$, and thus quantifies dissipation in the system. In the steady state, $dS_{sys}/dt = 0$, and, consequently, $dS_{total}/dt = dS_{med}/dt$. dS_{med}/dt denotes the rate of entropy exchange between the system and the reservoir.

$$\frac{dS_{med}}{dt} = \left(w_1^3 p_3 - w_3^1 p_1\right)\ln\left[\frac{w_3^1}{w_1^3}\right] + \left(w_1^2 p_2 - w_2^1 p_1\right)\ln\left[\frac{w_1^2}{w_2^1}\right] + \left(w_3^2 p_2 - w_2^3 p_3\right)\ln\left[\frac{w_2^3}{w_3^2}\right] \tag{14.21}$$

When the detailed balance condition is obeyed the right hand side of Eq. (14.21) vanishes. This implies that dS_{total}/dt vanishes as well in this situation, *i.e.*, the total entropy of the system (S_{total}) does not change. Thus, the

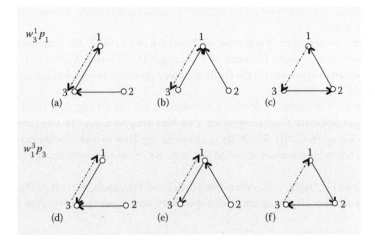

Figure 14.9 Graphs contributing to the first term in Eq. (14.21). **(a)–(c)** Shows the graphs that contribute to $w_3^1 p_1$. **(d)–(f)** Graphs contributing to $w_1^3 p_3$. The dash-dot lines with arrowheads in the graphs represent the terms in that arise due to the multiplication of w_3^1 or w_1^3 to p_1 or p_3, respectively. The graph in **(a)** or **(b)** is identical to that in **(d)** or **(e)** respectively. This implies that the contribution of these graphs in the terms $w_3^1 p_1$ and $w_1^3 p_3$ will cancel for any values of the rates. Transitions occur in reverse directions in graphs in **(c)** and **(f)**. The presence of the microscopic reversibility (Eq. (14.5)) ensures that the contribution of the graph in **(c)** to $w_3^1 p_1$ and in the graph in **(f)** to $w_3^1 p_3$ are identical. This results in vanishing of the first term in Eq. (14.21).

system kinetics does not generate any dissipation. Its easy see how the detailed balance condition will lead to the vanishing of dS_{med}/dt. We will show this graphically by using the solution (Eq. (14.16)) of the Master equation derived in the previous section. Consider the graphs (Figure 14.9) that correspond to the first term in Eq. (14.21). Visual inspection of Figure 14.9 shows that the contribution of $w_3^1 p_3$ matches exactly with $w_3^1 p_1$ when the Kolmogorov criterion in Eq. (14.17) is obeyed (see Figure 14.9 and the legend for details). This renders the first term zero. Similarly, it can be easily shown that the other terms in Eq. (14.21) vanish in the presence of the detailed balance condition.

ACKNOWLEDGMENTS

The author acknowledges the funding R56AI108880–01 from NIAID and thanks Ashok Prasad for a critical reading of the chapter.

REFERENCES

Altan-Bonnet, G., and Germain, R.N. (2005). Modeling T cell antigen discrimination based on feedback control of digital ERK responses. *PLoS Biol 3*, e356.

Chakraborty, A.K., and Weiss, A. (2014). Insights into the initiation of TCR signaling. *Nat Immunol 15*, 798-807.

Das, J. (2013). Positive feedback produces broad distributions in maximum activation attained within a narrow time window in stochastic biochemical reactions. *J Chem Phys 138*, 015101.

Das, J. (2016). Limiting Energy Dissipation Induces Glassy Kinetics in Single-Cell High-Precision Responses. *Biophys J 110*, 1180-1190.

Das, J., Ho, M., Zikherman, J., Govern, C., Yang, M., Weiss, A., Chakraborty, A.K., and Roose, J.P. (2009a). Digital signaling and hysteresis characterize ras activation in lymphoid cells. *Cell 136*, 337-351.

Das, J., Kardar, M., and Chakraborty, A.K. (2009b). Positive feedback regulation results in spatial clustering and fast spreading of active signaling molecules on a cell membrane. *J Chem Phys 130*, 245102.

Del Vecchio, D., Ninfa, A.J., and Sontag, E.D. (2008). Modular cell biology: Retroactivity and insulation. *Mol Syst Biol 4*, 161.

Dirac, P.A.M. (1935). *The principles of quantum mechanics* (2d ed.). Oxford: The Clarendon Press.

Faeder, J.R., Hlavacek, W.S., Reischl, I., Blinov, M.L., Metzger, H., Redondo, A., Wofsy, C., and Goldstein, B. (2003). Investigation of early events in FcεRI-mediated signaling using a detailed mathematical model. *J Immunol 170*, 3769-3781.

Feng, Y., Brazin, K.N., Kobayashi, E., Mallis, R.J., Reinherz, E.L., and Lang, M.J. (2017). Mechanosensing drives acuity of alphabeta T-cell recognition. *Proc Natl Acad Sci U S A 114*, E8204-E8213.

Ferrell Jr, J.E., and Xiong, W. (2001). Bistability in cell signaling: How to make continuous processes discontinuous, and reversible processes irreversible. *Chaos: An Interdisciplinary Journal of Nonlinear Science 11*, 227-236.

François, P., Voisinne, G., Siggia, E.D., Altan-Bonnet, G., and Vergassola, M. (2013). Phenotypic model for early T-cell activation displaying sensitivity, specificity, and antagonism. *Proc Natl Acad Sci U S A 110*, E888-E897.

Ge, H., and Qian, H. (2010). Physical origins of entropy production, free energy dissipation, and their mathematical representations. *Phys Rev E 81*.

Goel, N.S., and Dyn, N. (1974). *Stochastic models in biology.* New York, NY: Academic Press.

Govern, C.C., Paczosa, M.K., Chakraborty, A.K., and Huseby, E.S. (2010). Fast on-rates allow short dwell time ligands to activate T cells. *Proc Natl Acad Sci U S A 107*, 8724-8729.

Gunawardena, J. (2014). Models in biology: "Accurate descriptions of our pathetic thinking". *BMC Biol 12*, 29.

Hoffmann, A., Levchenko, A., Scott, M.L., and Baltimore, D. (2002). The IkappaB-NF-kappaB signaling module: temporal control and selective gene activation. *Science 298*, 1241-1245.

Hopfield, J.J. (1974). Kinetic proofreading: A new mechanism for reducing errors in biosynthetic processes requiring high specificity. *Proc Natl Acad Sci U S A 71*, 4135-4139.

Huang, J., Zarnitsyna, V.I., Liu, B., Edwards, L.J., Jiang, N., Evavold, B.D., and Zhu, C. (2010). The kinetics of two-dimensional TCR and pMHC interactions determine T-cell responsiveness. *Nature 464*, 932-936.

Huse, M., Klein, L.O., Girvin, A.T., Faraj, J.M., Li, Q.-J., Kuhns, M.S., and Davis, M.M. (2007). Spatial and temporal dynamics of T cell receptor signaling with a photoactivatable agonist. *Immunity 27*, 76-88.

Huse, M., Lillemeier, B.F., Kuhns, M.S., Chen, D.S., and Davis, M.M. (2006). T cells use two directionally distinct pathways for cytokine secretion. *Nat Immunol 7*, 247-255.

Imparato, A., and Peliti, L. (2007). The distribution function of entropy flow in stochastic systems. *J Stat Mech-Theory E*.

Iversen, L., Tu, H.L., Lin, W.C., Christensen, S.M., Abel, S.M., Iwig, J., Wu, H.J., Gureasko, J., Rhodes, C., Petit, R.S. *et al.* (2014). Molecular kinetics. Ras activation by SOS: Allosteric regulation by altered fluctuation dynamics. *Science 345*, 50-54.

Jarzynski, C. (2011). Equalities and inequalities: Irreversibility and the second law of thermodynamics at the nanoscale. *Annu Rev Conden Ma P 2*, 329-351.

Jun, J.E., Rubio, I., and Roose, J.P. (2013). Regulation of Ras exchange factors and cellular localization of Ras activation by lipid messengers in T cells. *Front Immunol 4*, 239.

Kampen, N.G.v. (1992). *Stochastic processes in physics and chemistry* (Rev. and enl. ed.) Amsterdam, New York, NY: North-Holland.

Kochanczyk, M., Kocieniewski, P., Kozlowska, E., Jaruszewicz-Blonska, J., Sparta, B., Pargett, M., Albeck, J.G., Hlavacek, W.S., and Lipniacki, T. (2017). Relaxation oscillations and hierarchy of feedbacks in MAPK signaling. *Sci Rep 7*, 38244.

Lever, M., Lim, H.-S., Kruger, P., Nguyen, J., Trendel, N., Abu-Shah, E., Maini, P.K., van der Merwe, P.A., and Dushek, O. (2016a). Architecture of a minimal signaling pathway explains the T-cell response to a 1 million-fold variation in antigen affinity and dose. *Proc Natl Acad of Sci U S A*, 201608820.

Lever, M., Lim, H.S., Kruger, P., Nguyen, J., Trendel, N., Abu-Shah, E., Maini, P.K., van der Merwe, P.A., and Dushek, O. (2016b). Architecture of a minimal signaling pathway explains the T-cell response to a 1 million-fold variation in antigen affinity and dose. *Proc Natl Acad Sci U S A 113*, E6630-E6638.

Ma, W., Trusina, A., El-Samad, H., Lim, W.A., and Tang, C. (2009). Defining network topologies that can achieve biochemical adaptation. *Cell 138*, 760-773.

Margarit, S.M., Sondermann, H., Hall, B.E., Nagar, B., Hoelz, A., Pirruccello, M., Bar-Sagi, D., and Kuriyan, J. (2003). Structural evidence for feedback activation by Ras. GTP of the Ras-specific nucleotide exchange factor SOS. *Cell 112*, 685-695.

Mathews, J., and Walker, R.L. (1970). *Mathematical methods of physics* (2d ed.). New York, NY: W. A. Benjamin.

McKeithan, T.W. (1995). Kinetic proofreading in T-cell receptor signal transduction. *Proc Natl Acad Sci U S A 92*, 5042-5046.

Mor, A., and Philips, M.R. (2006). Compartmentalized Ras/MAPK signaling. *Annu Rev Immunol 24*, 771-800.

Mukherjee, S., Rigaud, S., Seok, S.-C., Fu, G., Prochenka, A., Dworkin, M., Gascoigne, N.R., Vieland, V.J., Sauer, K., and Das, J. (2013a). In silico modeling of Itk activation kinetics in thymocytes suggests competing positive and negative IP4 mediated feedbacks increase robustness. *PloS one 8*, e73937.

Mukherjee, S., Zhu, J., Zikherman, J., Parameswaran, R., Kadlecek, T.A., Wang, Q., Au-Yeung, B., Ploegh, H., Kuriyan, J., Das, J. *et al.* (2013b). Monovalent and multivalent ligation of the B cell receptor exhibit differential dependence upon Syk and Src family kinases. *Sci Signal 6*, ra1.

Munsky, B., and Khammash, M. (2006). The finite state projection algorithm for the solution of the chemical master equation. *J Chem Phys 124*, 044104.

Murphy, K., and Weaver, C. (2016). *Janeway's immunobiology*. Garland Science.

Murray, J.D. (1989). *Mathematical biology*. Berlin; New York: Springer-Verlag.

Nelson, P.C., Bromberg, S., Hermundstad, A., and Prentice, J. (2015). *Physical models of living systems*. WH Freeman.

Ninio, J. (1975). Kinetic amplification of enzyme discrimination. *Biochimie 57*, 587-595.

Phillips, R. (2017). Musings on mechanism: Quest for a quark theory of proteins? *FASEB J 31*, 4207-4215.

Qi, S., Krogsgaard, M., Davis, M.M., and Chakraborty, A.K. (2006). Molecular flexibility can influence the stimulatory ability of receptor-ligand interactions at cell-cell junctions. *Proc Natl Acad Sci U S A 103*, 4416-4421.

Rényi, A.D. (2007). *Probability theory* (Dover ed.). New York, NY: Dover Publications.

Schnakenberg, J. (1976). Network Theory of Microscopic and Macroscopic Behavior of Master Equation Systems. *Rev Mod Phys 48*, 571-585.

Seifert, U. (2012). Stochastic thermodynamics, fluctuation theorems and molecular machines. *Rep Prog Phys 75*.

Swain, P.S., Elowitz, M.B., and Siggia, E.D. (2002). Intrinsic and extrinsic contributions to stochasticity in gene expression. *Proc Natl Acad Sci U S A 99*, 12795-12800.

Trudeau, R.J. (2013). *Introduction to graph theory*. New York, NY: Dover Publications.

Zia, R.K.P., and Schmittmann, B. (2007). Probability currents as principal characteristics in the statistical mechanics of non-equilibrium steady states. *J Stat Mech-Theory E*.

Modeling and inference of cell population dynamics

MICHAEL FLOSSDORF AND THOMAS HÖFER

15.1 INTRODUCTION: MODELS OF CELL POPULATION DYNAMICS AND PARAMETER IDENTIFIABILITY

Compartment models are the most common approach for describing the dynamics of immune cell populations. Compartments are distinguished by cell type (e.g., naïve, effector, and memory T cells) or/and spatial location (e.g., spleen, lymph nodes, and effector sites). The processes connecting compartments are cell differentiation (for cell-type compartments) and migration or transport (for spatial compartments). Within the compartments, cell proliferation and death may take place. Thus, the cell number in compartment of type i, n_i, is governed by a differential equation of the general form

$$\frac{dn_i}{dt} = j_i - (\alpha_i + \delta_i - \lambda_i)n_i \tag{15.1}$$

where j_i is the influx (by immigration of cells or differentiation of precursor cells giving rise to type i), λ_i and δ_i are the per capita rates of cell proliferation and death, respectively, and α_i is the per capita rate of onward differentiation or spatial efflux (Figure 15.1). In general, these rates are not constants but are affected by the cell numbers in the system and by external stimuli. This regulation is mediated by cell-contact-dependent or soluble signals, such as cytokines, or by competition for common resources. Hence, population dynamic models that take these regulatory effects into account consist of systems of nonlinear

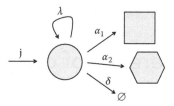

Figure 15.1 Basic processes determining the dynamics of cell numbers in a compartment of interest (round cell): Influx j; proliferation rate λ, differentiation rates α, and loss (death) rate δ. If the compartment represents a branch point in a lineage differentiation pathway, there is more than one differentiation rate (here: into two different cell types symbolized by square and hexagon). Thus, the inference of the corresponding differentiation rates α_1 and α_2 from the data also carries information on the topology of the pathway.

differential equations. Nevertheless, for many practical applications, the approximation of constant rates is appropriate. Then the differential equations become mathematically simple: they are linear with (usually) constant coefficients. However, even in this case, the inference of rates from data is often a formidable problem. This can be readily appreciated by recognizing that proliferation, death, differentiation, and export rates all enter a single effective rate constant, $k_i = \alpha_i + \delta_i - \lambda_i$, and thus straightforward measurements of the cell number over time, $n_i(t)$, will not suffice to separately identify the parameters making up k_i. In the context of steady-state hematopoiesis, Busch et al. (2015) have termed $1/k_i$ the *residence time* of a compartment because it provides a theoretical estimate for the time taken by the compartment to run dry if its influx were switched off.

In this chapter, we will systematically introduce approaches for parameterizing population-dynamic models of the form of Equation 15.1. We will emphasize the information on parameters contained in different kinds of experimental data. Indeed, statistically sound parameterization of population dynamic models will usually benefit from careful planning of the corresponding experiments. In this context, we will emphasize the importance of measuring absolute numbers of the cell types of interest, in addition to the more customary measurements of cell-type frequencies readily made by flow cytometry. The numbers of cells of different types and their changes over time are more informative on the causes of these changes than mere cell-type frequencies. The chapter is broadly divided into two parts: first considering deterministic models for measurements of average cell numbers followed by stochastic approaches for addressing single-cell-based fate-mapping data. The emphasis is on methodology; we will briefly review biological insights gained, but for more in-depth information in this regard, we refer the reader to the literature cited. A recurring idea is that the accurate identification of parameters for a given model will often also allow one to discriminate between alternative models for a given system, thus gaining mechanistic insight that extends beyond mere model parameterization.

15.2 IDENTIFYING RATES FROM POPULATION-LEVEL DATA

15.2.1 INTRODUCTION

Deterministic models describing average cell numbers, as exemplified by Eq. 15.1, are the most common type of population dynamic models in practical applications. This is foremost due to the fact that most experimental measurements sample cell populations. However, techniques for analyzing clonal progenies of individual precursor cells are increasingly becoming available (Buchholz et al. 2016), and associated mathematical approaches will be discussed in Section 15.3. Two principal situations can be distinguished: (1) The system overall is in *steady state*; that is, the cell numbers in the compartments of interest do not change in time. (2) The system is in a *transient* state, with at least some cell numbers changing. We will consider prototypical examples of steady state and transient dynamics: the formation of blood cells during unperturbed hematopoiesis in the healthy adult organism and the response of T cells following an acute infection.

15.2.2 PARAMETER INFERENCE FROM MEASURING ABSOLUTE CELL NUMBERS OVER TIME: T-CELL IMMUNE RESPONSES

During the course of an adaptive immune response, antigen-specific T lymphocytes expand massively and diversify into distinct functional subsets that are distinguished using cell-surface markers. In particular, short-lived effector cells develop that kill, and help other cells killing, the invading pathogen, whereas long-lived memory cells provide protection against reinfection by the same pathogen. The population of memory T cells further subdivides into functionally distinct subsets. Central memory T cells recirculate through secondary lymphoid organs and proliferate vigorously upon rechallenge, while effector memory T cells reside in peripheral organs and can mount immediate effector function following stimulation. A key question concerns the developmental pathways by which short-lived effector cells and precursors of memory cells emerge out of the pool of activated naïve cells (see Section 15.3). As an example, we will here consider a very simple two-population version of the so-called *progressive differentiation model* in which the central memory precursor subset (CM) develops first and then gives rise to T cells of effector function (E) (Buchholz et al. 2016; Gattinoni et al. 2017). For clarity, we make the simplifying assumption that the activation of naïve T cells is so fast that its kinetics need not be considered explicitly. During the expansion phase of the T-cell response, we can further assume exponential growth leading us to the following dynamic equations:

$$\frac{dn_{CM}}{dt} = (\lambda_{CM} - \delta_{CM} - \alpha_{CM})n_{CM} \tag{15.2.1}$$

$$\frac{dn_{E}}{dt} = \alpha_{CM}n_{CM} + (\lambda_{E} - \delta_{E} - \alpha_{E})n_{E}, \tag{15.2.2}$$

where we made use of the nomenclature introduced in Equation 15.1.

A common technique to experimentally assess cell dynamics *in vivo* is the adoptive transfer of genetically labeled cells. At various time points post transfer, the heritable labels are used to distinguish the progeny of the transferred cells from the endogenous cells of the recipient. Examples for such labels comprise allelic variants of surface markers distinguishable by flow cytometry and genetic barcodes that can be identified by DNA sequencing. Experiments of the first kind have been used extensively to study the dynamics of activated T cells responding to an infection. To understand how such measurements can be used to study T-cell responses on a quantitative basis, the explicit solution of Eqs. 15.2.1 and 15.2.2 is illustrative. Defining the effective proliferation rates to be $\lambda_{CM}^{eff} = \lambda_{CM} - \delta_{CM} - \alpha_{CM}$ and $\lambda_{E}^{eff} = \lambda_{E} - \delta_{E}$, we find

$$n_{CM}(t) = n_{CM,0}\, e^{\lambda_{CM}^{eff} t} \tag{15.3.1}$$

$$n_{E}(t) = n_{CM,0}\frac{\alpha_{CM}}{\lambda_{CM}^{eff} - \lambda_{E}^{eff}}\left(e^{\lambda_{CM}^{eff} t} - e^{\lambda_{E}^{eff} t}\right), \tag{15.3.2}$$

where $n_{CM,0}$ is the initial central memory precursor compartment size, i.e., the number of those naïve T cells that successfully engrafted following transplantation and got recruited into the immune response at $t = 0$. As expected, the solution is not explicitly dependent on proliferation or death rates but only on differences between the two—the effective proliferation rates. In particular, time-resolved measurements of the absolute cell numbers in the CM compartment allow us to assess both the initial compartment size $n_{CM,0}$ and the effective proliferation rate of this compartment (Eq. 15.3.1).

The growth of the effector compartment at large times $\left(t \gg 1/\left|\lambda_{CM}^{eff} - \lambda_E^{eff}\right|\right)$ depends on whichever effective proliferation rate is bigger (Eq. 15.3.2). In the case that $\lambda_{CM}^{eff} < \lambda_E^{eff}$ (which is the case for cytotoxic T cells; Buchholz et al. 2013), we can use measurements at such time points to estimate λ_E^{eff} and the factor $F = \alpha_{CM}/\left(\lambda_{CM}^{eff} - \lambda_E^{eff}\right)$, which effectively enables us to estimate all parameters of Eqs. 15.3.1 and 15.3.2. On the other hand, if $\lambda_{CM}^{eff} > \lambda_E^{eff}$, the effector compartment will asymptotically be growing proportional to $e^{\lambda_{CM}^{eff} t}$ (which we already know from the $n_{CM}(t)$ data). In this case, kinetic measurements of the number of effector cells $n_E(t)$ at relatively late time points would not be informative on the proliferation rate of this compartment but only yield additional information on F. Thus, for $\lambda_{CM}^{eff} > \lambda_E^{eff}$, an independent estimation of λ_E^{eff} and α_{CM} based just on cell numbers at late time points in the response is not possible (see below for a quantitative estimate of "late"). If one, nevertheless, attempted parameter estimation from such data, one would find variable estimates for λ_E^{eff} and α_{CM}, with (negative) correlations such that the estimate of F stays approximately constant. This example illustrates that the identifiability of rate parameters from a given set of data may depend on the actual values these parameters have: For $\lambda_{CM}^{eff} < \lambda_E^{eff}$, both central memory precursor and effector net proliferation rates and the differentiation rate are identifiable from time course measurements of the cell numbers in the two compartments, whereas for $\lambda_{CM}^{eff} > \lambda_E^{eff}$, this is not the case if the data are measured at too late time points.

To understand whether data measured at earlier time points $\left(t < 1/\left|\lambda_{CM}^{eff} - \lambda_E^{eff}\right|\right)$ add information on the parameters, it is useful to consider the relative size of the CM compartment:

$$\rho_{CM}(t) = \frac{n_{CM}(t)}{n_{CM}(t) + n_E(t)} = \frac{1}{1 + F\left(1 - e^{-\Delta\lambda^{eff}t}\right)}, \tag{15.4}$$

where we defined $\Delta\lambda^{eff} = \lambda_{CM}^{eff} - \lambda_E^{eff}$ as the excess proliferation rate of the first compartment (CM). Note that for cytotoxic T cells in practice, $\lambda_{CM}^{eff} < \lambda_E^{eff}$ (Buchholz et al. 2013), but for other cases of one cell compartment giving rise to another, $\Delta\lambda^{eff}$ may indeed be positive. In this latter case ($\Delta\lambda^{eff} > 0$), both compartments approach a constant cell number ratio at late time points, $\rho_{CM}(t) \approx 1/(1 + F)$. The speed with which this proportionality is reached contains information about $\Delta\lambda^{eff}$. Therefore, measurements at both early and late time points are pivotal to identify all kinetic parameters when the precursor compartment proliferates faster than the product. Note that Eq. 15.4 is true irrespective of λ_{CM}^{eff} being bigger or smaller than λ_E^{eff}. In the latter case, which we discussed before, early time point data also provide additional information about F and $\Delta\lambda^{eff}$, resulting in more precise estimates of all parameters.

What are "early" and "late" time points in practice? Buchholz et al. (2013) give approximately $\lambda_{CM}^{eff} = 0.8$ per day and $\lambda_E^{eff} = 1.6$ per day for an acute immune response to *Listeria* presenting the SIINFEKL peptide to OT-I T cells. Hence, $1/\left|\lambda_{CM}^{eff} - \lambda_E^{eff}\right| = 1.25$ days. Experimental measurements of T-cell immune responses *in vivo* at such early time points after pathogen challenge are very rare, due to the small cell numbers that would need to be recovered from the experimental animal, but would be informative in quantitative terms.

In general, differentiation between the two compartments may not be unidirectional. Our simple model can still be treated analytically if a "backward" differentiation rate α_E from E to CM is introduced:

$$n_{CM}(t) = \frac{1}{2}CM_0 e^{\frac{1}{2}\left(\lambda_{CM}^{eff} + \lambda_E^{eff}\right)t}\left(e^{\frac{1}{2}rt} + e^{-\frac{1}{2}rt}\right) + \frac{\Delta\lambda^{eff}}{2\alpha_{CM}}n_E \tag{15.5.1}$$

$$n_E(t) = CM_0 \frac{\alpha_{CM}}{r} e^{\frac{1}{2}\left(\lambda_{CM}^{eff} + \lambda_E^{eff}\right)t}\left(e^{\frac{1}{2}rt} - e^{-\frac{1}{2}rt}\right), \tag{15.5.2}$$

where $r = \sqrt{4\alpha_{CM}\alpha_E + \Delta\lambda^{eff^2}}$. Interestingly, α_E only enters these equations through the lumped rate parameter r (this asymmetry with α_{CM} is due to the initial condition $n_E(0) = 0$). For $t \ll 1/r$, Taylor expansion shows that the absolute cell numbers of both compartments no longer depend on r, implying that measurements at both early and late time points are necessary to estimate the model parameters including α_E.

Population dynamic models are usually more complex than the two-compartment model discussed here. However, the analytical insights afforded by this simple example illustrate several points of practical importance. First, parameter identifiability depends on the available data, and the selection of time points for the measurements can be critical. For assessing parameter identifiability in practice, the profile likelihood method is a useful tool (Venzon and Moolgavkar 1988; Raue et al. 2009). Second, cell number measurements, in addition to relative compartment sizes, are key to parameter estimation. For practical purposes, it can be beneficial to explicitly use relative compartment sizes in the parameter estimation procedure due to their usually small measurement error when determined by flow cytometry, complemented by separate measurements of the total cell number. It is intuitively clear that proliferation rates cannot be determined without knowing time courses of cell numbers. However, even the inference of differentiation rates generally requires such information. To illustrate this point, we note that Equation 15.4 reduces to $\rho_{CM}(t) = e^{-\alpha_{CM}t}$ only if the difference between proliferation and death rates is equal for both compartments (and $\alpha_E = 0$), so that in this special case, α_{CM} could be estimated from the fraction of progenitor (CM) cells. However, in general, $\rho_{CM}(t)$ will also depend on $\Delta\lambda^{eff}$ (and α_E).

15.2.3 CELL-CYCLE-DEPENDENT LABELS

In this section, we will briefly introduce two experimental techniques that are commonly used to quantify cell division of lymphocytes *in vivo*. For a more thorough discussion of the quantification of lymphocyte turnover, see the review by De Boer and Perelson (2013). The first technique is based on oral administration or injection of bromodeoxyuridine (BrdU), which is an analogue of the DNA nucleoside desoxythymidine. Following its incorporation into newly synthesized DNA, BrdU can be detected in cells that recently divided, using antibody staining and flow cytometry. As long as BrdU is available, every unlabeled cell results in two labeled daughter cells. This results in the following model for the dynamics of the number of BrdU labeled (n_L) and unlabeled (n_U) cells during the labeling phase:

$$\frac{dn_U}{dt} = -(\lambda + \delta)n_U \tag{15.6.1}$$

$$\frac{dn_L}{dt} = 2\lambda n_U + (\lambda - \delta)n_L \tag{15.6.2}$$

Here λ denotes the proliferation rate and δ denotes the loss rate from the compartment under consideration (sum of death, onward differentiation, and emigration rates). For the fraction of BrdU-positive cells $f^+ = n_L/(n_L + n_U)$, one then obtains

$$\frac{df^+}{dt} = 2\lambda(1 - f^+). \tag{15.7}$$

Considering that $f^+(t_L) = 0$ at the time point of labeling t_L, this is solved by

$$f^+ = 1 - e^{2\lambda(t-t_L)}. \tag{15.8}$$

If the labeling duration is small compared to the mean interdivision time $1/\lambda$, the fraction of BrdU-positive cells grows linearly with time: $f^+ \approx 2\lambda(t - t_L)$. Thus, the fraction of labeled cells is independent of loss rates, and its measurement allows direct inference of the proliferation rate. Possible complications that we neglected here include the fact that, depending on the availability of BrdU, not all cell divisions might result in labeled daughter cells and that the concentration of BrdU will not be constant over time (De Boer and Perelson 2013). During delabeling, the BrdU label gets halved with every division, resulting in a decline of the measured fraction of BrdU-positive cells f^+ that is dependent not only on the proliferation rate but also on the threshold BrdU intensity below which a cell is detected as BrdU negative (Ganusov and De Boer 2013). A fine detail of interpreting BrdU labeling data relates to the fact that BrdU given over a certain time period labels cells that are initially already in the S phase of the cell cycle and cells that enter the S phase during this period. Strictly speaking, only the latter are relevant for estimating the proliferation rate, and dual pulse labeling, using distinguishable desoxythymidine analogues (such as BrdU and EdU; Bradford and Clarke 2011), may give more accurate results.

Another widely used technique to monitor lymphocyte proliferation is based on carboxyfluorescein succinimidyl ester (CFSE), which is a fluorescent dye that irreversibly enters cells and then becomes diluted approximately twofold upon cell division (a number of further dyes of this kind are available). For T cells, up to seven to eight divisions can be identified by measuring the CFSE intensity of individual cells before the fluorescence intensity gets indistinguishable from the autofluorescence background. This results in experimental estimates for the number of cells n_i in each generation. For a simple proliferation–death model, the corresponding dynamical equations read

$$\frac{dn_0}{dt} = -(\lambda + \delta)n_0 \tag{15.9.1}$$

$$\frac{dn_i}{dt} = 2\lambda n_{i-1} - (\lambda + \delta)n_i. \; i = 1, 2, \ldots \tag{15.9.2}$$

Iteratively solving these differential equations yields for the fraction of cells in each generation:

$$f_i = \frac{(2\lambda t)^i}{i!} e^{-2\lambda t}. \tag{15.10}$$

Thus, the relative number of cell divisions in this model is Poisson-distributed with mean $2\lambda t$. For more complicated population dynamic models, CFSE and BrdU data contain information that helps to disentangle cell division and death rates.

Several other labels that are taken up by cells and then diluted by cell divisions have been used for estimating cell proliferation rates, including stable isotypes (e.g., deuterated water or deuterated glucose, both of which can be used with human subjects; Ahmed et al. 2015) or fluorescently tagged histones expressed from a transgene in mice (Foudi et al. 2009). A specialty of T cells exploited for estimating proliferation rates are T-cell receptor excision circles (TRECs), small DNA circles generated through the recombination of the T-cell receptor genes in the thymus that are subsequently not replicated. Combining stable isotype labeling and TREC dynamics, den Braber et al. (2012) quantitatively defined the role of thymic output for maintaining the naïve T-cell compartment in juvenile and adult mice and humans.

15.2.4 STEADY-STATE DYNAMICS: HEMATOPOIESIS

Unlike acute immune responses, where lymphocyte numbers grow over time, during maintenance mode, cellular compartments are approximately in a steady state, which is determined by the balance of cell influx, proliferation, and loss. To provide a concrete example, we consider hematopoiesis—the process by which hematopoietic stem cells (HSCs) give rise to a plethora of blood and immune cell types. Cell differentiation from HSCs to mature cells proceeds through various progenitor cell states during which cell numbers are amplified to meet demand. To illustrate this, consider an adult mouse, which has of the order of 10^4 HSC in the bone marrow and overall about 10^7 granulocytes. Granulocytes are very short-lived leukocytes that are pivotal to the innate immune defense; they have an average lifetime in the blood of less than 1 day [accurately determined in humans (Lahoz-Beneytez et al. 2016) but likely to be similar in the mouse]. Hence, a mouse should produce of the order of 10 million granulocytes every day, or about 100 granulocytes per second. This production rate could not be sustained directly by 10,000 HSC and requires intermediary amplifying compartments. Cell production rates for humans are naturally even larger. For example, humans have of the order of 10^{13} erythrocytes (Bianconi et al. 2013), with a lifetime of 100–120 days. Hence, we need to produce approximately 10^6 new red blood cells per second (HSC numbers in humans are not well known, but may, in fact, not be so different from the numbers in mice; Abkowitz et al. 2002).

Quantitative considerations on overall hematopoietic productivity have been made in considerable detail (Mackey 2001). However, experimental tools for measuring the activity of unperturbed hematopoietic stem and progenitor cells, producing downstream progeny in the adult bone marrow, have only recently become available (Busch et al. 2015). The key idea is to label HSC, using a genetically heritable label that is passed on to all progeny of a labeled HSC without dilution, theoretically over an infinite number of generations (contrasting with proliferation-dependent labels discussed in Section 15.2.3). Sophisticated, noninvasive techniques for generating such heritable labels in specific cell types have been developed to map the fate of cells in development and establish precursor–product relationships (reviewed for hematopoiesis in Höfer et al. 2016a). Busch et al. (2015) have developed a mathematical approach to derive differentiation and proliferation rates from such fate-mapping data. Here we consider a typical experiment that measures labeled cells in successive compartments $i = 0,1,2, \ldots$, e.g., the label is introduced in HSC ($i = 0$) and then propagates to progenitor cell stages (usually referred to as short-term HSC or ST-HSC, $i = 1$, multipotent progenitors or MPP, $i = 2$, and so on). Downstream of ST-HSC, there is a fundamental branching in this differentiation pathway between lymphoid development (yielding T, B, and NK cells) and erythromyeloid development. For the moment, we disregard branching, yielding the following basic equations for the cell numbers in the different compartments:

$$n_0(t) = \text{const.} \tag{15.11.1}$$

$$\frac{dn_i}{dt} = \alpha_{i-1} n_{i-1} - (\alpha_i + \delta_i - \lambda_i) n_i, \tag{15.11.2}$$

where the HSC number is taken as conserved. It turns out that the propagation dynamics of the fate-mapping label do not suffice to separately identify proliferation rates λ_i and death rates δ_i; hence we define

$$\beta_i = \lambda_i - \delta_i \tag{15.12}$$

as the net or excess proliferation. For adult mice, Eqs. 15.11.1 and 15.11.2 can be considered to be in steady state, $dn_i/dt = 0$, yielding

$$\frac{n_i}{n_{i-1}} = \frac{\alpha_{i-1}}{\alpha_i - \beta_i} \tag{15.13}$$

Note that the cell number ratio between a precursor–product pair of compartments (left-hand side of Eq. 15.13) can be measured by flow cytometry; this measurement constrains the values the rate parameters can take.

At $t = 0$, heritable label is introduced in the HSC, and hence the labeled cells are not in steady state. They obey

$$n_0^*(t) = \text{const.} \tag{15.14.1}$$

$$\frac{dn_i^*}{dt} = \alpha_{i-1} n_{i-1}^* - (\alpha_i - \beta_i) n_i^*. \tag{15.14.2}$$

Note that the rate constants are not altered by the presence of the label. Absolute cell numbers from the bone marrow cannot easily be measured with high accuracy, whereas the labeling frequency, the ratio of labeled to unlabeled cells $f_i = n_i^* / n_i$, can. Using this definition and Eq. 15.13, we find from Eq. 15.14 the label propagation equation:

$$\frac{\mathrm{d}f_i}{\mathrm{d}t} = (\alpha_i - \beta_i)(f_{i-1} - f_i).$$

(15.15)

It implies that the labeling frequency in the product compartment will equilibrate with the labeling frequency in the precursors. Therefore, eventually, the entire hematopoietic system derived from the HSC should attain the labeling frequency that was initially induced in the HSC. The characteristic time for the equilibration depends only on the parameters of the product:

$$\tau_i = \frac{1}{\alpha_i - \beta_i}.$$

(15.16)

The residence time τ_i (Busch et al. 2015) provides a measure of the degree of self-renewal in the compartment. A compartment with a large residence time can almost compensate cell loss (by onward differentiation and death) through proliferation, whereas a compartment with a small residence time depends predominantly on cell influx from its precursor.

Consider the deviation of the label frequency from its steady-state value relative to the HSC labeling frequency:

$$\varphi_i = 1 - \frac{f_i}{f_0}.$$

The characteristic waiting time for the label accumulation in the ith compartment can then be defined as

$$T_i = \int_0^\infty \varphi_i(t)\,\mathrm{d}t,$$

(15.17)

yielding

$$T_i = \sum_{j=1}^{i} \tau_j.$$

(15.18)

The delay for label accumulation in a downstream compartment is given by the sum of the residence times along the differentiation pathway. In particular, a nearly self-renewing compartment presents a bottleneck for the propagation of fate mapping label.

Eqs. 15.13 and 15.15 form the basis for the inference of the steady-state parameters, differentiation rates α_i, and net proliferation rates β_i, from time-resolved fate mapping data (Busch et al. 2015). The measurement of labeling frequencies over time, $f_i(t)$, allows the determination of τ_i and hence the self-renewal capacities of the measured compartments in steady state. Together with additional data on the cell number ratios (Eq. 15.13), the label propagation data yield estimates of α_i and β_i. Busch et al. (2015) derive these rates, together with the flux ratio at the branch point between erythromyeloid and lymphoid developmental pathways from experimental data. In adult mice, HSCs contribute only rarely to differentiated progeny during unchallenged hematopoiesis—on average about once in 3–4 months. Accordingly, progenitor compartments immediately downstream of HSCs are very close to self-renewal in unperturbed hematopoiesis. Unperturbed hematopoiesis differs from the dynamics of the system after transplantation in important aspects (Busch and Rodewald, 2016; Höfer et al. 2016a). Recent experimental advances now allow the noninvasive barcoding of single HSC *in situ* (Pei et al., 2017), thus setting the stage for applying model selection approaches to hematopoiesis that are described in Chapter 3.

15.3 SINGLE-CELL-BASED FATE MAPPING AND MODEL SELECTION

15.3.1 INTRODUCTION

Thus far, we have been concerned with the inference of rate parameters from experimental data, where the connections between compartments were given (principally by differentiation rates or migration). However, there are many areas of research where the "topology" of lineage differentiation and migration pathways itself is under study (e.g., Buchholz et al. 2013; Perié et al. 2014). Rate inference and study of lineage topology are related. Consider, for example, a situation where a cell compartment i forms a branch point from which several differentiation pathways into distinct lineages emerge. Equation 15.1 then becomes

$$\frac{\mathrm{d}n_i}{\mathrm{d}t} = j_i - \left(\sum_j \alpha_{ij} + \delta_i - \lambda_i\right)n_i.$$

Thus, if one could infer from data which differentiation rates α_{ij} are nonzero, one would, at the same time, deduce lineage pathways. Recent theoretical work has addressed new experimental techniques that allow the measurement of cell numbers emerging from single labeled progenitors, here called single-cell progenies (Buchholz et al. 2013). These data contain information on both rate parameters and lineage topologies.

15.3.2 ADDED VALUE OF SINGLE-CELL PROGENY DATA

The cell numbers of single-cell progenies contain valuable information on the underlying differentiation and proliferation dynamics. As an example, consider again a simple birth-and-death process in which cells divide and die with constant rates λ and δ, respectively. If there are n_0 cells at time point zero, then the mean value follows a simple exponential growth:

$$\mu = n_0 e^{(\lambda-\delta)t}. \tag{15.19}$$

Thus, as we already saw in Section 15.2.2, only n_0 and the difference between proliferation and death rates can be identified by measurements of the time evolution of the mean population size. However, evaluating single-cell progeny statistics beyond the mean yields more information. For example, the coefficient of variation (CV) for the cell numbers reads for $t \gg 1/(\lambda - \delta)$

$$CV = \frac{1}{\sqrt{n_0}}\sqrt{\frac{\lambda+\delta}{\lambda-\delta}} \tag{15.20}$$

and the probability of extinction is

$$P_0 = \left(\frac{\delta}{\lambda}\right)^{n_0} \tag{15.21}$$

(e.g., Bharucha-Reid 2010). Measurements of CV or P_0 together with the dynamics of the mean cell number allow separate identification of λ and δ.

However, initial population sizes in the experiments other than one imply two important complications. First, the effect of experimental noise on CV or P_0 becomes harder to evaluate. Second, if n_0 is not constant, but itself a random number, then Eq. 15.20 still holds when n_0 is replaced by its mean, whereas both the CV and the probability of extinction will depend on higher-order properties of the n_0 distribution. For transplant experiments of labeled cells, this means that the—generally unknown—experimental variability in the number of engrafted cells constitutes a confounding factor and usually precludes the use of measured CV or P_0 for parameter estimation.

This problem can be appreciated by considering the measured overall variability in the absolute cell number, quantified by the coefficient of variation CV_T, which contains contributions both from the variable number of engrafted cells (CV_E) as well as the stochasticity of the underlying proliferation model (CV_S):

$$CV_T^2 = CV_E^2 + CV_S^2$$

For the same reason, the pairwise correlations between the absolute cell numbers of cellular progenies in two compartments cannot be utilized for parameter estimation when n_0 is distributed. By contrast, if it can be ensured that all measured progenies arise from a single cell, we will see in the next section that such correlations offer rich information about the underlying differentiation process.

The above arguments generalize to more realistic models of cell population dynamics where the coefficient of variation and P_0 (among other quantities) have been successfully utilized for parameter estimation and model discrimination using *in vivo* single-cell-based fate mapping (Buchholz et al. 2013; Kaiser et al. 2013; Perié et al. 2014).

15.3.3 ILLUSTRATIVE EXAMPLE: BRANCHED VERSUS LINEAR DIFFERENTIATION PATHWAYS

As perhaps the simplest example of lineage topology, we consider two schemes, a branching pathway and a linear pathway, connecting three cell subsets A, B, and C (Figure 15.2a). Suppose we would like to distinguish between these alternatives experimentally. Figure 15.2b illustrates that mean value kinetics, even if measured nearly continuously, are not informative on the question of pathway topology: The differentiation and proliferation rates of both models can be chosen in such a way that they generate almost identical dynamics of the mean absolute cell number in each subset. In particular, in this example also the cell division rates of both models are similar; hence, proliferation monitoring (see Section 15.2.3) would not help discriminate between these two lineage topologies.

By contrast, consider the outcome of two hypothetical single-cell-based fate-mapping experiments depicted in Figure 15.2c. Shown are the pairwise correlations between the absolute cell numbers of the three subsets at a single time point for the linear (upper row) and branched (lower row) pathways. These data were simulated using the same parameters as in Figure 15.2b; specifically, the proliferation rate of cell type A is smaller than those of B and C, which were chosen to be similar. For the linear differentiation model, this hierarchy of proliferation rates implies a strong correlation between the cell numbers of cell types B and C, while the compartment size of subset A is almost uncorrelated with the other two subsets. On the other hand, for the branched pathway model, the small correlations between the cell numbers of subsets A and B as well as between A and C imply an even smaller correlation between B and C. This example illustrates how single-cell progeny data, even if measured only at a single time point, can be used to discriminate between different pathway topologies (Höfer et al. 2016b).

15.3.4 CD8+ T-CELL DIVERSIFICATION DURING ACUTE IMMUNE RESPONSES

Buchholz et al. (2013) applied these ideas on single-cell progenies to infer the pathway of the diversification of cytotoxic T cells into memory precursor subsets and short-lived effector cells; for further work on

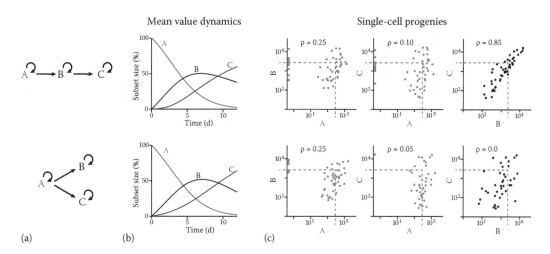

Figure 15.2 Single-cell-based fate mapping can be used to distinguish between different model topologies. **(a)** Schematic depictions of a linear and a branched pathway topology connecting three hypothetical subsets A, B, and C. **(b)** Parameters of both models were chosen to generate almost identical mean cell number dynamics for all three subsets (upper row: linear pathway; lower row: branched pathway). **(c)** Pairwise correlations between the absolute cell numbers of the three subsets at a single time point for the linear (upper row) and branched (lower row) pathways. Data were simulated using the same parameters as in **(b)**. (Figure redrawn from Höfer T et al., *Curr Opin Biotechnol* 39, 150–156, 2016.)

hematopoietic differentiation pathways and bacterial infection dynamics, see Perié et al. (2014) and Kaiser et al. (2013), respectively. The experimental data report the numbers of central memory precursors (TCMp, identified as CD27⁺ CD62L⁺ activated T cells), effector memory precursors (TEMp, identified as CD27⁺ CD62L⁻ activated T cells), and short-lived effector cells (CD27⁻ CD62L⁻ T cells) in single-cell progenies at day 8 of an immune response to *Listeria monocytogenes*, an intracellular bacterium, in mice. The used bacteria are genetically engineered to express the protein ovalbumin (OVA), and the tracked cytotoxic T cells carry a T-cell receptor that is specific for an OVA-derived peptide (OT-I T cells). The data show great variability in cell numbers (over four orders of magnitude) and, at the same time, characteristic correlations between certain subsets (Figure 15.3a).

To rationalize these single-cell progeny data, Buchholz et al. (2013) set up a stochastic model of the population dynamics, writing a master equation for the probability $P(n_{\mathrm{CMp}}, n_{\mathrm{EMp}}, n_{\mathrm{EF}})$ to find n_{CMp} TCMp cells, n_{EMp} TEMp cells, and n_{EF} effector T cells within a progeny at a given time:

$$\frac{\mathrm{d}}{\mathrm{d}t}P = M(\alpha,\lambda)P. \qquad (15.22)$$

The transition matrix M depends on the vectors of proliferation and differentiation rates λ and α, respectively. The authors assumed constant, subset-specific proliferation rates. The number and identity of differentiation rates depend on the assumed differentiation pathway connecting the initial naïve cell from which a progeny arises and the three activated subsets. Standard theory shows how the subset means (μ_{CMp}, μ_{EMp}, μ_{EF}), coefficients of variation (CV_{CMp}, CV_{EMp}, CV_{EF}), and pairwise correlation coefficients ($CC_{\mathrm{CMp,EMp}}$, $CC_{\mathrm{CMp,EF}}$, $CV_{\mathrm{EMp,EF}}$) are obtained by solving a system of ordinary differential equations. Thus, estimates for the rate parameters, including profile-likelihood-based confidence bounds, were obtained by minimizing an objective function based on means, coefficients of variation, and correlations. This efficient approach at parameter estimation for the stochastic dynamical system (Eq. 15.22) allowed the authors to systematically examine all possible lineage topologies that generate all three subsets from a naïve precursor (as borne out by the data; Figure 15.3b). Remarkably, only two lineage topologies provided reasonable fits to the single-cell progeny data measured at a single time point, further augmented by a time course of the subset means

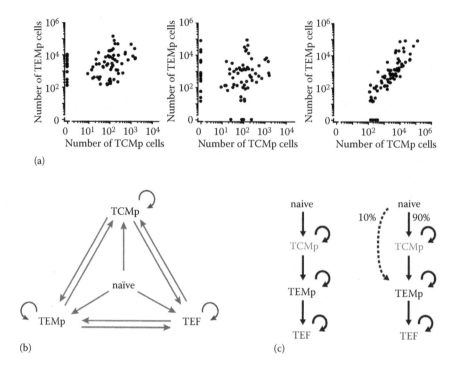

(a)

(b)   (c)

Figure 15.3 Progressive differentiation model of cytotoxic T-cell diversification into short-lived effector and memory subsets follows from single-cell progeny data. **(a)** Numbers of central memory precursors (TCMp), effector memory precursors (TEMp), and short-lived effector T cells (TEF) in single-cell progenies at day 8 after infection of mice with *Listeria*. The two-dimensional plots emphasize the extent of subset correlations. **(b)** Unbiased scheme of differentiation pathways, with subset-specific proliferation rates. There are 304 distinct subgraphs (differentiation pathway topologies) of the directed graph shown that produce all three subsets from a naïve precursor. **(c)** Fitting all 304 models to the single-cell progeny data and to the mean subset size kinetics selects two pathways; their core is the progressive differentiation model naïve T cell → TCMp → TEMp → TEF. (Redrawn from Buchholz VR et al., *Science* 340, 630–635, 2013.)

(Figure 15.3c); all other topologies were incompatible with the data (for details of the model selection, see the original paper). Thus, the single-cell progeny data provide a highly informative basis for model selection. Further modeling work has also examined the potential role of asymmetric cell division in subset specification (Flossdorf et al. 2015).

The two selected model topologies share as a common feature the early origin of central memory precursor cells. Indeed the model implies that these memory precursors have the potential to develop further into effector memory precursors and short-lived effector cells or develop into central memory cells after the acute response has subsided. In this model, central memory T cells can be viewed as a stem-cell-like compartment from which memory immune responses are generated. This prediction of stemness has indeed been corroborated by elegant transfer experiments of single cytotoxic central memory T cells (Graef et al. 2014). Thus, the specification of memory and effector subsets appears to take place by progressive differentiation, passing through stem-cell-like stages (Buchholz et al. 2013; Restifo and Gattinoni 2013; Buchholz et al. 2016; Cho et al. 2017). Of note, the traditional effector–memory dichotomy is not a fitting terminology for this model, as central memory precursors also display effector properties during the acute response. The progressive differentiation model of cytotoxic T-cell subsets has important practical implications for adoptive T-cell therapies of cancer and immunodeficiency (Busch et al. 2016; Gattinoni et al. 2017).

REFERENCES

Abkowitz JL, Catlin SN, McCallie MT, Guttorp P (2002) Evidence that the number of hematopoietic stem cells per animal is conserved in mammals. *Blood* 100, 2665–2667.

Ahmed R, Westera L, Drylewicz J, Elemans M, Zhang Y, Kelly E, Reljic R, Tesselaar K, de Boer RJ, Macallan DC, Borghans JA, Asquith B (2015) Reconciling estimates of cell proliferation from stable isotope labeling experiments. *PLoS Comput Biol* 11:e1004355.

Bharucha-Reid AT (2010) *Elements of the Theory of Markov Processes and Their Applications.* Dover Publications.

Bianconi E, Piovesan A, Facchin F, Beraudi A, Casadei R, Frabetti F, Vitale L, Pelleri MC, Tassani S, Piva F, Perez-Amodio S, Strippoli P, Canaider S (2013) An estimation of the number of cells in the human body. *Ann Hum Biol* 40, 463–471.

Bradford JA, Clarke ST (2011) Dual-pulse labeling using 5-ethynyl-2′-deoxyuridine (EdU) and 5-bromo-2′-deoxyuridine (BrdU) in flow cytometry. *Curr Protoc Cytom* Chapter 7:Unit 7.38.

Buchholz VR, Flossdorf M, Hensel I, Kretschmer L, Weissbrich B, Gräf P, Verschoor A, Schiemann M, Höfer T, Busch DH (2013) Disparate individual fates compose robust CD8+ T cell immunity. *Science* 340, 630–635.

Buchholz VR, Schumacher TN, Busch DH (2016) T cell fate at the single-cell level. *Annu Rev Immunol* 34, 65–92.

Busch DH, Fräßle SP, Sommermeyer D, Buchholz VR, Riddell SR (2016) Role of memory T cell subsets for adoptive immunotherapy. *Semin Immunol* 28, 28–34.

Busch K, Klapproth K, Barile M, Flossdorf M, Holland-Letz T, Schlenner SM, Reth M, Höfer T, Rodewald HR (2015) Fundamental properties of unperturbed haematopoiesis from stem cells in vivo. *Nature* 518, 542–546.

Busch K, Rodewald HR (2016) Unperturbed vs. post-transplantation hematopoiesis: Both in vivo but different. *Curr Opin Hematol* 23, 295–303.

Cho YL, Flossdorf M, Kretschmer L, Höfer T, Busch DH, Buchholz VR (2017) TCR signal quality modulates fate decisions of single CD4+ T cells in a probabilistic manner. *Cell Rep* 20, 806–818.

De Boer RJ, Perelson AS (2013) Quantifying T lymphocyte turnover. *J Theor Biol* 327, 45–87.

den Braber I, Mugwagwa T, Vrisekoop N, Westera L, Mögling R, de Boer AB, Willems N, Schrijver EH, Spierenburg G, Gaiser K, Mul E, Otto SA, Ruiter AF, Ackermans MT, Miedema F, Borghans JA, de Boer RJ, Tesselaar K (2012) Maintenance of peripheral naive T cells is sustained by thymus output in mice but not humans. *Immunity* 36, 288–297.

Flossdorf M, Rössler J, Buchholz VR, Busch DH, Höfer T (2015) CD8+ T cell diversification by asymmetric cell division. *Nat Immunol* 16, 891–893.

Foudi A, Hochedlinger K, Van Buren D, Schindler JW, Jaenisch R, Carey V, Hock H (2009) Analysis of histone 2B-GFP retention reveals slowly cycling hematopoietic stem cells. *Nat Biotechnol* 27, 84–90.

Ganusov VV, De Boer RJ (2013) A mechanistic model for bromodeoxyuridine dilution naturally explains labelling data of self-renewing T cell populations. *J R Soc Interface* 10:20120617.

Gattinoni L, Speiser DE, Lichterfeld M, Bonini C (2017) T memory stem cells in health and disease. *Nat Med* 23, 18–27.

Graef P, Buchholz VR, Stemberger C, Flossdorf M, Henkel L, Schiemann M, Drexler I, Höfer T, Riddell SR, Busch DH (2014) Serial transfer of single-cell-derived immunocompetence reveals stemness of CD8+ central memory T cells. *Immunity* 41, 116–126.

Höfer T, Barile M, Flossdorf M (2016b) Stem-cell dynamics and lineage topology from in vivo fate mapping in the hematopoietic system. *Curr Opin Biotechnol* 39, 150–156.

Höfer T, Busch K, Klapproth K, Rodewald HR (2016a) Fate mapping and quantitation of hematopoiesis in vivo. *Annu Rev Immunol* 34, 449–478.

Kaiser P, Slack E, Grant AJ, Hardt WD, Regoes RR (2013) Lymph node colonization dynamics after oral *Salmonella typhimurium* infection in mice. *PLoS Pathog* 9:e1003532.

Lahoz-Beneytez J, Elemans M, Zhang Y, Ahmed R, Salam A, Block M, Niederalt C, Asquith B, Macallan D (2016) Human neutrophil kinetics: Modeling of stable isotope labeling data supports short blood neutrophil half-lives. *Blood* 127, 3431–3438.

Mackey MC (2001) Cell kinetic status of haematopoietic stem cells. *Cell Prolif* 34, 71–83.

Pei W, Feyerabend TB, Rössler J, Wang X, Postrach D, Busch K, Rode I, Klapproth K, Dietlein N, Quedenau C, Chen W, Sauer S, Wolf S, Höfer T, Rodewald HR (2017) Polylox barcoding reveals haematopoietic stem cell fates realized in vivo. *Nature* 548, 456–460.

Perié L, Hodgkin PD, Naik SH, Schumacher TN, de Boer RJ, Duffy KR (2014) Determining lineage pathways from cellular barcoding experiments. *Cell Rep* 6, 617–624.

Raue A, Kreutz C, Maiwald T, Bachmann J, Schilling M, Klingmüller U, Timmer J (2009) Structural and practical identifiability analysis of partially observed dynamical models by exploiting the profile likelihood. *Bioinformatics* 25, 1923–1929.

Restifo NP, Gattinoni L (2013) Lineage relationship of effector and memory T cells. *Curr Opin Immunol* 25, 556–563.

Venzon DJ, Moolgavkar SH (1988) A method for computing profile-likelihood-based confidence intervals. *J Roy Stat Soc* 37, 87–94.

Population dynamics of host and pathogens

AMBER M. SMITH, RUY M. RIBEIRO, AND ALAN S. PERELSON

16.1 INTRODUCTION

Infectious diseases are among the top causes of death and morbidity in the world. The majority of the world's population lives in low-income countries where infectious diseases are the predominant cause of death, particularly lower respiratory tract infections (LRTI), HIV/AIDS, tuberculosis, and malaria. Worldwide, LRTI are the fourth leading cause of death and HIV/AIDS is the 6th (WHO, 2014). Even in the United States, influenza and pneumonia together are the 8th leading cause of death, responsible for over 50,000 deaths yearly (Heron, 2015).

Understanding the dynamic, of host-pathogen interactions can have a substantial impact in our fight against infectious diseases. In this regard, kinetic models are a robust means of analyzing experimental results and explaining biological phenomena without testing every scenario experimentally. By considering the dynamical interactions of populations of viruses, cells susceptible to infection ("target cells"), infected cells, and cells involved in the immune response, various aspects of the biology of infections have been quantified and elucidated. This modeling approach, termed "viral dynamics", has been successfully used in many viral infections such as HIV, hepatitis C virus, hepatitis B virus, cytomegalovirus, and influenza virus (Perelson and Nelson, 1999; Emery et al., 1999; Ciupe, Ribeiro, and Perelson, 2014; Baccam et al., 2006; Reluga, Dahari, and Perelson, 2009). Substantial insights into the dynamics and pathogenesis of these infections have been gained through the development of mathematical models that describe host-pathogen interactions, allowing quantification of the rates of virus production and clearance and infected cell lifespans (Ho et al., 1995; Wei et al., 1995; Perelson et al., 1996; Perelson et al., 1997; Perelson, 2002; Bonhoeffer et al., 1997). In turn, this has facilitated the investigation of treatment strategies and predictions about how quickly drug resistant variants appear (Ribeiro and Bonhoeffer, 2000; Ribeiro, Bonhoeffer, and Nowak, 1998). Here, we discuss the power of this approach and use influenza viral dynamics and the effect of bacterial coinfection as case studies.

16.2 BIOLOGY OF INFLUENZA VIRUSES

Influenza viruses are negative sense, single stranded RNA segmented viruses of the orthomyxoviridae family (Shaw and Palese, 2013). The influenza A virus (IAV) genome has eight gene segments (PB1, PB2, PA, M, NP, NS, NA, and HA) that code for ~12–14 proteins. The HA and NA segments are important antigenic determinants because they elicit antibodies that are essential for immunity. There are at least 18 different HAs (H1-H18) and 11 different NAs (N1-N11) that define the influenza subtypes, e.g., H1N1, H3N2, or H7N9. IAV genome replication occurs in the nucleus of the infected cell, whereas virion assembly occurs at the apical surface of the infected cell after sufficient production of the viral proteins. In humans, IAV infects epithelial cells of the upper and lower respiratory tract and results in an acute, self-limiting, respiratory illness, characterized by inflammation of the pharynges, trachea, bronchia, and, in some cases, the lower airways.

Influenza viruses cause seasonal epidemics each year between October and April in the U.S. Over 40 million (M) individuals are infected each year, which results in ~1M hospitalizations and ~30,000–50,000 deaths (CDC, 2015). The illness ranges from mild to severe and is often exacerbated in children, the elderly, and in those with underlying health conditions. In contrast with these seasonal epidemics, influenza pandemics occur when a new strain with a novel antigenic profile (e.g., new type of HA and/or NA) emerges and infects a significant proportion of individuals who are naïve to the new strain. The "Spanish Flu" pandemic in 1918-1919 is the most deadly influenza pandemic to date with over 40M deaths worldwide (Potter, 1998). While the virus itself caused severe primary viral pneumonia, ~95% of the fatalities were associated with secondary bacterial infections (Morens, Taubenberger, and Fauci, 2008). More recently in 2009, a novel H1N1 virus infected over 60M people in the U.S. (Shrestha et al., 2011) and resulted in ~200,000 deaths worldwide (Dawood et al., 2012). This strain was associated with lower levels of mortality and secondary bacterial infections (~45% of deaths) (Weinberger et al., 2011) than in previous pandemics (Louria et al., 1959; Morens, Taubenberger, and Fauci, 2008), but the economic cost was substantial.

Relatively little is known about the time course of IAV infections, how various immune responses contribute to morbidity and mortality, how different IAV strains interact with the host immune response, or how the virus interacts with bacterial pathogens. A better quantitative understanding of the dynamics of the virus infection and coinfection with bacterial pathogens within the host could contribute to the development of better therapeutics and management of the disease.

16.3 INFLUENZA VIRUS INFECTION KINETICS

16.3.1 BASIC MODEL OF VIRAL DYNAMICS

The basic or standard viral dynamics model (see for example (Perelson, 2002; Nowak and May, 2000)) describes a virus infection using three state populations: target cells (T), infected cells (I), and free virus (V).

$$\frac{dT}{dt} = s - dT - \beta TV \tag{16.1}$$

$$\frac{dI}{dt} = \beta TV - \delta I \tag{16.2}$$

$$\frac{dV}{dt} = pI - cV \tag{16.3}$$

In this model, susceptible cells, called target cells, are supplied at constant rate s, die at per capita rate d, and become infected at rate βV. Infected cells are lost at per capita rate δ, virion production occurs at rate p per infected cell per day, and virions are cleared at rate c per day. Each of these terms represents multiple biological processes. For example, cell loss with rate δ can be due to apoptosis, viral cytopathic effects, killing of the cell by an immune effector, or loss of the infected state by non-cytolytic effects. In this latter case, the cell could again become a target for infection, in which case a term $+\delta I$ should be added to Eq. (16.1), or the cell could become resistant to infection (i.e., refractory) and a new equation for this cell class could be included (Pawelek et al., 2012; Saenz et al., 2010).

Numerical solution of these non-linear equations shows that the virus initially grows exponentially, as long as the target cell population remains relatively constant. In this case, the growth rate is r_0 (i.e., $V \sim V_0 e^{r_0 t}$), where r_0 is the leading eigenvalue of the linearized system at the beginning of infection (with $T(0) = s/d$, $I(0) = 0$ and $V(0) = V_0$). This eigenvalue can be obtained by solving $r_0^2 + (c+\delta)r_0 - c\delta(R_0 - 1) = 0$, where $R_0 = \beta ps/c\delta d$ quantifies the number of infected cells that arise from each infected cell when target cells are not limiting and is called the basic reproductive number (Nowak and May 2000). Following the initial period of exponential growth, target cells are depleted and the virus reaches a peak before beginning to decline. If $s>0$ and $R_0>1$, then a positive steady state is reached following a period of viral decay ($V^* = (\beta ps - c\delta d)/\beta c\delta$). This describes a persistent infection. However, if target cell regeneration is delayed such that $s \approx 0$ prior to clearance of virus, then viral loads asymptotically decay according to $e^{-\delta t}$ (see "Approximate Solutions" below for further explanation) following the peak and the infection is cleared. This describes an acute infection.

Equations (16.1)–(16.3) form the basis of the first simple model used to analyze IAV infection in human volunteers (Baccam et al., 2006). To more accurately reflect the underlying biology of IAV infection, two modifications of the basic model are necessary. First, the birth (s) and death (d) rates of target cells are set to 0 due to little regeneration and natural loss of target cells during the short time of an acute infection (~1 week). Second, to account for the delay in virus production after a cell becomes infected, i.e., an eclipse phase, the infected cell class is split into populations of cells that are newly infected and not yet producing virus (I_1) and cells that are producing virus (I_2). Cells transition between these two classes at rate k. It is assumed that no infected cells are lost during the eclipse phase (I_1). This can be justified by assuming that these cells have similar properties to uninfected cells prior to virus production, i.e., they die at rate d, which is set to 0 in this model. However, it is possible that intracellular immune mechanisms can detect infection prior to viral production and lead to death of the cell. In this case, a term $-\delta_1 I_1$ should be added to Eq. (16.5) below, where δ_1 could be different from δ. This model adds biological realism and includes an exponentially distributed delay (with mean duration $1/k$) between the start of infection and the initial growth of the virus. Other types of delays with different distributions can also be modeled, for instance by adding more intermediate compartments (Mittler et al., 1998; Holder and Beauchemin, 2011) or by using a fixed time delay (Herz et al., 1996). This model has been termed the "target-cell limited" model and is defined by Eqs. (16.4)–(16.7). The model dynamics are summarized in Figure 16.1a.

$$\frac{dT}{dt} = -\beta TV \tag{16.4}$$

$$\frac{dI_1}{dt} = \beta TV - kI_1 \tag{16.5}$$

$$\frac{dI_2}{dt} = kI_1 - \delta I_2 \tag{16.6}$$

$$\frac{dV}{dt} = pI_2 - cV \tag{16.7}$$

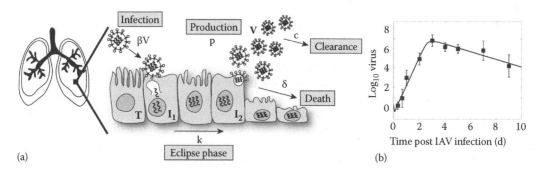

Figure 16.1 Schematic and Output of the Target Cell Limited Model. **(a)** In the target cell limited model (Baccam et al. 2006) (Eqs. (16.4)–(16.7)), target cells (*T*) are infected with virus (*V*) at rate β*V*. Newly infected cells (*I₁*) enter an eclipse phase and transition to producing virus at rate *k*. Productive infected cells (*I₂*) produce virus at rate *p* and are cleared at rate δ. Virus is cleared at rate c. **(b)** Fit of the target cell limited model to viral titer data from the lungs of mice infected with influenza A/Puerto Rico/34/8 (PR8). The data and model solution were reproduced from (Smith et al., 2011). (a. From Baccam, P. et al., *Journal of Virology*, 80, 7590–7599, 2006; b. The data and model solution were reproduced from Smith, A.M. et al., *PLoS Computational Biology*, 7, e1001081, 2011.)

The model given by Eqs. (16.4)–(16.7) has been used to analyze IAV infection data *in vitro* and *in vivo* in mice, ferrets, horses, and humans (reviewed in (Smith and Perelson, 2011; Beauchemin and Handel, 2011; Boianelli et al., 2015)). Typically, the model is solved numerically and the predicted $\log_{10}$ viral levels ($\log_{10} V(t)$) are fitted to the $\log_{10}$ viral load data to estimate the parameter values. Figure 16.1b shows a representative fit of the model to viral load data from the lungs of IAV infected mice (Smith et al., 2011).

Several considerations have to be taken into account in these fits, including sparsity of the data, uncertainty in the parameter estimates, identifiability of the parameters, and the model structure. Parameters are often correlated or cannot be defined by the available data. One way to help identify these parameters is to use ensemble fitting methods and examine two-dimensional projections of the parameters (see, for example, Figure 16.2d) (Smith et al., 2013; Smith et al., 2011). In doing so, it becomes easy to see that the parameters *c* and δ are correlated and the confidence interval for *c* is large. Although this may seem problematic, robust conclusions can still be made (Gutenkunst et al., 2007). However, a thorough investigation of how the model solution is affected by changes in the parameter values must be completed. This can be done by performing a detailed sensitivity analysis and/or attempting to find an analytical solution.

16.3.2 Approximate solutions

Equations (16.4)–(16.7) are nonlinear and cannot be solved analytically. However, approximations can be made to linearize the system. Doing so identifies how each parameter affects the kinetics of viral growth and decay (Smith, Adler, and Perelson, 2010). This information can then be paired with parameter estimates obtained from fitting the model to data, which allows for more robust interpretation of the viral dynamics (Smith et al., 2011).

To find approximate analytical solutions, the observation that the viral dynamics splits into two phases can be used. That is, (i) virus grows exponentially during initial infection (Phase I) and (ii) declines exponentially as the infection resolves (Phase II). There is an additional phase between Phases I and II when virus growth slows and viral loads peak. The solutions to Phases I and II can be derived by assuming that the target cell (*T*) level, and thus the total number of cells (*Z*), remains relatively constant with $T \approx T_0 \rightarrow Z(t) = T(t) + I_1(t) + I_2(t) \approx I_1(t) + I_2(t)$ in Phase I; and $T \approx 0 \rightarrow Z(t) = T(t) + I_1(t) + I_2(t) \approx I_2(t) \approx I_1(t) + I_2(t)$ in Phase II. This linearizes Eqs. (16.4)–(16.7), which can then be easily solved to yield:

$$\text{Phase I: } V_1(t) = \alpha_1 e^{\lambda t} \tag{16.8}$$

$$\text{Phase II: } V_2(t) = \alpha_2 e^{-\delta t} + \alpha_3 e^{-ct} + \alpha_4 e^{-kt}, \tag{16.9}$$

where λ is the dominant eigenvalue of the linearized system and the α_i's are combinations of the parameters (Smith, Adler, and Perelson, 2010). While all model parameters are involved in the initial growth phase,

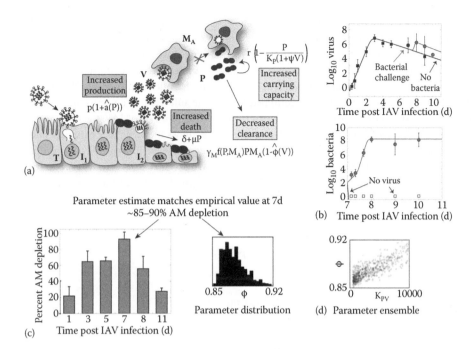

Figure 16.2 Schematic, Output, and Experimental Validation of the Coinfection Model. **(a)** In the IAV-SP coinfection model (Eqs. (16.19)–(16.23)), the target cell limited model (Eqs. (16.4)–(16.7)) is paired with a pneumococcal model (Eq. (16.18)) by including two interaction terms for bacteria (P) effects and two interaction terms for virus (V) effects): (i) an increase in virus production ($\hat{a}(P) = aP^z$), (ii) an increase in cell death (μP), (iii) an increase in the carry capacity (ψV), and (iv) a decrease in phagocytosis of bacteria ($\hat{\phi}(V) = \phi V/(K_{PV} + V)$). **(b)** Fit of the coinfection model to viral and bacterial titer data from the lungs of mice infected with influenza PR8 followed 7d later by pneumococcus D39. **(c)** The dynamics of alveolar macrophages and the correlation to the estimate of ϕ. **(d)** Correlation of the parameter estimates for ϕ and K_{PV}. Each dot represents a value within the 95% confidence interval. (From Smith, A.M. et al., *PLoS Pathogens*, 9, e1003238, 2013. a. From Smith, A.M. et al., *PLoS Pathogens*, 9, e1003238, 2013; b. From Smith, A.M. et al., *PLoS Pathogens*, 9, e1003238, 2013; c. The dynamics of alveolar macrophages: Adapted from Ghoneim, H.E. et al., *The Journal of Immunology*, 191, 1250–1259, 2013; Smith, A.M., and Smith, A.P., *Scientific Reports*, 6, 38703, 2016. The correlation to the estimate of ϕ: Smith, A.M. et al., *PLoS Pathogens*, 9, e1003238, 2013. The data, model solutions, and parameters were adapted from Smith, A.M. et al., *PLoS Pathogens*, 9, e1003238, 2013 [panels b, c, and d] and Smith, A.M., and Smith, A.P., *Scientific Reports*, 6, 38703, 2016 [panel c].)

the exponential decay phase is dominated by the smallest of k, c and δ. In most parameter regimes (reviewed in (Smith and Perelson, 2011)), the infected cell death rate δ controls the rate of decay. Further, because the solution is asymptotically log-linear (i.e., $V(t) \approx V_p e^{-\delta t}$ in Phase II, where V_p is the peak viral load), the slope of a linear regression can provide an estimate of δ. Each phase lasts for a set amount of time, which can be defined as the point when the approximate solutions deviate from the numerical solution by ~10%. In doing so, it can be seen that exponential growth lasts for ~2 days (d), followed by a 12-hour (h) intermediate phase where growth is slowing down at which point the exponential decay phase dominates until infection resolution (Smith, Adler, and Perelson, 2010).

16.3.3 Drug treatment

Currently there are two classes of FDA-approved antivirals used to treat IAV infections: (i) M2 inhibitors (M2I), which block the ion-channel activity of the M2 protein and disrupt virion uncoating (Ison, 2011; Gubareva and Hayden, 2006) and (ii) neuraminidase (NA) inhibitors (NAI), which block the action of viral neuraminidase on the cell surface and prevent virions from budding from the cell (Ison, 2011).

M2Is block successful infection of cells, which can be modeled either by changing the infection rate, β, to $(1-\varepsilon)\beta$ or by changing the eclipse phase rate, k, to $(1-\varepsilon)k$. Likewise, NAIs work to block virus production and can be modeled by changing the viral production rate, p, to $(1-\varepsilon)p$. In both cases, ε describes the effectiveness of the drug in blocking the corresponding step of the viral lifecycle and is equal to 0 in the absence of drug and to 1 when the drug is 100% effective. Antivirals are typically ineffective if they are administered after the first 2 d of infection (Hayden, 1996). This is because these processes have little effect during the later stages of the infection, as indicated by the Phase II solution in Eq. (16.9) (Smith, Adler, and Perelson, 2010; Smith, 2016).

Even when one of these antivirals is administered early in infection, drug resistance can arise rapidly (Perelson, Rong, and Hayden 2012). This is due to the high mutation rate of IAV, the rapid production and clearance of the virus, and the plasticity of its genome, which allows the virus to accumulate mutations that have little impact on viral fitness and thus may lead to resistance. Indeed, multiple IAV strains that have been in circulation are resistant to one or more of the available drugs (Hurt, 2014). To determine the biological processes that drive the emergence of drug resistance and assess the rate at which resistant mutants arise, classes of viruses that are sensitive to antivirals (V_s) or resistant (V_r) to antivirals can be included and modeled by Eqs. (16.10)–(16.16).

$$\frac{dT}{dt} = -\beta T (V_s + V_r) \tag{16.10}$$

$$\frac{dI_{1s}}{dt} = \beta T V_s - k_s I_{1s} \tag{16.11}$$

$$\frac{dI_{1r}}{dt} = \beta T V_r - k_r I_{1r} \tag{16.12}$$

$$\frac{dI_{2s}}{dt} = k_s I_{1s} - \delta I_{2s} \tag{16.13}$$

$$\frac{dI_{2r}}{dt} = k_r I_{1r} - \delta I_{2r} \tag{16.14}$$

$$\frac{dV_r}{dt} = (1 + \mu)\, p I_{2r} - \mu p I_{2s} - c V_r \tag{16.15}$$

$$\frac{dV_s}{dt} = (1 - \mu)\, p I_{2s} + \mu p I_{2r} - c V_s \tag{16.16}$$

Here, it is assumed that the drug effect is in blocking the infected cell transition from the eclipse phase (I_1) to productive infection (I_2), and thus resistance is manifested by including different transition rates, k_s and k_r corresponding to the drug sensitive and resistant virus, respectively. The model also includes the possibility that each virus produced by a cell infected with a drug sensitive virus, I_{2s}, or drug resistant virus, I_{2r}, can mutate at rate μ. The model allows for analysis of the relative production of sensitive and resistance viruses prior to when the strong effect of selection due to drug is imposed on the system. The relative frequency of sensitive and resistant strains within the host can then be calculated before and after drug treatment (Ribeiro, Bonhoeffer, and Nowak, 1998).

16.3.4 IMMUNE RESPONSES

The model in Eqs. (16.4)–(16.7) does a remarkable job of describing the initial growth and control of the virus, and has been shown to fit viral titer data quite well in different types of experiments (reviewed in (Smith and Perelson, 2011; Beauchemin and Handel, 2011; Boianelli et al., 2015)). This is the case even without including explicit immune responses. However, it is well known that the immune response against IAV infection can be vigorous, including several innate and adaptive mechanisms, and is essential in clearing the infection.

Early in IAV infection, infected cells and resident immune cells (e.g., alveolar macrophages) release pro-inflammatory cytokines and chemokines that limit virus replication and recruit other cells (e.g., neutrophils, macrophages, and natural killer (NK) cells) to the infection site (reviewed in (Iwasaki and Pillai, 2014)). Within 2-4 d after infection, the innate immune response controls virus replication and signals the adaptive response. Cytotoxic T cells enter at ~5-6 d post-infection and work to remove the remaining infected cells (reviewed in (Braciale, Sun, and Kim, 2012)).

Specific immune responses can be incorporated into Eqs. (16.4)–(16.7) in various ways, including by allowing parameters to vary as a function of time or as a function of the state variables. Alternatively, additional equations for immune cell populations can be included. While different immune responses have been modeled (reviewed in (Smith and Perelson, 2011; Beauchemin and Handel, 2011; Boianelli et al., 2015)), the focus here will be on an important component of innate immunity: the type I interferon (IFN-α,β) response. Type I IFNs are thought to play a major role in limiting viral replication by three mechanisms (reviewed in (McNab et al., 2015)): (i) reducing virus production within infected cells, (ii) interacting with susceptible cells and rendering them resistant to infection, and (iii) enhancing the effect of cytotoxic cells that remove infected cells. The simplest way to model the effect of IFN in decreasing virus production from infected cells is to make the rate of viral production a function of time, $p(t)$. Although the form of this function is unknown, it is likely a decreasing function of time. Another way to model the IFN effect is based on the fact that infected cells can produce type I IFNs, which means that virus production should decline as the number of infected cells and the amount of IFN increases. Thus, p could also be made a decreasing function of the concentration of infected cells or the integral over all infected cells.

A more mechanistic way to model the effect of IFN is to write an equation for the concentration of IFN (F),

$$\frac{dF}{dt} = \alpha I_2 - d_F F \tag{16.17}$$

where α is the rate of IFN production and d_F is the rate of IFN decay. Because IFN levels do not begin to rise until after virus has surpassed Phase I of exponential growth (~2 d), a time delay (τ) is often included such that the equation becomes $dF/dt = \alpha I_2(t - \tau) - d_F F$ (Baccam et al., 2006). The reduction in virus replication in infected cells can then be included by changing the viral production rate to $p = \hat{p}/(1 + \varepsilon_1 F)$ and/or the rate of exiting the eclipse phase to $k = \hat{k}/(1 + \varepsilon_2 F)$, where $\hat{p}$ and $\hat{k}$ are the rates of these processes in the absence of IFN. The efficiency of IFN in inhibiting these processes is reflected by the parameters ε_1 and ε_2 (Baccam et al., 2006). Type I IFNs also act by placing cells in an antiviral state, which can be modeled by including an equation for cells refractory to infection (Saenz et al., 2010). IFNs can also enhance the activity of cytotoxic cells, such as NK cells, which can be modeled by including an additional death term (i.e., $-\kappa I_2 F$) in Eq. (16.6) (Pawelek et al., 2012).

16.4 BACTERIAL COINFECTION DURING INFLUENZA INFECTION

As IAV infection progresses and immune responses work to clear the virus, host epithelial cells die, inflammation increases, and the respiratory tract is damaged. Bacterial pathogens, like *Streptococcus pneumoniae* (SP) and *Staphylococcus aureus* (SA), can take advantage of this damage and easily invade the injured lung (reviewed in (Smith and McCullers, 2014; McCullers, 2014; Short et al., 2012; Metzger and Sun, 2013)). These secondary bacterial infections are a common complication of IAV infections and have accounted for 40–95% of influenza-related mortality in past pandemics (Morens, Taubenberger, and Fauci, 2008; Louria et al., 1959; Dawood et al., 2012; Weinberger et al., 2011).

IAV-SP coinfection pathogenesis has been extensively studied in the laboratory due to the availability of well-characterized animal models (reviewed in (Smith and McCullers, 2014)). These studies have elucidated numerous pathogenic and immunological components that contribute to the acquisition, pathogenicity, and lethality of coinfection (reviewed in (Smith and McCullers, 2014; McCullers, 2014; Short et al., 2012;

Metzger and Sun, 2013)). With such complexity, it is difficult to decipher the role and regulation of each identified factor with traditional experimental approaches. In contrast, modeling coinfection dynamics has been able to unravel some of the complex host-pathogen interactions and identify important mechanisms that drive bacterial establishment after IAV infection (Smith et al., 2013; Smith and Smith, 2016).

Data collected from mice indicates that the maximum lethality from IAV-SP coinfection occurs when the bacterial infection is initiated 7 d into the IAV infection (McCullers and Rehg, 2002). This time point is ~2–4 d after the virus peak when viral loads are declining (Figure 16.1). Once the bacterial infection begins, viral loads rebound briefly and bacterial titers rapidly grow to high levels (Figure 16.2). To investigate the mechanisms that produce these kinetics, Smith et al. (2011) developed a model for pneumococcal infection that could then be coupled to a model of IAV infection, such as that in Eqs. (16.4)–(16.7).

16.4.1 PNEUMOCOCCAL INFECTION KINETICS

Pneumococcus is a gram-positive bacterium that often resides in the nasopharynx of healthy individuals without manifestation of disease. However, some strains of pneumococci are more virulent and can spread to other locations of the body causing pneumonia, meningitis, otitis media, or septicemia. This is particularly true when the host is immunocompromised, such as in the elderly or after an IAV infection.

Because this bacterium grows extracellularly, a target-cell limited type of model is not appropriate. Here, the immune response needs to be taken into consideration in order to accurately reflect bacterial loads after infection and do so for different doses (Smith, McCullers, and Adler, 2011). In the case of pneumococcus, alveolar macrophages (AMs) that reside in the respiratory tract act as the initial defense in controlling this pathogen (Dockrell et al., 2003). Neutrophils infiltrate shortly after and aid bacterial clearance until new macrophages are recruited (Bergeron et al. 1998). While a detailed model that includes the dynamics of AMs, neutrophils, recruited macrophages, and the cytokine signaling between them has been developed (Smith, McCullers, and Adler, 2011), corresponding models describing these populations during IAV infection have not. Thus, we restrict our attention to modeling the AM response.

To model how AMs control pneumococci, pneumococci (P) are assumed to grow logistically with a maximum rate r and tissue carrying capacity K_P, and are phagocytosed by AMs (M_A) at rate $\gamma_M f(P,M_A)M_A$ per bacterium (Smith, McCullers, and Adler, 2011). Here, γ_{MA} is the maximum rate of phagocytosis and the function $f(P,M_A)$ represents the decrease in the efficiency of phagocytosis as the pneumococcal population grows. Although it is possible that pneumococci induce AM death, we neglect the turnover of these cells during the early stages of the infection and assume their population size remains constant. The equation representing these dynamics is given by

$$\frac{dP}{dt} = rP\left(1 - \frac{P}{K_P}\right) - \gamma_M f(P,M_A)PM_A, \tag{16.18}$$

where

$$f(P,M_A) = \frac{n^2 M_A}{n^2 M_A + P^2},$$

and n represents the maximum number of bacterial colony forming units (CFU) simultaneously phagocytosed per AM. The model in Eq. (16.18) has been shown to match initial bacterial titer data from mice infected with pneumococcus at three different doses (Smith, McCullers, and Adler, 2011).

16.4.2 IAV-SP COINFECTION KINETICS

To pair the models in Eqs. (16.4)–(16.7) and Eq. (16.18), terms that describe proposed mechanisms of interaction are included (Smith et al., 2013). It is not readily apparent which terms in the individual models should be modified or how they should be changed to mimic coinfection. However, testing specific hypotheses (e.g., viral-induced impairment of bacterial phagocytosis) and knowledge of how each parameter affects the viral titer curve during Phases I and II (Eqs. (16.8)–(16.9)) of the IAV infection provide reasonable starting places.

The hypothesis that bacterial pathogens invade during influenza infection because they can more easily attach to exposed receptors and to virus-infected epithelial cells (Ahmer et al. 1999; Peltola and Mccullers, 2004) can be examined by assuming that more available infection sites means a larger carrying capacity (K_P). Thus, multiplying K_P by a factor of ($1+\psi V$) in Eq. (16.18). However, another possible consequence of this improved attachment to infected cells is that bacterial toxins, such as pneumolysin, can increase the rate at which these cells (I_1 and I_2) die (Fischetti et al., 2006). This is included in the model by adding $-\mu P I_{1,2}$ to Eqs. (16.5)–(16.6), respectively. A similar term can also be added to Eq. (16.4), but doing so has little effect on the dynamics because the target cell population is near zero when the bacterial infection is initiated (7 d post-influenza).

Another hypothesis that can be examined with Eqs. (16.4)–(16.7) and (16.18) is that IAV infection may alter bacterial clearance by impairing the protective ability of AMs (Sun and Metzger, 2008). To represent this effect in the simplest way, the clearance term in Eq. (16.18) can be adjusted to $-\gamma_{MA} f(P,M_A)PM_A(1-\hat{\phi}(V))$, where $\hat{\phi}(V)$ is a function that is dependent on the amount of virus present and describes how the phagocytosis rate is reduced. One functional form that has been used is a Hill-type function, $\hat{\phi}(V)=\phi V/(K_{PV}+V)$, where ϕ is the maximal reduction of the phagocytosis rate and K_{PV} is the half-saturation constant (Smith et al., 2013).

In developing a model, building equations that can reproduce the data may require inclusion of terms for which there is no pre-determined hypothesis or experimental evidence. In the case of IAV-SP coinfections, the rebound in viral titers could be reproduced by modifying the rate of virus production (p) to $pI_2(1+\hat{a}(P))$, where $\hat{a}(P)$ is a function that is dependent on the amount of bacteria present and describes how the virus production rate is increased. The functional form $\hat{a}(P)=aP^z$ has been used to describe this effect (Smith et al., 2013).

Other processes that could be altered in the model include the rates of viral infectivity (βV), viral clearance (c), and infected cell loss (δ). Based on the Phase I and II solutions (Eqs. (16.8)–(16.9)), β and c most influence the model solution in the first 2-3 d but have little effect in the later stages of infection. Thus, potential alterations to these processes can be excluded. The infected cell loss (δ), on the other hand, dictates the viral decay. However, this decline is exponential and modifying the rate can at most slow the decay rather than increase the viral load in the non-linear fashion observed in the data. Thus, effects on these terms of the equations are not considered. Taken together, the following equations (shown schematically in Figure 16.2a) describe the processes proposed above.

$$\frac{dT}{dt} = -\beta TV \tag{16.19}$$

$$\frac{dI_1}{dt} = \beta TV - kI_1 - \mu PI_1 \tag{16.20}$$

$$\frac{dI_2}{dt} = kI_1 - \delta I_2 - \mu PI_2 \tag{16.21}$$

$$\frac{dV}{dt} = pI_2(1+\hat{a}(P)) - cV \tag{16.22}$$

$$\frac{dP}{dt} = rP\left(1 - \frac{P}{K_P(1+\psi V)}\right) - \gamma_M f(P,M_A)PM_A(1-\hat{\phi}(V)) \tag{16.23}$$

Figure 16.2b shows the simultaneous fit of Eqs. (16.19)–(16.23) to the viral and bacterial lung titers in mice from an IAV infection followed 7 d later by a pneumococcal infection. The dynamics generated are in good agreement with data and indicate that two independent mechanisms are at play. First, a reduced rate (~85–90%) of bacterial phagocytosis by AMs in the presence of IAV can lead to rapid bacterial growth. Based on the change in slope in the bacterial dynamics at 10 h post-bacterial infection (Figure 16.2b), clearance by unimpaired AMs diminishes quickly. Second, additional virions can be released from infected cells in the presence of SP. Further, model fits to the data suggest that although bacteria may adhere to epithelial cells better in IAV-infected individuals, that this does not affect the viral and bacterial load dynamics.

16.4.3 Initial dose threshold

It can be easily seen by simulating Eqs. (16.19)–(16.23) with values for ϕ between 0 and 1 that ϕ is a bifurcation parameter dictating whether bacteria grow to their carrying capacity or are cleared (Smith and Smith 2016). These two outcomes are stable steady states of the system, and the unstable steady state that helps define the separatrix between them can be derived analytically. This separatrix is dependent on ϕ and predicts an initial dose threshold (Figure 16.3a) (Smith and Smith, 2016). This means that the bacterial dose needed for successful bacterial invasion during IAV infection is correlated with the changes in AMs and varies rapidly as the rate of bacterial phagocytosis declines (i.e., as $\phi \rightarrow 100\%$). For a bacterial infection 7 d post-influenza, $\phi \approx 87\%$ and thus any dose greater than 1 CFU could support bacterial growth (Figure 16.3A). The point where any dose will elicit a bacterial infection can be calculated from where the unstable steady state changes from being a real root to a complex root and is defined by $\hat{\phi}_{crit} = 1 - r/(\gamma_M M_A)$ (Smith and Smith, 2016).

16.5 EXPERIMENTALLY VALIDATING MODEL PREDICTIONS

In modeling host-pathogen dynamics, we attempt to make robust predictions that can be subjected to experimental examination. This is not always possible due to technical limitations, but the predictions from the IAV-SP model have recently been examined and verified. With regards to the model prediction that bacteria increase the rate of virus production, results from an *in vitro* experiment that investigated molecular changes during coinfection found that IAV replicates more efficiently due to bacterial inhibition of IFN signaling in IAV infected cells (Warnking et al., 2015). With regards to the model prediction

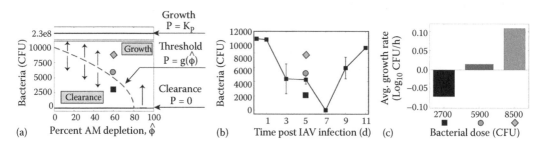

Figure 16.3 Initial Dose Threshold and Experimental Validation. **(a)** Bacterial steady states (solid horizonal lines) for the coinfection model for different values of AM depletion: clearance (0 CFU) or growth to maximum carrying capacity (K_P). The nonlinear threshold (dashed line) dictates if bacteria increase or decrease. The square, circle, and triangle (panels **a** and **b**) indicate 3 of the 20 combinations of AM depletion and bacterial doses that were examined to validate the threshold prediction (see panel **c**). **(b)** Estimated initial dose requirement throughout IAV infection calculated using the degree of AM depletion at the indicated time point (see **c**) and the threshold in panel **a**. **(c)** Average bacterial growth rate in the first 4 h for infection with influenza PR8 followed 5d later with pneumococcus D39 at the indicated doses. Bacterial loads decay for doses below the threshold, remain relatively constant for doses near the threshold, and grow for doses above the threshold. (From Smith, A.M., and Smith, A.P., *Scientific Reports*, 6, 38703, 2016. a. From Smith, A.M., and Smith, A.P., *Scientific Reports*, 6, 38703, 2016; b. From Smith, A.M., and Smith, A.P., *Scientific Reports*, 6, 38703, 2016. The data and models in all panels were reproduced from Smith, A.M., and Smith, A.P., *Scientific Reports*, 6, 38703, 2016.)

that IAV reduces phagocytosis by AMs, results from an experiment that tracked the AM population with a labeling dye and standard flow cytometry techniques found that these cells become depleted during IAV infection (Ghoneim, Thomas, and McCullers, 2013). In addition, this study found that the minimum number of AMs occurs on day 7 of the IAV infection (Figure 16.2c). This minimum was 85–90% lower than baseline, which is consistent with the model's estimate of $\phi = 0.87$ that resulted from fitting Eqs. (16.19)–(16.23) to the data (Figure 16.2b). These results help explain the laboratory evidence that bacterial coinfections are most lethal 7 d after influenza (McCullers and Rehg, 2002) and gave important insight into immune cell dynamics during IAV infection.

Importantly, these new data on the AM population validate the added $1 - \hat{\phi}(V)$ term in Eq. (16.23) and its dependency on the virus concentration (V). However, the chosen functional form, $\hat{\phi}(V) = \phi V / (K_{PV} + V)$, may be incorrect. Nevertheless, approximating $\hat{\phi}(V)$ in this way and assuming that the AM population remains constant still produced robust predictions. Another remarkable observation from the experiments that validated the model is that a precise estimate for the value of ϕ was possible even when this parameter was correlated to K_{PV} (Figure 16.2d) (Smith et al., 2013; Ghoneim, Thomas, and McCullers, 2013).

With the knowledge about the fate of AMs during IAV infection, new analysis of the model in Eqs. (16.19)–(16.23) is possible (Smith and Smith, 2016). The time-dependent dynamics of AM depletion and the evidence that ϕ is an estimate of this depletion suggests that the initial dose threshold for successful invasion of the bacteria, which is a function of ϕ (i.e., AM depletion), is dynamic. An estimate of the dose requirement to initiate bacterial growth throughout IAV infection can be calculated (Figure 16.3b) and the results have been tested in the laboratory (Figure 16.3c) (Smith and Smith, 2016). Indeed, experiments that examined bacterial growth for doses above and below the threshold at different initiation times for the bacterial coinfection verified the model prediction (Smith and Smith, 2016).

16.6 CONCLUDING REMARKS

The dynamics of host-pathogen interactions are complex. Over the last several years, the technical capabilities to measure living systems in more quantitative detail have improved and allowed for a large amount of data to be generated in an attempt to gain a deeper understanding of infectious disease pathogenesis. However, interpreting the data requires developing mathematical models that can explain the observations and provide important insights into the biology of these systems. These models readily assess the rate, magnitude, and effectiveness of host-pathogen interactions and the dynamic feedback of variables, which are often nonlinear and occur on various time scales.

Here, we discussed some examples of mechanistic models that have been used to investigate the complex interactions between the host and viral and bacterial pathogens. We also highlighted multiple examples of how experiments that test the model predictions can verify model accuracy and yield additional biological insight. Importantly, the approach we described is not based on including every biological detail in the analyses, but rather provides a simplification or approximation to the underlying dynamics and is used to identify the most important components driving the kinetics. Model complexity is then increased step-by-step as the data supports it and as each model reveals its own successes and failures at explaining the data. This approach, beginning with the basic model (Eqs. (16.1)–(16.3)), has been used with great success in investigating infectious disease dynamics. For example, this model has been used to study acute infections, such as with influenza virus (reviewed in (Smith and Perelson, 2011; Beauchemin and Handel, 2011; Boianelli et al., 2015)), West Nile virus (Banerjee et al., 2016), Zika virus (Best et al., 2017), chronic infections, such as primary HIV infection (Stafford et al., 2000), treatment of HIV, HBV, HCV, or IAV infection (e.g., (Neumann, 1998; Perelson et al., 1996; Ribeiro, Lo, and Perelson, 2002; Smith, 2016; Baccam et al., 2006)), and viral-bacterial coinfections (Smith and Smith, 2016; Smith et al., 2013).

Importantly, further work is still needed in developing mechanistic models that assess the host immune response and the synergism or antagonism of simultaneous or sequential infections. The examples discussed here are only the beginning and will facilitate the new collaborative efforts between experimental scientists and modelers with the goal of gaining new insights into infectious disease pathogenesis.

ACKNOWLEDGMENTS

This work was supported by NIH grants K25-AI100946, R56-AI125324, R01-AI104373, R01-AI028433 and R01-OD011095 and by ALSAC. We gratefully acknowledge the support of the U.S. Department of Energy through the LANL/LDRD Program (20160054DR). Portions of this work were done under the auspices of the U.S. Department of Energy under contract DE-AC52-06NA25396.

REFERENCES

Ahmer, O.R., Raza, M.W., Ogilvie, M.M., Weir, D.M., and Blackwell, C.C. (1999). Binding of Bacteria to HEp-2 Cells Infected with Influenza A Virus. *FEMS Immunology & Medical Microbiology 23*, 331-341.

Baccam, P., Beauchemin, C., Macken, C.A., Hayden, F.G., and Perelson, A.S. (2006). "Kinetics of Influenza A Virus Infection in Humans. *Journal of Virology 80*, 7590-7599.

Banerjee, S., Guedj, J., Ribeiro, R.M., Moses, M., and Perelson, A.S. (2016). Estimating Biologically Relevant Parameters under Uncertainty for Experimental within-Host Murine West Nile Virus Infection. *Journal of The Royal Society Interface 13*, 20160130.

Beauchemin, C.A.A., and Handel, A. (2011). A Review of Mathematical Models of Influenza A Infections within a Host or Cell Culture: Lessons Learned and Challenges Ahead. *BMC Public Health 11*, S7.

Bergeron, Y., Ouellet, N., Deslauriers, A.-M., Simard, M., Olivier, M., and Bergeron, M.G. (1998). Cytokine Kinetics and Other Host Factors in Response to Pneumococcal Pulmonary Infection in Mice. *Infection and Immunity 66*, 912-922.

Best, K., Guedj, J., Madelain, V., Lamballerie, X.D., Lim, S.-Y., Osuna, C.E., Whitney, J. and Perelson, A.S. (2017). Zika plasma virus dynamics in nonhuman primates provide insights into early infection and antiviral strategies. *Proceedings of the National Academy of Sciences of the United States of America 114*, 8847-8852.

Boianelli, A., Nguyen, V., Ebensen, T., Schulze, K., Wilk, E., Sharma, N., Stegemann-Koniszewski, S. et al. (2015). Modeling Influenza Virus Infection: A Roadmap for Influenza Research. *Viruses 7*, 5274-5304.

Bonhoeffer, S., May, R.M., Shaw, G.M., and Nowak, M.A. (1997). Virus Dynamics and Drug Therapy. *Proceedings of the National Academy of Sciences 94*, 6971-6976.

Braciale, T.J., Sun, J., and Kim, T.S. (2012). Regulating the Adaptive Immune Response to Respiratory Virus Infection. *Nature Reviews Immunology 12*, 295-305.

CDC. (2015). Estimated Influenza Illnesses and Hospitalizations Averted by Vaccination—United States, 2014-15 Influenza Season. MMWR.

Ciupe, S.M., Ribeiro, R.M., and Perelson, A.S. (2014). Antibody Responses during Hepatitis B Viral Infection. R. R. Regoes (Ed.). *PLoS Computational Biology 10*, e1003730.

Dawood, F.S., Iuliano, A.D., Reed, C., Meltzer, M.I., Shay, D.K., Cheng, P., Bandaranayake, D. et al. (2012). Estimated Global Mortality Associated with the First 12 Months of 2009 Pandemic Influenza A H1N1 Virus Circulation: A Modelling Study. *The Lancet Infectious Diseases 12*, 687-695.

Dockrell, D.H., Marriott, H.M., Prince, L.R., Ridger, V.C., Ince, P.G., Hellewell, P.G., and Whyte, M.K.B. (2003). Alveolar Macrophage Apoptosis Contributes to Pneumococcal Clearance in a Resolving Model of Pulmonary Infection. *Journal of Immunology 171*, 5380-5388.

Emery, V.C., Cope, A.V., Bowen, E.F., Gor, D., and Griffiths, P.D. (1999). The Dynamics of Human Cytomegalovirus Replication in Vivo. *The Journal of Experimental Medicine 190*, 177-182.

Fischetti, V.A., Novick, R.P., Ferretti, J.J., Portnoy, D.A., and Rood, J.I. (2006). *Gram-Positive Pathogens.* ASM Press.

Ghoneim, H.E., Thomas, P.G., and McCullers, J.A. (2013). Depletion of Alveolar Macrophages during Influenza Infection Facilitates Bacterial Superinfections. *The Journal of Immunology 191*, 1250-1259.

Gubareva, L.V., and Hayden, F.G. (2006). M2 and Neuraminidase Inhibitors: Anti-Influenza Activity, Mechanisms of Resistance, and Clinical Effectiveness. *Influenza Virology: Current Topics*, 169-202.

Gutenkunst, R.N., Waterfall, J.J., Casey, F.P., Brown, K.S., Myers, C.R., and Sethna, J.P. (2007). Universally Sloppy Parameter Sensitivities in Systems Biology Models. *PLoS Computational Biology 3*, e189.

Hayden, F.G. (1996). Safety and Efficacy of the Neuraminidase Inhibitor GG167 in Experimental Human Influenza. *JAMA: The Journal of the American Medical Association 275*, 295.

Heron, M. (2015). Deaths: Leading Causes for 2012. *National Vital Statistics Reports*.

Herz, A.V., Bonhoeffer, S., Anderson, R.M., May, R.M., and Nowak, M.A. (1996). Viral Dynamics in Vivo: Limitations on Estimates of Intracellular Delay and Virus Decay. *Proceedings of the National Academy of Sciences of the United States of America 93*, 7247-7251.

Ho, D.D., Neumann, A.U., Perelson, A.S., Chen, W., Leonard, J.M., and Markowitz, M. (1995). Rapid Turnover of Plasma Virions and CD4 Lymphocytes in HIV-1 Infection. *Nature 373*, 123-126.

Holder, B.P., and Beauchemin, C.A.A. (2011). Exploring the Effect of Biological Delays in Kinetic Models of Influenza within a Host or Cell Culture. *BMC Public Health 11*, S10.

Hurt, A.C. (2014). The Epidemiology and Spread of Drug Resistant Human Influenza Viruses. *Current Opinion in Virology 8*, 22-29.

Ison, M.G. (2011). Antivirals and Resistance: Influenza Virus. *Current Opinion in Virology 1*, 563-573.

Iwasaki, A., and Pillai, P.S. (2014). Innate Immunity to Influenza Virus Infection. *Nature Reviews Immunology 14*, 315-328.

Louria, D.B., Blumenfeld, H.L., Ellis, J.T., Kilbourne, E.D., and Rogers, D.E. (1959). Studies on Influenza in the Pandemic of 1957-1958. II. Pulmonary Complications of Influenza. *Journal of Clinical Investigation 38*, 213-265.

McCullers, J.A. (2014). The Co-Pathogenesis of Influenza Viruses with Bacteria in the Lung. *Nature Reviews Microbiology 12*, 252-262.

McCullers, J.A., and Rehg, J.E. (2002). Lethal Synergism between Influenza Virus and *Streptococcus Pneumoniae*: Characterization of a Mouse Model and the Role of Platelet-Activating Factor Receptor. *The Journal of Infectious Diseases 186*, 341-350.

McNab, F., Mayer-Barber, K., Sher, A., Wack, A., and O'Garra, A. (2015). Type I Interferons in Infectious Disease. *Nature Reviews Immunology 15*, 87-103.

Metzger, D.W., and Sun, K. (2013). Immune Dysfunction and Bacterial Coinfections Following Influenza. *The Journal of Immunology 191*, 2047-2052.

Mittler, J.E., Sulzer, B., Neumann, A.U., and Perelson, A.S. (1998). Influence of Delayed Viral Production on Viral Dynamics in HIV-1 Infected Patients. *Mathematical Biosciences 152*, 143-163.

Morens, D.M., Taubenberger, J.K., and Fauci, A.S. (2008). Predominant Role of Bacterial Pneumonia as a Cause of Death in Pandemic Influenza: Implications for Pandemic Influenza Preparedness. *The Journal of Infectious Diseases 198*, 962-970.

Neumann, A.U. (1998). Hepatitis C Viral Dynamics in Vivo and the Antiviral Efficacy of Interferon-Therapy. *Science 282*, 103-107.

Nowak, M.A., and May, R.M. (2000). *Virus Dynamics: Mathematical Principles of Immunology and Virology*. Oxford: Oxford University Press.

Pawelek, K.A., Huynh, G.T., Quinlivan, M., Cullinane, A., Rong, L., and Perelson, A.S. (2012). Modeling Within-Host Dynamics of Influenza Virus Infection Including Immune Responses. *PLoS Computational Biology 8*, e1002588.

Peltola, V.T., and Mccullers, J.A. (2004). Respiratory Viruses Predisposing to Bacterial Infections: Role of Neuraminidase. *The Pediatric Infectious Disease Journal 23*, S87-S97.

Perelson, A.S. (2002). Modelling Viral and Immune System Dynamics. *Nature Reviews Immunology 2*, 28-36.

Perelson, A.S., Essunger, P., Cao, Y., Vesanen, M., Hurley, A., Saksela, K., Markowitz, M., and Ho, D.D. (1997). Decay Characteristics of HIV-1-Infected Compartments during Combination Therapy. *Nature 367*, 188-191.

Perelson, A.S., and Nelson, P.W. (1999). Mathematical Analysis of HIV-1 Dynamics in Vivo. *SIAM Review 41*, 3-44.

Perelson, A.S., Neumann, A.U., Markowitz, M., Leonard, J.M., and Ho, D.D. (1996). HIV-1 Dynamics in Vivo: Virion Clearance Rate, Infected Cell Life-Span, and Viral Generation Time. *Science 271*, 1582-1586.

Perelson, A.S., Rong, L., and Hayden, F.G. (2012). Combination Antiviral Therapy for Influenza: Predictions From Modeling of Human Infections. *Journal of Infectious Diseases 205*, 1642-1645.

Potter, C.W. (1998). Chronicle of Influenza Pandemics. *Textbook of Influenza*. Oxford: Blackwell Science.

Reluga, T.C., Dahari, H., and Perelson, A.S. (2009). Analysis of Hepatitis C Virus Infection Models with Hepatocyte Homeostasis. *SIAM Journal on Applied Mathematics 69*, 999-1023.

Ribeiro, R.M., and Bonhoeffer, S. (2000). Production of Resistant HIV Mutants during Antiretroviral Therapy. *Proceedings of the National Academy of Sciences 97*, 7681-7686.

Ribeiro, R.M., Bonhoeffer, S., and Nowak, M.A. (1998). The Frequency of Resistant Mutant Virus before Antiviral Therapy. *AIDS (London, England) 12*, 461-465.

Ribeiro, R.M., Lo, A., and Perelson, A.S. (2002). Dynamics of Hepatitis B Virus Infection. *Microbes and Infection 4*, 829-835.

Saenz, R.A., Quinlivan, M., Elton, D., MacRae, S., Blunden, A.S., Mumford, J.A., Daly, J.M. et al. (2010). Dynamics of Influenza Virus Infection and Pathology. *Journal of Virology 84*, 3974-3983.

Shaw, M.L., and Palese, P. (2013). Orthomyxoviridae. In *Fields Virology*. Philadelphia, PA: Lippincott Williams and Wilkins.

Short, K.R., Habets, M.N., Hermans, P.W.M., and Diavatopoulos, D.A. (2012). Interactions between *Streptococcus Pneumoniae* and Influenza Virus: A Mutually Beneficial Relationship? *Future Microbiology 7*, 609-624.

Shrestha, S.S., Swerdlow, D.L., Borse, R.H., Prabhu, V.S., Finelli, L., Atkins, C.Y., Owusu-Edusei, K. et al. (2011). Estimating the Burden of 2009 Pandemic Influenza A (H1N1) in the United States (April 2009-April 2010). *Clinical Infectious Diseases 52*, S75-S82.

Smith, A.M. (2016). Quantifying the Therapeutic Requirements and Potential for Combination Therapy to Prevent Bacterial Coinfection during Influenza. *Journal of Pharmacokinetics and Pharmacodynamics 44*, 81-93.

Smith, A.M., Adler, F.R., McAuley, J.L., Gutenkunst, R.N., Ribeiro, R.M., McCullers, J.A., and Perelson, A.S. (2011). Effect of 1918 PB1-F2 Expression on Influenza A Virus Infection Kinetics. *PLoS Computational Biology 7*, e1001081.

Smith, A.M., Adler, F.R., and Perelson, A.S. (2010). An Accurate Two-Phase Approximate Solution to an Acute Viral Infection Model. *Journal of Mathematical Biology 60*, 711-726.

Smith, A.M., Adler, F.R., Ribeiro, R.M., Gutenkunst, R.N., McAuley, J.L., McCullers, J.A., and Perelson, A.S. (2013). Kinetics of Coinfection with Influenza A Virus and Streptococcus Pneumoniae. *PLoS Pathogens 9*, e1003238.

Smith, A.M., and McCullers, J.A. (2014). Secondary Bacterial Infections in Influenza Virus Infection Pathogenesis. In R.W. Compans and M.B.A. Oldstone (Eds.), *Influenza Pathogenesis and Control - Volume I* (327-356). Cham: Springer International Publishing.

Smith, A.M., McCullers, J.A., and Adler, F.R. (2011b). Mathematical Model of a Three-Stage Innate Immune Response to a Pneumococcal Lung Infection. *Journal of Theoretical Biology 276*, 106-116.

Smith, A.M., and Perelson, A.S. (2011a). Influenza A Virus Infection Kinetics: Quantitative Data and Models. *Wiley Interdisciplinary Reviews: Systems Biology and Medicine 3*, 429-445.

Smith, A.M., and Smith, A.P. (2016). A Critical, Nonlinear Threshold Dictates Bacterial Invasion and Initial Kinetics During Influenza. *Scientific Reports 6*, 38703.

Stafford, M.A., Corey, L., Cao, Y., Daar, E.S., Ho, D.D., and Perelson, A.S. 2000. Modeling Plasma Virus Concentration during Primary HIV Infection. *Journal of Theoretical Biology 203*, 285-301.

Sun, K., and Metzger, D.W. (2008). Inhibition of Pulmonary Antibacterial Defense by Interferon-γ during Recovery from Influenza Infection. *Nature Medicine 14*, 558-564.

Warnking, K., Klemm, C., Löffler, B., Niemann, S., van Krüchten, A., Peters, G., Ludwig, S., and Ehrhardt, C. (2015). Super-Infection with *Staphylococcus Aureus* Inhibits Influenza Virus-Induced Type I IFN Signalling through Impaired STAT1-STAT2 Dimerization: Influenza Virus- and *S. Aureus* -Mediated Signalling. *Cellular Microbiology 17*, 303-317.

Weinberger, D.M., Simonsen, L., Jordan, R., Steiner, C., Miller, M., and Viboud, C. (2011). Impact of the 2009 Influenza Pandemic on Pneumococcal Pneumonia Hospitalizations in the United States. *Journal of Infectious Diseases 205*, 458-465.

Wei, X., Ghosh, S.K., Taylor, M.E., Johnson, V.A., Emini, E.A., Deutsch, P., Lifson, J.D., Bonhoeffer, S., Nowak, M.A., and Hahn, B.H. (1995). Viral Dynamics in Human Immunodeficiency Virus Type 1 Infection. *Nature 373*, 117-122.

WHO. (2014). The Top 10 Causes of Death. Factsheet 310. http://www.who.int/mediacentre/factsheets/fs310/en/.

Viral fitness landscapes
A physical sciences perspective

GREGORY R. HART AND ANDREW L. FERGUSON

17.1 INTRODUCTION

Viruses are the most prevalent biological agents on Earth, occupying every ecological niche, infecting all known forms of life, and outnumbering cellular organisms by at least an order of magnitude [1–4]. Derived from the Latin meaning "venom" [5,6], viruses are often considered organisms "on the edge of life" carrying hereditary genetic material and subject to natural selection, but which are themselves unable to reproduce, instead reliant on hijacking the replication machinery of an infected host [5,7,8]. Viruses exist as small pathogenic particles tens to hundreds of nanometers in size known as *virions* [1]. A virion comprises a single or double stranded RNA or DNA genome shrouded in a proteinaceous coat known as a capsid, which itself may be encapsulated by a lipid bilayer envelope containing additional proteins and/or carbohydrates [1,8,9]. Viruses are communicated by many means, including air, water, sexual contact, and vectors such as mosquitos. Common viruses infecting humans include influenza, hepatitis B virus (HBV), hepatitis C virus (HCV), human immunodeficiency virus (HIV), and Zika virus. Upon entering the body, innate and adaptive immune responses seek to destroy the virus and prevent an infection, which—depending on the viral strain, health of the host, intensity of infection, and efficacy of treatment—can induce symptoms ranging from mild discomfort, to organ failure, to death.

Upon infecting a susceptible cell, a virus releases its genetic material and proteins to coopt the host replication machinery and produce daughter virions that are released to go on and infect other cells. Infection damages host tissues by inducing pathological changes to the host cell, and ultimately cell death by lysis or apoptosis (programmed cell death) [5]. Some viruses, however, can remain dormant within infected cells for years, providing a latent reservoir of infection [5]. Most viruses, RNA viruses in particular, are highly error prone in copying their genetic material, introducing random mutations into the genome of the daughter virions [8,10]. Most mutations are deleterious to the virus by impairing the activity of viral proteins, others are neutral having negligible impact on viral function, while a small number may be beneficial by enabling the virus to escape from host immune pressure or develop resistance to an antiviral drug. Mutation rates are a strong function of genome size, and can vary between $10^{-8} - 10^{-6}$ substitutions per nucleotide per cell infection for DNA viruses to $10^{-6} - 10^{-4}$ for RNA viruses [11,12]. Together with high virion production rates, the genetic diversity of viral strains within an infected host can be exceedingly high, enabling rapid escape from host immune responses. In hepatitis C virus, for example, a high mutation rate of $\sim 1.2 \times 10^{-4}$ substitutions per nucleotide per cell infection conspires with a high virion production rate of $\sim 10^{12}$ viral progeny per day to produce all possible point mutations at all positions in the 9600-nucleotide genome every single day [11,13,14]. Data-driven models of viral mutation and evolution based on physical sciences principles can provide new fundamental understanding of the relationship between viral sequence and infection outcome, and guide and accelerate the design of new antiviral vaccines and drugs.

17.2 SEQUENCE SPACE AND VIRAL FITNESS LANDSCAPES

The *genotype* of each viral strain—the genetic sequence of its RNA or DNA genome—determines, together with its interaction with its environment, its *phenotype*—the characteristics and performance of the virus [10]. The phenotype, in turn, dictates the viral *fitness* [10,15–17]. The definition of fitness can be somewhat slippery [15,18,19]. For viral replication within an infected host the *replicative fitness* is the appropriate measure, and has been succinctly defined as "the capacity of a virus to produce infectious progeny in a given environment" [15,17]. (This should be distinguished from transmission fitness describing the capacity of a viral strain to jump between hosts and the epidemiological fitness defining the capacity of a particular viral strain to come to dominate within a particular host population [15].) The replicative fitness is a positive real number that can be empirically measured *in vitro* or *in vivo* [15,19–22].

For a viral genome of length M nucleotides, each position can be occupied by one of four nucleobases, leading to 4^M possible distinct viral strains. Alternatively, for a N-residue proteome in which each position can be occupied by one of 20 naturally occurring amino acids, there are 20^N distinct sequences. For hepatitis C virus, $M \approx 9600$ and $N \approx 3000$, such that there are more than 10^{5700} distinct viral genomes and 10^{3900} distinct proteomes [14]. For comparison, there are "only" around 10^{80} protons in the universe [8,23,24]. The size of the known universe may be astronomically big, but the sequence space accessible to the virus is "genomically" large [25]!

Mathematically, the ensemble of viral genomes or proteomes define a set S. Distances between sequences are naturally measured by the *Hamming distance*, d_H, quantifying the number of point mutations by which a pair of sequences differ. The set S and distance d_H together define a M-dimensional metric space (S,d_H) known as *sequence space* [8,10,12,26]. The sequence space can be conceived as a M-dimensional hypercube with genome sequences residing on the vertices and edges connecting nearest neighbors differing by a single point mutation [10,12]. This space is high-dimensional, highly-connected, and dense [8] (Figure 17.1).

Superposing the (replicative) fitness of each strain onto the sequence space defines a $(M+1)$-dimensional *fitness landscape* [8,10,26,27]. First posited by Sewall Wright in the 1930s [24] and refined by J. Maynard Smith [28], Manfred Eigen, and Peter Schuster [29,30] in the 1970s, the fitness landscape is a cornerstone of population genetics coupling the key concepts of sequence space and differential fitness. In essence, the fitness landscape can be considered the "playing field" over which the virus is constrained to evolve, defining a quantitative map describing how its fitness changes as point mutations arise by the error prone replication machinery. Replicatively fit strains that rapidly produce progeny reside at the peaks of the fitness landscape, whereas unfit strains containing mutations that impair protein function reside in low-fitness valleys [31,32]. Viral evolution is the process of mutational motion over the fitness landscape under applied selective pressure [28].

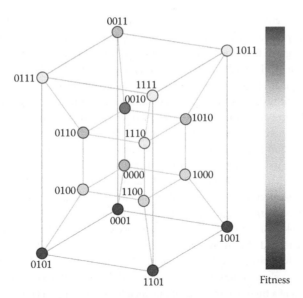

Figure 17.1 Illustrative fitness landscape for a hypothetical M = 4 position virus, each of which can take on z = 2 values {0,1}. The K = z^M = 2^4 = 16 distinct viral genomes comprising the sequence space S define the nodes of a 4-dimensional hypercube (tesseract) with edges linking genomes differing by a single point muta-tion (Hamming distance, d_H = 1). Superposing the fitness of each mutant over the sequence space defines the (M+1)-dimensional fitness landscape represented here as a heat map. Although low-dimensional pictures provide "a very inadequate representation of such a field" [24], the mathematical concept indicated by this schematic straightforwardly generalizes to arbitrary M and z.

17.3 QUASISPECIES THEORY

For rapidly mutating viruses, the picture of viral evolution as a hill-climbing process in which the virus seeks to maximize fitness is not quite correct [18,27]. Due to the high rate at which mutations are introduced during viral replication, a viral strain residing in sequence space at a particular vertex of the *M*-dimensional hyper-cube does not generate identical copies of itself, but produces daughter progeny that "leak" along the edges of the hypercube into neighboring mutational states. Recognizing the importance of this effect upon natural selection, Manfred Eigen and Peter Schuster proposed that the unit of natural selection was not a particular viral strain, but a swarm of closely related mutant strains known as a *quasispecies* that arises from a balance between mutation and selection [29,30]. The deterministic evolution of the quasispecies over the fitness land-scape in the infinite population size limit is specified by a first order nonlinear differential equation known as Eigen's equation, or the quasispecies equation [8,10,29,30,33–35],

$$\dot{n}_i = \sum_{j=1}^{K} n_j f_j q_{ij} - \phi(\{n_k\}) n_i \tag{17.1}$$

where there are *K* distinct genomes *i* = 1..*K*, n_i is the fraction of the population with genome *i* and the popu-lation fractions are normalized such that $\sum_{i=1}^{K} n_i = 1$, $\dot{n}_i$ is the rate of change of the fraction of strain *i*, f_i is the relative replicative fitness of strain *i*, q_{ij} is the mutational probability that replication of strain *j* produces strain *i* under replication and are normalized such that $\sum_{i=1}^{K} q_{ij} = 1$, and $\phi(\{n_k\}) = \sum_{i=1}^{K} n_i f_i$ is the average fitness of the population defining the fitness-independent removal rate of each strain to keep the total popula-tion size fixed. This equation may be succinctly expressed in matrix-vector form as [35],

$$\dot{n} = QFn - (n.f)n, \tag{17.2}$$

where $n = [n_1, n_2, ..., n_K]^T$ is a column vector specifying the instantaneous structure of the viral population, $\dot{n}$ is the rate of change of the population structure, $Q = [q_{ij}]$ is the left stochastic mutation matrix, $f = [f_1, f_2, ..., f_K]^T$, and $F = \text{diag}(f)$ is the diagonal fitness matrix. The nonlinear quasispecies equation can be transformed into a linear differential equation and solved exactly using path integrals [36,37]. This treatment represents the time evolution of the viral population as a sum over all possible mutational trajectories from the initial to the final population structures, and rests on similar principles and mathematics as the path integral formulation of quantum mechanics due to Paul Dirac and Richard Feynman [38]. In the limit of perfect replication fidelity (i.e., a diagonal mutation matrix), the quasispecies equation reduces to the standard replicator equation [10].

The quasispecies equation is central to the study of viral dynamics, and makes a number of important predictions (Figure 17.2). First, it asserts that for rapidly mutating viruses, natural selection acts on the level of the quasispecies rather than the individual strain [12,29,30]. Second, it predicts that while at low mutation rates the equilibrium quasispecies will be centered on the global fitness maximum, at sufficiently high mutation rates it may sacrifice a narrow high peak in favor of a broad lower peak [8,10,29,30]. This result can be understood as natural selection on the level of the quasispecies, which seeks to maximize the mean fitness of the swarm of closely related strains. A virus with a low-error rate can exist as a tight cloud of member strains within a narrow high fitness peak, resulting in a high mean fitness of the population. A high-error rate virus exists as a diffuse cloud of strains due to mutational "leakage" along the edges of the sequence space hypercube. In the region of a high narrow peak, many members of the high-error rate ensemble will exist in low fitness states outside the peak, pulling down the mean fitness of the population. In the region of a lower but broader peak, more members of the quasispecies occupy high fitness states, leading to a net elevation of the mean fitness. This phenomenon has been termed "survival of the flattest" [39,40]. Third, it predicts the existence of a maximum error rate beyond which the quasispecies loses cohesion and cannot adapt to the

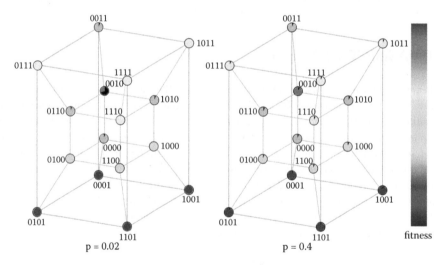

Figure 17.2 Equilibrium quasispecies distribution n^* over the sequence space as a function of mutation rate. Continuing the example of a $M = 4$ position virus with $z = 2$ values {0,1} per position, we can simulate its quasispecies dynamics over its $K = 16$ state fitness landscape in Figure 17.1. The fitness landscape is specified by the (relative) fitness vector $f = [0.7, 0.1, 0.9, 0.7, 0.5, 0.1, 0.7, 0.6, 0.5, 0.1, 0.7, 0.6, 0.5, 0.1, 0.6, 0.6]^T$ with elements arranged in standard order (i.e., 1 = 0000, 2 = 0001, ..., 15 = 1110, 16 = 1111). The mutation matrix is specified as $Q = [q_{ij}]$, where $q_{ij} = p^{H_{ij}}(1-p)^{(M-H_{ij})}$ (Eq. 17.3), H_{ij} is the Hamming distance between strains i and j, and p is the mutation rate per position per replication cycle. We solve for the equilibrium quasispecies distribution over the sequence space by solving for the steady state solution of the quasispecies equation (Eq. 17.2) as a function of mutation rate [35]. In the left panel we reproduce the fitness landscape illustrated in Figure 17.1 superposed with pie segments indicating the equilibrium fraction of the quasispecies population partitioning into each mutational state at a low mutation rate of $p = 0.02$. Under these conditions, the virus possesses relatively high copying fidelity and the quasispecies localizes around the fitness peak at state [0010], with a small fraction of the population leaking into the neighboring strains. In the right panel we illustrate the equilibrium distribution at an elevated mutation rate of $p = 0.4$, where the quasispecies has experienced an error catastrophe such that it cannot adapt to the topography of the fitness landscape and has delocalized across sequence space.

fitness landscape [8,10,33,41–44]. This *error catastrophe* can be shown to be analogous to a first order phase transition in a finite system [45], corresponding to a loss of locality of the quasispecies within sequence space [46–50]. Evidence suggests that many RNA viruses possess mutation rates close to the error threshold, which is thought to provide a survival advantages to the virus by offering a reservoir of viral phenotypes, enhancing adaptability, and aiding in the development of immunological escape mutations [8,43,51,52]. Drug therapies that elevate the viral mutation rate above the error threshold are under investigation as novel treatments for HIV [53–56].

Despite the central importance of quasispecies theory in the theoretical understanding of viral evolution, it has not enjoyed strong experimental support largely due to the technical difficulties associated with sequencing a substantial fraction of the strains constituting the quasispecies [34]. Nevertheless, support exists for the existence of the error catastrophe [57], and recent advances in deep sequencing and ultra-deep sequencing are expected to enable more rigorous testing of its predictions [34]. One significant deficiency of the theory is that it is inherently deterministic, therefore pertaining to formally infinite viral populations. Viruses can have relatively small effective population sizes, such that stochastic effects can play an important role in their evolutionary dynamics [33,50]. Numerical population genetics simulations provide a means to explicitly account for stochasticity and also straightforwardly incorporate other effects such as co-infection, recombination, spatial heterogeneity, and drug or immune pressure [33,50,58–61]. Finally, we note the ingenious observation by Guy Sella and Aaron Hirsh of an isomorphism – under relatively restrictive conditions – between population genetics and equilibrium statistical thermodynamics [62]. Similar analogies to statistical mechanics and information theory have been made by Michael Deem, Arup Chakraborty, Bill Bialek, Hendrik Richter, and ourselves [26,31,32,49,59,63–68].

A prerequisite to simulating viral dynamics using either quasispecies theory or numerical simulations is specification of the fitness landscape f and the mutation matrix Q. The mutation matrix is typically assumed to be non-negative, symmetric, and stochastic [35]. Assuming independent identically distributed (*iid*) mutations, the mutation matrix $Q = [q_{ij}]$ can be straightforwardly specified as [8,35],

$$q_{ij} = \left(\frac{p}{z-1}\right)^{H_{ij}} (1-p)^{(M-H_{ij})}, \tag{17.3}$$

where q_{ij} is the mutational probability that replication of strain j produces strain i, p is the mutation rate per position per replication cycle, z is the size of the alphabet at each position ($z = 4$ for genomes, $z = 20$ for proteomes), M is the number of positions in the strain, and H_{ij} is the Hamming distance (i.e., number of substitutions) between strains i and j. For $p = 0$, the Q matrix becomes the identity matrix corresponding to perfect replication fidelity. For sufficiently small values of p, daughter strains containing two or more mutations within the same replication cycle ($H_{ij} \geq 2$) may be considered vanishingly rare. Accordingly, Q may be approximated as $q_{ii} = (1-p)^M$, $q_{ij} = \left(\frac{p}{z-1}\right)(1-p)^{(M-1)}$ for $H_{ij} = 1$, and $q_{ij} = 0$ for $H_{ij} \geq 2$, corresponding to a situation in which the progeny of any viral strain can contain at most one point mutation and multi-mutant hops along the edges of the sequence space hypercube are forbidden. More complex models may allow, for example, for correlated mutations, differential probabilities in mutating from a purine to a pyrimidine nucleobase on the level of the genome, or accounting for synonymous and non-synonymous mutations in the three-base amino acid codon on the level of the proteome. Specification of the fitness landscape defined by the fitness vector f is a more involved problem that is the subject of Section 17.4.

17.4 VIRAL FITNESS LANDSCAPES FROM EXPERIMENT AND THEORY

The genotype of a viral strain within a particular environment specifies its phenotype that, in turn, dictates its replicative fitness. The fitness landscape is the convolution of this double mapping from genotype to phenotype to fitness [10,23,26,27]. This mapping can be conceived as a (complicated) function of the viral sequence, which integrates over the characteristics and performance of the virus within its environment to produce a non-negative real number specifying its replicative competency. Fitness landscapes have typically been defined by one of two methods: sparse experimental fitness measurements of very limited regions of sequence space, or theoretical models designed to reproduce the statistical properties of real landscapes [69,70]. The former pertain to one particular viral system and therefore can be used to make fitness predictions, but have proven difficult to both define and to generalize. The latter are designed to be statistical abstractions that are generic to some class of viruses, but necessarily sacrifice predictive accuracy of the fitness of any particular virus.

Experimental determination of comprehensive fitness landscapes is rendered extremely challenging by the vast size of viral sequence space. For a viral proteome comprising N amino acids there are 20^N distinct viral sequences, meaning that experimental measurements of the replicative capacity can only probe a vanishingly small fraction of the sequence space [23]. Taking hepatitis C virus as an example, $N \approx 3000$ meaning that there are 10^{3900} distinct proteomes [14]. Fewer than around 1 in 10^{3897} strains would have to be represented in meaningful quantities during infection to define a sequence space sufficiently small to be comprehensively probed by experimental fitness assays. Nevertheless, advances in next-generation sequencing and high-throughput automated assays has led to a growing body of experimental studies designed to probe general features of fitness landscapes by measuring the fitness of a limited subset of tens to hundreds of mutant strains [23,27,69,71–73]. For example, Qi et al. coupled saturation mutagenesis with deep sequencing to measure the fitness of all 1720 possible point mutants within an 86-residue region of the hepatitis C virus protein NS5A known to be a target for replication inhibitors [74]. Nonetheless, experimental determination of comprehensive fitness landscapes remains inherently intractable for even the smallest viruses, offering only a "glimpse…within the immense genotype space" [23].

A more scalable approach is offered by using limited experimental data to fit statistical or regression fitness models that may then be extrapolated to predict the fitness of strains that were not directly assayed [23,27,72,73,75–78]. For example, Hayashi et al. combined molecular evolution experiments with infectivity assays to fit the parameters of an NK-model [76]. Hinkley et al. fitted a regularized regression model to *in vitro* fitness measurements of 70,081 mutant strains of HIV incorporating pairwise interactions that was capable of explaining 54.8% of the variance in the measured fitness [73]. Segal et al. employed decision tree-based approaches to predict HIV-1 replicative capacity as a function of the amino acid sequence of the protease and reverse transcriptase viral proteins [77]. In all cases, however, the time, labor, and expense associated with *in vitro* fitness measurements means that models are fit to a sparse library of fitness measurements sampling an infinitesimally small fraction of sequence space. The fitted models are therefore subject to significant bias and possess large extrapolation errors for mutant strains dissimilar to those upon which the model was trained [75].

A number of theoretical fitness landscape models have been proposed that seek to reproduce the statistical features and correlations observed in real landscapes. These models have proved extremely useful in gaining insight into viral dynamics and adaptation over archetypal landscapes, and as baseline models containing parameters that may be tuned to experiment. Epistasis—nonlinear effects due to interaction of two or more mutational loci—gives rise to non-additive fitness landscapes and appears to play a critical role in the function, dynamics, and evolution of viruses [23,31,34,49,79–81]. One of the first and most popular fitness models explicitly designed to capture epistasis is Kaufmann's "tuneably rugged" (i.e., "tuneably epistatic") NK-model [23,26,70,76,82–84]. This model specifies fitness as the sum of random variables corresponding to the fitness contributions from N positions, each of which depends on the mutational state of K other positions. Specifically, the mutational state of an organism is described by a vector $\boldsymbol{x} = [x_1, x_2, \ldots, x_n]$, where $x_i = \{0, 1, \ldots, (p_i - 1)\}$ denote the p_i possible allelic states of mutational locus i. The organismal fitness is given by the sum of the fitness contributions of the N loci $f(x) = \sum_{i=1}^{N} \phi\left(x_i, \{x_j\}_{j \in \omega i}\right)$, where ϕ is a function specifying the fitness contribution of position i which depends on both its mutational state x_i and the mutational states of K other positions $\{x_j\}_{j \in \omega i}$ with which position i interacts. The set of K interaction partners ω_i for each position i may be defined randomly or based on some measure of proximity. The fitness contributions

$\phi\left(x_i,\{x_j\}_{j\in\omega i}\right)$ are typically specified as independent identically distributed (iid) random variables drawn from a distribution over its $K + 1$ arguments. In the limit $K = 0$, there is no epistasis (i.e., all positions have independent fitness contributions) and the landscape is unfrustrated and smooth, the so-called "Mount Fiji" model [23]. The limit of $K = (N-1)$ corresponds to all-to-all epistasis, producing a highly rugged and frustrated landscape containing many local fitness maxima known as a "house of cards" model that is isomorphic to a random energy spin glass [23,85,86]. Generalizations of the NK-model accounting for protein structure and binding interactions have subsequently been proposed [63,87]. The "rough Mount Fiji" model superposes onto the NK-model a fitness contribution that falls off with Hamming distance away from a reference (usually the wild-type) strain [23,33,88]. An alternative model is provided by Motoo Kimura's neutral theory of evolution, which envisages mutations to be either neutral or lethal [89]. The corresponding fitness landscape is binary, containing viable strains of equal fitness residing on a neutral plateau fissured by valleys of unviable mutant strains [88]. Since the unviable strains are considered to be mutationally inaccessible (i.e., have zero fitness), this has been described as a "holey" fitness landscape that is isomorphic to a percolation problem over the sequence space hypercube [26,88].

17.5 DATA-DRIVEN VIRAL FITNESS LANDSCAPES

Very recently, data-driven approaches have emerged as a third way to determine empirical fitness landscapes from databases of viral sequences [31,32,35,64,90,91]. These approaches adopt a Bayesian perspective to determine fitness landscapes consistent with observations of viral strains sequenced from infected hosts by assuming a relationship between strain fitness and the relative prevalence of correlated mutational patterns within the sequence database [75]. Although the predictions of such models may be validated against *in vitro* fitness assays, these techniques are distinguished from the fitting of fitness models to experimental measurements in that they require only a library of observed viral sequences and do not appeal to experimental fitness measurements for their construction. This is a critical distinction, since modern low-cost, high-throughput sequencing technologies has made these approaches massively more scalable than those predicated on laborious and time consuming fitness assays [34,92].

In 2013, one of us (Andrew L. Ferguson) together with Arup Chakraborty pioneered a data-driven approach to reconstruct viral fitness landscapes from viral sequence databases [31]. Subsequent works have produced sophistications, analyses, and validations of the approach, and applications to both hepatitis C virus and HIV [32,49,59,64,65]. The essence of the approach is to regard the viral strains within a sequence database as observations over an unknown fitness landscape and perform Bayesian inference to solve the "inverse problem" and reconstruct the most probable fitness landscape from which the strains were drawn. Provided that founder effects are weak such that the virus rapidly anneals to the immune response of a newly infected host and that the sequence databases of observed viral strains are sufficiently large and represent hosts with diverse immunological genotypes, we have demonstrated by both theory and empiricism that the fitness landscapes we compute quantify the intrinsic molecular fitness of the virus uncorrupted by "footprints" of adaptive immunity [31,32,59,64,93]. In effect, the diversity of possible immune responses means that particular positions within the viral genome are subject to mutational pressure from a small subset of the hosts constituting the database, and particular immune responses act as a small perturbation when averaged over sufficiently many hosts [59]. The fitness landscapes determined by our approach reflect the *intrinsic* replicative capacity of the virus in the absence of immune pressure, and can be straightforwardly adapted to reflect the *effective* fitness landscape experienced by the virus in any particular host by superposing the adaptive immune responses as an external perturbation [31,32,59].

17.5.1 RELATIONSHIP TO OTHER WORK

In 2015, Niko Beerenwinkel and co-workers proposed an elegant framework to estimate intrahost fitness landscapes from next generation sequencing data of the viral quasispecies within an infected host [34,35,92].

This approach shares similarities with our own in that it employs a Bayesian inference approach to reconstruct fitness landscapes from observations of viral strains, but has some important distinguishing differences. First, the approach is based on intrahost sequencing data and therefore calculates fitness landscapes that are the convolution of the intrinsic fitness (i.e., in the absence of immune pressure) with the adaptive immune responses of the particular host. The authors used their approach to recover the fitness landscape for HIV protein p7 in two hosts, and found the landscapes to be quite different. Containing the "footprints" of host immune pressure [93], it is a challenge to generalize these fitness landscapes to new environments (e.g., different immune responses, drug pressure, *in vitro* culture). Second, the approach postulates that the ensemble of strains should follow the equilibrium distribution predicted by quasispecies theory to provide a model linking strain fitness to prevalence in the sequencing data. Due to the immense size of sequence space, it is necessary to operate in a reduced subset of sequence space in which low fitness viral strains are neglected [35]. Moreover, the fitness landscape f and mutation matrix Q are not independently identifiable (Eq. 17.2) [35,94], meaning that the inference problem requires the specification of a particular Q upon which the inferred f then depends. In contrast, our approach is non-parametric in the sense that it does not appeal to quasispecies theory nor assume an *a priori* functional form for the fitness landscape, instead seeking the least biased (i.e., maximum entropy) model consistent with the data. The authors devise a Monte Carlo approach to perform the Bayesian inference, and have made this available for free public download at http://www.cbg.ethz.ch/software/quasifit.

We also observe the relationship of our approach to earlier work by Beerenwinkel et al. in 2005 and Deforche et al. in 2008 that coupled cross-sectional sequence data (i.e., sequence data from different infected hosts at different times) from treated and untreated cohorts of HIV patients with *in vivo* evolutionary models to estimate the effect of drug therapy upon viral fitness and mutation [90,91]. The more recent work by Beerenwinkel and ourselves seeks not differential fitness responses to drug therapy, but rather the complete fitness landscape either in the presence [35] or absence [31] of host immune pressure.

Our methodology also shares commonalities with innovative work by Bill Bialek and co-workers who employed data-driven spin glass models to quantify antibody diversity in zebrafish, the activity of ensembles of neurons in salamander retinae, and the flocking behavior of birds [66,68,95–98], and Martin Weigt, Terry Hwa, José Onuchic, and co-workers who used data-driven spin glass models to identify coevolving amino acid residues or nucleotides to predict putative protein and RNA tertiary structure contacts [99–103].

17.5.2 MATHEMATICAL AND COMPUTATIONAL DETAILS

Given a multiple sequence alignment (MSA) of viral sequences drawn from multiple infected hosts, we have developed an approach to determine the least biased model capable of recapitulating the relative prevalence of viral strains within the database [31,32,59,64]. We choose to work with viral proteomes, but the approach is equally applicable for viral genomes. Since the viral strains are drawn from amongst the population of infected hosts and not from within a single host, we assume that the viral *prevalence landscape* on the level of the infected population is a good proxy for the *fitness landscape* on the level of a single host. We also make the simplifying assumption that the sequences within the database are independent and identically distributed (iid). We have demonstrated by both analytical theory and experimental comparisons that both of these assumptions are valid for sufficiently large and diverse clinical sequence databases containing strains that are phylogenetically proximate (e.g., belong to the same viral subtype) [31,32,59,64]. We seek the maximum entropy model consistent with the two lowest moments of the amino acid distribution [104,105], namely the frequency with which the 20 amino acids are observed at each single position and each of the $20 \times 20 = 400$ pairs of amino acids are observed in each pair of positions. The resulting model is the simplest non-trivial fitness landscape capable of capturing epistasis at the level of pairs. A natural extension would be to include higher order epistatic effects (e.g., triplets, quads, etc.). It has been shown, however, that the exponential explosion in the model parameters associated with higher order terms quickly degrades both the numerical stability and predictive performance of the model [73]. By terminating the expansion at second order, we determine not the *intrinsic* one- and two-body coefficients, but *effective* coefficients that implicitly capture higher-order correlations and which we have shown to reproduce both the three- and four-body amino acid frequencies [31,32]. This is consistent with observations that effective pairwise interaction models can reproduce higher order correlations from the emergent interactions of the constitutive pairs [68,75,96,97].

The maximum entropy model that emerges from this analysis is the infinite-range Potts spin glass from statistical physics [32,64,106]. The Potts model can be considered a multistate generalization of the Ising model, describing a system of N pairwise interacting spins that each take on one of q discrete states. The model is infinite range in the sense that each spin interacts with all other spins, and the energy assigned to a particular configuration of the system contains one-body contributions from each of the N spins, and two-body contributions from the $N(N-1)/2$ pairwise interactions. The parameters of the model specify the character of these interactions and can generically lead to highly rugged and non-trivial energy landscapes [106]. Given an N-residue viral proteome in which each position can be occupied by one of $q = 20$ naturally occurring amino acids, $\vec{A} = \{A_i\}_{i=1}^{N}$, where A_i specifies the identity of the amino acid residue in position i, the Potts model specifies the probability of observing that sequence as [32,64],

$$P(\vec{A}) = \frac{1}{z} e^{-E(\vec{A})}, \quad E(\vec{A}) = \sum_{i=1}^{N} h_i(A_i) + \sum_{i=1}^{N} \sum_{j=i+1}^{N} J_{ij}(A_i, A_j), \tag{17.4}$$

where E is a fictitious dimensionless "energy", $E(\vec{A})$ is the spin glass Hamiltonian specifying the mapping from sequence to energy, and the normalizing factor $Z = \sum_{\vec{A}} e^{-E(\vec{A})}$ is the partition function. The Hamiltonian comprises N 20-element vectors $\{h_i\}$ specifying the contribution of each amino acid in each single position to the sequence energy, and $N(N-1)/2$ 20×20 matrices $\{J_{ij}\}$ specifying the contributions of each pair of amino acids in each pair of positions. Since we fit our model against population level sequence databases, $P(\vec{A})$ should be interpreted as the probability of observing a particular strain within the ensemble of infected hosts. We, and others, have demonstrated using analytical theory [59,62], computer simulations [59], and comparisons against *in vitro* and *in vivo* data [31,32,64] that the prevalence of a strain at the population level $P(\vec{A})$ is a good proxy for intrinsic viral replicative capacity within an infected host $f(\vec{A})$. The Potts Hamiltonian therefore defines the (relative) replicative fitness landscape f of the virus as $f(\vec{A}) \propto e^{-E(\vec{A})}$. If absolute fitness values are required, the constant of proportionality can be determined by fitting against experimental fitness measurements for a small number of mutant strains [32,64].

The model parameters $\{h_i, J_{ij}\}$ are fitted such that Eq. 17.4 reproduces the one- and two-body amino acid frequencies observed in the MSA, and may be computed in many ways, including mean field and post-mean field approximations [100,107–111], message passing [99], adaptive cluster expansions [64,112], pseudo-likelihood maximization [113], minimum probability flow [114], and Monte Carlo sampling [95,115]. We have developed an approach employing iterative gradient descent and Monte Carlo evaluation of model probabilities that provides highly accurate parameter fits. We accelerate convergence using a combination of Bayesian regularization, initial mean field parameter estimates, and parallel Monte Carlo chains exploiting CPU or GPU multicore architectures. Full details of our methodology and a freely available C++ implementation of our code are provided in Ref. [64]. We have also made a user-friendly MATLAB implementation suitable for computing fitness landscapes for small viral proteins available for free download at https://bitbucket.org/andrewlferguson/viralfitness_matlab.

17.6 APPLICATIONS

To illustrate our approach, we first demonstrate its application to a cartoon two-residue virus as the simplest possible model system capable of exhibiting epistatic couplings between residues. We then describe its application to determine the fitness landscape of the hepatitis C virus RNA-dependent RNA polymerase (protein NS5B) and show how this landscape may be used for *in silico* design of vaccine immunogens. We have also employed our approach to determine fitness landscapes for multiple proteins of both hepatitis C virus and HIV, perform *in silico* design cytotoxic T cell vaccine immunogens, and make the first theoretical prediction of a viral error catastrophe in an empirically-defined viral fitness landscape for the p6 HIV protein [31,32,49,59,64].

17.6.1 A TOY MODEL OF A TWO-RESIDUE VIRUS

We first consider a toy virus comprising precisely two amino acid residues. This is the simplest possible system capable of exhibiting epistasis, and possesses the appealing property that the fitness landscape can be easily visualized in three dimensions. We specify the fitness landscape of this virus by fiat, and demonstrate the capacity of our approach to correctly infer the fitness landscape from sufficiently many observations of viral strains over the *a priori* unknown fitness landscape.

Identifying the particular amino acid residue in position $i = \{1,2\}$ by an index $A_i = \{1,2,...,20\}$ arbitrarily ordering the 20 natural amino acids, we adopt as the "true" fitness landscape for the cartoon virus the Potts spin glass (Eq. 17.4) with $\{h_i, J_{ij}\}$ parameters specified as,

$$h_1(A_1) = \frac{(A_1 - 1)}{4}, \quad h_2(A_2) = \frac{(A_2 - 1)}{8}, \tag{17.5a}$$

$$J_{12}(A_1, A_2) = 1.5\left(e^{-\left((A_1-4)^2+(A_2-4)^2\right)} - e^{-\left((A_1-9^2)+(A_2-8)^2\right)}\right). \tag{17.5b}$$

This fitness landscape was designed to possess a simple but non-trivial topography, possessing a global maximum at the sequence [1,1], a global minimum at [20,20], a local maximum at [9,8], and a local minimum at [4,4] (Figure 17.3). Since the form of the true fitness landscape and that inferred by our inference technique have the form of a Potts spin glass, our approach should be capable of accurately reproducing the one- and two-body amino acid frequencies and predicting strain fitness given sufficiently many observations of viral sequences over the landscape.

To test this hypothesis, we generated realizations of viral strains sampled over the landscape in proportion to their fitness using Markov chain Monte Carlo sampling [32]. We assembled strains generated in this manner into multiple sequence alignments containing different numbers of sequences, then used these

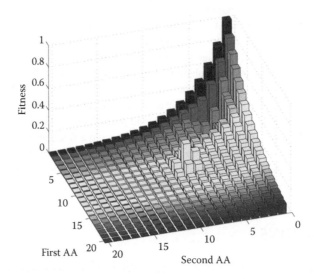

Figure 17.3 Fitness landscape of a cartoon viral protein possessing two amino acid residues specified by Eq. 17.5. We index the amino acid residues available to position *i* as $A_i = \{1,2,...,20\}$, but their ordering is arbitrary. A particular sequence $[A_i, A_j]$ can mutate into any other sequence in the same column by making a point mutation in the first residue, and to any other sequence in the same row by making a point mutation in the second. The fitness landscape was designed to possess a global maximum at the sequence [1,1], a global minimum at [20,20], a local maximum at [9,8], and a local minimum at [4,4].

alignments and our iterative gradient descent approach to infer the 40 $\{h_i\}$ and 400 $\{J_{ij}\}$ parameters from the data [32,64]. We report in Table 17.1 a quantitative assessment of the capacity of our inferred model to reproduce the one- and two-body amino acid frequencies observed in the MSA, and the agreement of the inferred model parameters with those of the true landscape. Containing just two mutating residues, the one- and two-body mutational frequencies of the true and fitted models can be computed analytically by enumerating over all viral mutants. We present in Figure 17.4 parity plots of the true and predicted fitness computed for all possible viral strains.

As anticipated, we find that the fitted model can reproduce the one- and two-body mutational frequencies and predict strain fitness to arbitrarily high fidelity given sufficiently many sequences in the MSA. The discrepancy between the inferred and true model parameters also decreases with the number of sequences in the MSA, but remains non-zero even for near-perfect reproduction of the one- and two-body mutational frequencies. This phenomenon appears to result from the existence of "null spaces" or "sloppy directions" within the $\{h_i, J_{ij}\}$ parameter space such that particular combinations of the parameters can be adjusted in concert without significantly perturbing the energy (i.e., fitness) of a strain or its one- and two-body mutational probabilities [116]. This simple toy problem indicates that it is possible to reconstruct fitness landscapes to high precision given sufficiently many sequences, but that care should be taken in assigning meaning to individual h_i and J_{ij} values.

Table 17.1 Quality of fitness landscape reconstruction for a cartoon 2-residue virus with a Potts spin glass fitness landscape with parameters specified by Eq. 17.5 for multiple sequence alignments containing various numbers of sequences. We report the Pearson correlation coefficient of the analytically computed one-body (ρ_{P1}) and two-body (ρ_{P2}) amino acid frequencies between the true and fitted fitness landscape. We also report the root mean squared error in the inferred $\{h_i\}$ and $\{J_{ij}\}$ parameters relative to their true values

MSA size	ρ_{P1} (p value)	ρ_{P2} (p value)	RMSE $\{h_i\}$	RMSE $\{J_{ij}\}$
10^0	0.47 (2.2×10^{-3})	0.22 (1.2×10^{-5})	14.7	19.6
10^1	0.52 (6.7×10^{-4})	0.25 (3.1×10^{-7})	17.2	40.9
10^2	0.72 (1.7×10^{-7})	0.37 (3.3×10^{-14})	23.1	93.5
10^3	0.93 (1.9×10^{-18})	0.81 (8.0×10^{-96})	14.7	81.3
10^4	0.99 (1.1×10^{-36})	0.97 (1.1×10^{-238})	2.6	48.5
10^5	1.00 (3.1×10^{-44})	1.00 ($<1.0 \times 10^{-308}$)	0.7	5.5

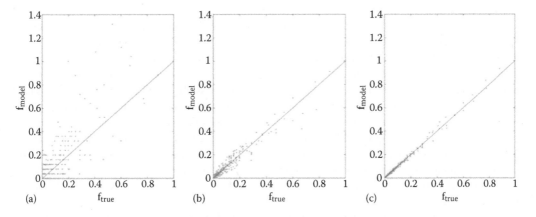

Figure 17.4 Parity plots of true versus reconstructed fitness for the cartoon $M = 2$ residue viral protein possessing the fitness landscape illustrated in Figure 17.3. The plots illustrate for the ensemble all $20^M = 400$ viral strains the true strain fitness specified by Eq. 17.5 against the fitness predicted by models reconstructed from multiple sequence alignments containing **(a)** 10^3, **(b)** 10^4, and **(c)** 10^5 viral strains.

17.6.2 HCV *IN SILICO* VACCINE DESIGN

Hepatitis C virus (HCV) is a 50 nm single-stranded RNA retrovirus that infects 170 million people worldwide—nearly 3% of the global population—and kills more than 350,000 annually [117–119]. The virus replicates within the hepatocytes of the liver, leading to fibrosis, cirrhosis, and ultimately hepatocellular carcinoma [120]. Known as the "silent killer" due to the fact that infected hosts remain asymptomatic until the onset of severe liver damage, HCV is the leading cause of liver transplantation in the industrialized world [117,121]. The anti-HCV drug Harvoni released by Gilead Sciences in 2014 is a dual-acting combination therapy targeting HCV proteins NS5A and NS5B with cure rates exceeding 95% [122]. The high cost of such treatments, however, makes them effectively inaccessible in the developing world, such that effective cure rates worldwide remain below 10% [118]. Prophylactic vaccination is "the most cost-effective and realistic method of controlling HCV globally" [121,123]. Although a cytotoxic T cell-based vaccine trial is in progress, a vaccine remains unavailable despite 20 years of work [124–126]. The definition of empirical fitness landscapes for HCV viral proteins presents a means to systematically identify regions of the viral proteome vulnerable to mutational pressure, informing the rational design of vaccine immunogens to prime the T cell and antibody responses capable of corralling the virus into low-lying valleys of the fitness landscape where its replicative capacity is compromised. In this manner, computational approaches can function as an efficient and inexpensive means to discover promising immunogen designs to guide capital and labor intensive experimental and clinical development efforts.

Considering the HCV subtype 1a that is the most prevalent viral clade in the United States, we applied our approach to the 591-residue RNA-dependent RNA polymerase—nonstructural protein 5B (NS5B)— that is responsible for the error-prone replication of the viral genome and is known to contain good targets for immune pressure and drug therapies [32]. We assembled an MSA comprising 976 clinically observed sequences of the NS5B region of HCV-1a. Only 283 positions were observed to mutate within the sequence ensemble, providing us with a ratio of sequences to mutating positions of 3.4:1. We fitted our model using the gradient descent approach detailed above using high-performance supercomputing hardware requiring approximately 12 CPU-months of calculation. As a numerical validation of the model, we verified that it not only accurately reproduced the one- and two-body amino acid frequencies in the MSA, but that it *predicted* the three-body correlations. As experimental validations, we demonstrated the fitness predictions of the model to be in excellent accord with *in vitro* replicative fitness measurements for 31 mutant viral strains, and to predict the documented high-fitness escape mutations. As a clinical validation, applications of our model to longitudinal sequencing data predict temporal fitness trajectories in good agreement with host immune responses, viral load, and maternofetal immune tolerance mechanisms. Full details of our application are provided in [32].

Immunodominance is the effect whereby cellular or humoral adaptive immune responses preferentially target particular antigenic epitopes within an invading pathogen [127,128]. Vaccine immunogens comprising complete viral proteins or sub-proteins may prime dominant immune responses against poor viral targets from which the virus can easily escape and can suppress subdominant responses against vulnerable targets that force mutations which cripple viral fitness [31,79,80,129]. Empirical fitness landscapes can reveal "soft spots" in the viral proteome particularly susceptible to immune targeting, offering a systematic means to determine which epitopes should be included in an epitope-based vaccine to elicit potent adaptive immune responses. The immune pressure can be conceived as an external perturbation over the viral fitness landscape that cripples the fitness of viral sequences recognized by adaptive immune responses, forcing the quasispecies to make deleterious escape mutations. Essentially, we seek to hit the virus where it hurts by priming immune responses to exclude it from high-fitness peaks and trap it in low-fitness valleys.

Having estimated and validated the empirical HCV-1a NS5B fitness landscape, we used it to exhaustively screen all 16,777,215 immunogen candidates comprising all possible combinations of the 24 cytotoxic T cell (CTL) epitopes targeted by the top 66 immunological haplotypes of North Americans. We evaluated each immunogen candidate by seeking to simultaneously optimize three design criteria: (i) maximize the

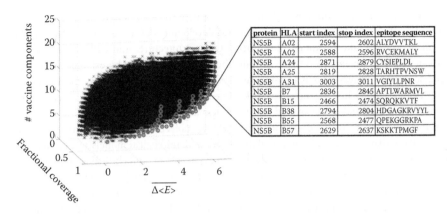

Figure 17.5 Scatter plot of all 16,777,215 HCV-1a immunogen candidates comprising all possible combinations of the 24 cytotoxic T cell epitopes targeted by the top 66 immunological haplotypes of North Americans. Each immunogen is evaluated along three design criteria: (i) the mean reduction in the fitness of the viral quasispecies over the empirical fitness landscape averaged over the vaccine recipient population, $\Delta\langle E \rangle$, (ii) the fraction of vaccine recipients capable of eliciting immune responses to at least one epitope within the vaccine immunogen, and (iii) the number of epitopes in the vaccine immunogen. Of all 16,777,215 immunogen candidates (crosses) there are 86 Pareto optimal candidates (circles) residing on the efficient frontier. These candidates are optimal in the sense that no design criterion can be improved without incurring a penalty in another. The particular candidate defining the global optimum depends on the relative importance assigned to each of the three criteria. We have illustrated the human leukocyte antigen (HLA) associations, locations within the HCV proteome, and sequences of the 10 epitopes comprising one particular candidate on the optimal frontier possessing $\Delta\langle E \rangle = 6.6$ and 71.2% fractional coverage.

mean reduction in the fitness of the viral quasispecies averaged over the North American population (i.e., the degree to which vaccine-induced immune responses are capable of ejecting the virus from the high-fitness peaks in the average vaccine recipient), (ii) maximize the fraction of the North American population responding to the vaccine (i.e., the fraction of vaccine recipients possessing at least one immune responses that can be primed by the vaccine), and (iii) minimize the size of the immunogen to control the cost and complexity of the vaccine [130]. We present in Figure 17.5 a scatter plot of all immunogen candidates within this 3D design space, and the 86 candidates residing on the Pareto (optimal) frontier [131]. These candidates are optimal in the sense that no one design criterion can be improved without incurring a penalty in another; candidates away from the frontier are non-optimal since one or more criteria can be improved without compromising another. This *in silico* design strategy enabled by data-driven fitness models provides a five orders of magnitude reduction in the combinatorial space of all possible immunogen candidates, presenting a means to guide and accelerate experimental vaccine design by focusing resources on the most promising candidates.

17.7 OUTLOOK AND CHALLENGES

The fitness landscape paradigm has a rich history dating back more than 85 years and is a cornerstone of theoretical population genetics [24,28–30]. The recent confluence of high-throughput sequencing technologies and high-performance computing has reinvigorated this concept in new and exciting ways by enabling the determination of empirical viral fitness landscapes from experimental and clinical sequence databases [26,31,32,34,35,64,70]. From a fundamental perspective, these quantitative models of the genotype-phenotype-fitness relationship furnish new understanding of viral dynamics and evolution. From an applied perspective, these mappings offer a powerful roadmap for rational *in silico* immunogen design to guide and accelerate the development of antiviral drugs and vaccines.

We envisage exciting opportunities and challenges for data-driven inference of viral fitness landscapes. Fitting models for large viral proteomes will require the development of computationally efficient algorithms and implementations to take advantage of multicore CPU architectures and GPU accelerators. Theoretical advances can also play an important role in reducing model complexity by establishing multi-resolution and/or coarse-grained fitness models to improve stability and reduce complexity, and to develop Bayesian procedures to incorporate heterogeneous prior knowledge such as tertiary protein structure, protein-protein interactions, mutational epistasis, and *in vitro* fitness assays into the model fitting procedure. We also anticipate the development of integrated models coupling molecular-level fitness landscapes to host-level models of viral quasispecies evolution to population-level epidemiological models as data-driven multiscale/multiphysics simulators of viral dynamics. Advances in experimental and clinical assays will play an important role in furnishing sequence data upon which these models are founded at both higher volume and higher quality, and in providing more rigorous and stringent tests of the model predictions. As next-generation sequencing becomes faster and cheaper, we envisage that it will become routine to determine empirical fitness landscapes for viral proteins and even entire proteomes. Calculating a full-proteome viral fitness landscape would represent an important milestone in virology and population dynamics, representing the first quantitative genotype-phenotype-fitness mapping for a complete organism. The definition of viral fitness landscapes is currently limited to relatively rapidly mutating viruses for which sufficiently high diversity in the viral quasispecies can be quantified to provide a good sampling of the accessible sequence space (e.g., HIV, HCV, dengue fever, influenza). Advances in deep and ultra-deep sequencing technologies capable of resolving more of the low-copy number members of the quasispecies ensemble will open the door to developing fitness models for less highly mutable viruses.

REFERENCES

Guide to the literature. Excellent and accessible introductions to the mathematical underpinnings of viral dynamics and evolution, including quasispecies theory, are provided in the books by Nowak and May [8] and Nowak [10]. The seminal works laying the foundational concepts of fitness landscapes are due to Wright [24], Smith [28], Eigen [29], and Eigen and Schuster [30], and summaries of contemporary theoretical and experimental efforts to develop model fitness landscapes are provided by de Visser and Krug [27] and Szendro et al. [23]. An excellent discussion of the error catastrophe in the context of antiviral therapies and the value of mathematical models of this phenomenon is provided in a commentary by Eigen [44]. The isomorphism from population dynamics to statistical thermodynamics is discussed by Sella and Hirsh [62]. A means to infer intrahost fitness landscapes from deep sequencing data is described by Siefert et al. [35]. Our approach to translate clinical sequence databases into intrinsic viral fitness landscapes and their use in rational vaccine design is described by Mann et al. [64] and Hart and Ferguson [32].

1. Knipe, D.M., and Howley, P.M. (Eds.). (2007). *Fields Virology – Volume 1* (5th ed.). Lippincott Williams and Wilkins.
2. Edwards, R.A., and Rohwer, F. (2005). Viral metagenomics. *Nature Reviews Microbiology 3*, 504-510.
3. Lawrence, C.M., Menon, S., Eilers, B.J., Bothner, B., Khayat, R., Douglas, T., and Young, M.J. (2009). Structural and functional studies of archaeal viruses. *Journal of Biological Chemistry 284*, 12599-12603.
4. Gargaud, M., Amils, R., Quintanilla, J.C., Cleaves II, H.J., Irvine, W.M., Pinti, D.L., and Viso, M. (Eds.). (2011). *Encyclopedia of Astrobiology*. Berlin: Springer-Verlag Berlin Heidelberg.
5. Kaminskyy, V., and Zhivotovsky, B. (2010). To kill or be killed: How viruses interact with the cell death machinery. *Journal of Internal Medicine 267*, 473-482.
6. Oxford English Dictionary Online. Oxford University Press. http://www.oed.com/view/Entry/223861 (Accessed: March 11, 2016).
7. Rybicki, E. (1990). The classification of organisms at the edge of life or problems with virus systematics. *South African Journal of Science 86*, 182-186.

8. Nowak, M.A. and May, R.M. (2000). *Virus Dynamics: Mathematical Principles of Immunology and Virology*. Oxford University Press.

9. Biswas, S.B. and Biswas, A. (1984). *An Introduction to Viruses* (4th ed.). Vani Educational Books.

10. Nowak, M.A. (2006). *Evolutionary Dynamics*. Harvard University Press.

11. Sanjuan, R., Nebot, M.R., Chirico, N., Mansky, L.M., and Belshaw, R. (2010). Viral mutation rates. *Journal of Virology 84*, 9733-9748.

12. Biebricher, C.K. and Eigen, M. (2005). The error threshold. *Virus Research 107*, 117-127.

13. Cubero, M., Esteban, J.I., Otero, T., Sauleda, S., Bes, M., Esteban, R., Guardia, J., and Quer, J. (2008). Naturally occurring NS3-protease-inhibitor resistant mutant A156T in the liver of an untreated chronic hepatitis C patient. *Virology 370*, 237-245.

14. Kim, C.W. and Chang, K.-M. (2013). Hepatitis C virus: Virology and life cycle. *Clinical and Molecular Hepatology 19*, 17-25.

15. Wargo, A.R. and Kurath, G. (2012). Viral fitness: Definitions, measurement, and current insights. *Current Opinion in Virology 2*, 538-545.

16. Domingo, E. and Holland, J. (1997). RNA virus mutations and fitness for survival. *Annual Reviews in Microbiology 51*, 151-178.

17. Domingo, E. (2010). Mechanisms of viral emergence. *Veterinary Research 41*, 38.

18. Orr, H.A. (2009). Fitness and its role in evolutionary genetics. *Nature Reviews Genetics 10*, 531-539.

19. Wu, H., Huang, Y., Dykes, C., Liu, D., Ma, J., Perelson, A.S., and Demeter, L.M. (2006). Modeling and estimation of replication fitness of human immunodeficiency virus type 1 in vitro experiments by using a growth competition assay. *Journal of Virology 80*, 2380-2389.

20. Hughes, D. and Andersson, D.I. (2015). Evolutionary consequences of drug resistance: Shared principles across diverse targets and organisms. *Nature Reviews Genetics 16*, 459-471.

21. Marée, A.F., Keulen, W., Boucher, C.A., and De Boer, R.J. (2000). Estimating relative fitness in viral competition experiments. *Journal of Virology 74*, 11067-11072.

22. Bonhoeffer, S., Barbour, A.D., and De Boer, R.J. (2002). Procedures for reliable estimation of viral fitness from time-series data. *Proceedings of the Royal Society of London B: Biological Sciences 269*, 1887-1893.

23. Szendro, I.G., Schenk, M.F., Franke, J., Krug, J., and De Visser, J.A.G. (2013). Quantitative analyses of empirical fitness landscapes. *Journal of Statistical Mechanics: Theory and Experiment 2013*, P01005.

24. Wright, S. (1932). The roles of mutation, inbreeding, crossbreeding, and selection in evolution. In D.F. Jones (Ed.), *Proceedings of the Sixth International Congress on Genetics – Volume 1 1932* (356-66).

25. Stephens, Z.D., Lee, S.Y., Faghri, F., Campbell, R.H., Zhai, C., Efron, M.J., Iyer, R., Schatz, M.C., Sinha, S., and Robinson, G.E. (2015). Big data: Astronomical or genomical? *PLOS Biology 13*, e1002195.

26. Richter, H., and Engelbrecht, A. (Eds.). (2014). *Recent Advances in the Theory and Application of Fitness Landscapes*. Berlin: Springer Berlin Heidelberg.

27. de Visser, J.A.G., and Krug, J. (2014). Empirical fitness landscapes and the predictability of evolution. *Nature Reviews Genetics 15*, 480-490.

28. Smith, J.M. (1970). Natural selection and the concept of a protein space. *Nature 225*, 563-564.

29. Eigen, M. (1971). Self-organization of matter and the evolution of biological macromolecules. *Naturwissenschaften 58*, 465-523.

30. Eigen, M., and Schuster, P. (1977). A principle of natural self-organization. *Naturwissenschaften 64*, 541-565.

31. Ferguson, A.L., Mann, J.K., Omarjee, S., Ndung'u, T., Walker, B.D., and Chakraborty, A.K. (2013). Translating HIV sequences into quantitative fitness landscapes predicts viral vulnerabilities for rational immunogen design. *Immunity 38*, 606-617.

32. Hart, G.R. and Ferguson, A.L. (2015). Empirical fitness models for hepatitis C virus immunogen design. *Physical Biology 12*, 066006.

33. Tripathi, K., Balagam, R., Vishnoi, N.K., and Dixit, N.M. (2012). Stochastic simulations suggest that HIV-1 survives close to its error threshold. *PLOS Computational Biology 8*, e1002684.

34. Seifert, D., and Beerenwinkel, N. (2015). Estimating Fitness of Viral Quasispecies from Next-Generation Sequencing Data. In E. Domingo, and P. Schuster (Eds.), *Quasispecies: From theory to experimental systems*. Springer International Publishing.

35. Seifert, D., Di Giallonardo, F., Metzner, K.J., Günthard, H.F., and Beerenwinkel, N. (2015). A framework for inferring fitness landscapes of patient-derived viruses using quasispecies theory. *Genetics 199*, 191-203.

36. Leuthäusser, I. (1987). Statistical mechanics of Eigen's evolution model. *Journal of Statistical Physics 48*, 343-360.

37. Saakian, D.B., Munoz, E., Hu, C.-K., and Deem, M. (2006). Quasispecies theory for multiple-peak fitness landscapes. *Physical Review E 73*, 041913.

38. Feynman, R.P., Hibbs, A.R., and Styer, D.F. (2010). *Quantum Mechanics and Path Integrals*. Courier Corporation.

39. Wilke, C.O., Wang, J.L., Ofria, C., Lenski, R.E., and Adami, C. (2001). Evolution of digital organisms at high mutation rates leads to survival of the flattest. *Nature 412*, 331-333.

40. Elena, S., Agudelo-Romero, P., Carrasco, P., Codoner, F., Martin, S., Torres-Barcelo, C., and Sanjuán, R. (2008). Experimental evolution of plant RNA viruses. *Heredity 100*, 478-483.

41. Nowak, M., and Schuster, P. (1989). Error thresholds of replication in finite populations mutation frequencies and the onset of Muller's ratchet. *Journal of Theoretical Biology 137*, 375-395.

42. Drake, J.W., and Holland, J.J. (1999). Mutation rates among RNA viruses. *Proceedings of the National Academy of Sciences of the United States of America 96*, 13910-13913.

43. Alonso, J., and Fort, H. (2010). Error catastrophe for viruses infecting cells: Analysis of the phase transition in terms of error *classes*. *Philosophical Transactions of the Royal Society of London A: Mathematical, Physical and Engineering Sciences 368*, 5569-5582.

44. Eigen, M. (2002). Error catastrophe and antiviral strategy. *Proceedings of the National Academy of Sciences of the United States of America 99*, 13374-13376.

45. Wales, D. (2003). *Energy Landscapes: Applications to Clusters, Biomolecules and Glasses*. Cambridge University Press.

46. Swetina, J., and Schuster, P. (1982). Self-replication with errors: A model for polynucleotide replication. *Biophysical Chemistry 16*, 329-345.

47. Tarazona, P. (1992). Error thresholds for molecular quasispecies as phase transitions: From simple landscapes to spin-glass models. *Physical Review A 45*, 6038-6050.

48. Eigen, M. (2000). Natural selection: A phase transition? *Biophysical Chemistry 85*, 101-123.

49. Hart, G.R., and Ferguson, A.L. (2015). Error catastrophe and phase transition in the empirical fitness landscape of HIV. *Physical Review E 91*, 032705.

50. Dixit, N.M., Srivastava, P., and Vishnoi, N.K. (2012). A finite population model of molecular evolution: Theory and computation. *Journal of Computational Biology 19*, 1176-1202.

51. Holmes, E.C. (2003). Error thresholds and the constraints to RNA virus evolution. *Trends in Microbiology 11*, 543-546.

52. Solé, R.V. (2003). Phase transitions in unstable cancer cell populations. *The European Physical Journal B – Condensed Matter and Complex Systems 35*, 117-123.

53. Dapp, M.J., Clouser, C.L., Patterson, S., and Mansky, L.M. (2009). 5-Azacytidine can induce lethal mutagenesis in human immunodeficiency virus type 1. *Journal of Virology 83*, 11950-11958.

54. Mullins, J.I., Heath, L., Hughes, J.P., Kicha, J., Styrchak, S., Wong, K.G., Rao, U., Hansen, A., Harris, K.S., Laurent, J.-P., Li, D., Simpson, J.H., Essigmann, J.M., Loeb, L.A., and Parkins, J. (2011). Mutation of HIV-1 genomes in a clinical population treated with the mutagenic nucleoside KP1461. *PLoS ONE 6*, e15135.

55. Smith, R.A., Loeb, L.A., and Preston, B.D. (2005). Lethal mutagenesis of HIV. *Virus Research 107*, 215-228.

56. Summers, J., and Litwin, S. (2006). Examining the theory of error catastrophe. *Journal of Virology 80*, 20-26.

57. Anderson, J.P., Daifuku, R., and Loeb, L.A. (2004). Viral error catastrophe by mutagenic nucleosides. *Annual Review of Microbiology 58*, 183-205.

58. Bauer, A.L., Beauchemin, C.A., and Perelson, A.S. (2009). Agent-based modeling of host-pathogen systems: The successes and challenges. *Information Sciences 179*, 1379-1389.

59. Shekhar, K., Ruberman, C.F., Ferguson, A.L., Barton, J.P., Kardar, M., and Chakraborty, A.K. (2013). Spin models inferred from patient-derived viral sequence data faithfully describe HIV fitness landscapes. *Physical Review E 88*, 062705.

60. Balloux, F. (2001). EASYPOP (version 1.7): A computer program for population genetics simulations. *Journal of Heredity 92*, 301-302.

61. Read, E.L., Tovo-Dwyer, A.A., and Chakraborty, A.K. (2012). Stochastic effects are important in intra-host HIV evolution even when viral loads are high. *Proceedings of the National Academy of Sciences of the United States of America 109*, 19727-19732.

62. Sella, G., and Hirsh, A.E. (2005). The application of statistical physics to evolutionary biology. *Proceedings of the National Academy of Sciences of the United States of America 102*, 9541-9546.

63. Deem, M.W. and Hejazi, P. (2010). Theoretical aspects of immunity. *Annual Review of Chemical and Biomolecular Engineering 1*, 247-276.

64. Mann, J.K., Barton, J.P., Ferguson, A.L., Omarjee, S., Walker, B.D., Chakraborty, A., and Ndung'u, T. (2014). The fitness landscape of HIV-1 gag: Advanced modeling approaches and validation of model predictions by in vitro testing. *PLoS Computational Biology 10*, e1003776.

65. Barton, J.P., Kardar, M., and Chakraborty, A.K. (2015). Scaling laws describe memories of host-pathogen riposte in the HIV population. *Proceedings of the National Academy of Sciences of the United States of America 112*, 1965-1970.

66. Castellana, M., and Bialek, W. (2014). Inverse spin glass and related maximum entropy problems. *Physical Review Letters 113*, 117204.

67. Tkacik, G., and Bialek, W. (2014). Information processing in living systems. *Annual Review of Condensed Matter Physics 7*, 89-117.

68. Mora, T., Walczak, A.M., Bialek, W., and Callan, C.G. (2010). Maximum entropy models for antibody diversity. *Proceedings of the National Academy of Sciences of the United States of America 107*, 5405-5410.

69. Rowe, W., Platt, M., Wedge, D.C., Day, P.J., Kell, D.B., and Knowles, J. (2010). Analysis of a complete DNA-protein affinity landscape. *Journal of The Royal Society Interface 7*, 397-408.

70. Manrubia, S. and Lázaro, E. (2015). Getting to know viral evolutionary strategies: Towards the next generation of quasispecies models. In E. Domingo, and P. Schuster (Eds.), *Quasispecies: From theory to experimental systems*. Springer International Publishing.

71. Acevedo, A., Brodsky, L., and Andino, R. (2014). Mutational and fitness landscapes of an RNA virus revealed through population sequencing. *Nature 505*, 686-690.

72. Kouyos, R.D., Leventhal, G.E., Hinkley, T., Haddad, M., Whitcomb, J.M., Petropoulos, C.J., and Bonhoeffer, S. (2012). Exploring the complexity of the HIV-1 fitness landscape. *PLoS Genetics 8*, e1002551.

73. Hinkley, T., Martins, J., Chappey, C., Haddad, M., Stawiski, E., Whitcomb, J.M., Petropoulos, C.J., and Bonhoeffer, S. (2011). A systems analysis of mutational effects in HIV-1 protease and reverse transcriptase. *Nature Genetics 43*, 487-489.

74. Qi, H., Olson, C.A., Wu, N.C., Ke, R., Loverdo, C., Chu, V., Truong, S., Remenyi, R., Chen, Z., Du, Y., Su, S.-Y., Al-Mawsawi, L.Q., Wu, T.-T., Chen, S.-H., Lin, C.-Y., Zhong, W., Lloyd-Smith, J.O., and Sun, R. (2014). A quantitative high-resolution genetic profile rapidly identifies sequence determinants of hepatitis C viral fitness and drug sensitivity. *PLoS Pathogens 10*, e1004064.

75. Otwinowski, J. and Nemenman, I. (2013). Genotype to phenotype mapping and the fitness landscape of the E. coli lac promoter. *PLoS ONE 8*, e61570.

76. Hayashi, Y., Aita, T., Toyota, H., Husimi, Y., Urabe, I., and Yomo, T. (2006). Experimental rugged fitness landscape in protein sequence space. *PLoS ONE 1*, e96.

77. Segal, M.R., Barbour, J.D., and Grant, R.M. (2004). Relating HIV-1 sequence variation to replication capacity via trees and forests. *Statistical Applications in Genetics and Molecular Biology 3*, 1-18.

78. Ma, J., Dykes, C., Wu, T., Huang, Y., Demeter, L., and Wu, H. (2010). vFitness: A web-based computing tool for improving estimation of in vitro HIV-1 fitness experiments. *BMC Bioinformatics 11*, 1.

79. Dahirel, V., Shekhar, K., Pereyra, F., Miura, T., Artyomov, M., Talsania, S., Allen, T.M., Altfeld, M., Carrington, M., Irvine, D.J., Walker, B.D., and Chakraborty, A.K. (2011). Coordinate linkage of HIV evolution reveals regions of immunological vulnerability. *Proceedings of the National Academy of Sciences of the United States of America 108*, 11530-11535.

80. Quadeer, A.A., Louie, R.H., Shekhar, K., Chakraborty, A.K., Hsing, I.-M., and McKay, M.R. (2014). Statistical linkage analysis of substitutions in patient-derived sequences of genotype 1a hepatitis C virus nonstructural protein 3 exposes targets for immunogen design. *Journal of Virology 88*, 7628-7644.

81. Neumann-Haefelin, C., Oniangue-Ndza, C., Kuntzen, T., Schmidt, J., Nitschke, K., Sidney, J., Caillet-Saguy, C., Binder, M., Kersting, N., Kemper, M.W., Power, K.A., Ingber, S., Reyor, L.L., Hills-Evans, K., Kim, A.Y., Lauer, G.M., Lohmann, V., Sette, A., Henn, M.R., Bressanelli, S., Thimme, R., and Allen, T.M. (2011). Human leukocyte antigen B27 selects for rare escape mutations that significantly impair hepatitis C virus replication and require compensatory mutations. *Hepatology 54*, 1157-1166.

82. Kauffman, S.A. and Weinberger, E.D. (1989). The NK model of rugged fitness landscapes and its application to maturation of the immune response. *Journal of Theoretical Biology 141*, 211-245.

83. Kauffman, S.A. (1993). *The Origins of Order: Self-organization and Selection in Evolution*. Oxford University Press.

84. Weinberger, E. (1996). NP Completeness of Kauffman's N-k Model, A Tuneably Rugged Fitness Landscape. SFI Working Paper: 1996-02-003.

85. Kingman, J. (1978). A simple model for the balance between selection and mutation. *Journal of Applied Probability 15*, 1-12.

86. Derrida, B. (1981). Random-energy model: An exactly solvable model of disordered systems. *Physical Review B 24*, 2613.

87. Perelson, A.S. and Macken, C.A. (1995). Protein evolution on partially correlated landscapes. *Proceedings of the National Academy of Sciences of the United States of America 92*, 9657-9661.

88. Franke, J., Klözer, A., de Visser, J.A.G., and Krug, J. (2011). Evolutionary accessibility of mutational pathways. *PLoS Computational Biology 7*, e1002134.

89. Kimura, M. (1983). *The Neutral Theory of Molecular Evolution*. Cambridge University Press.

90. Deforche, K., Camacho, R., Van Laethem, K., Lemey, P., Rambaut, A., Moreau, Y., and Vandamme, A.-M. (2008). Estimation of an in vivo fitness landscape experienced by HIV-1 under drug selective pressure useful for prediction of drug resistance evolution during treatment. *Bioinformatics 24*, 34-41.

91. Beerenwinkel, N., Däumer, M., Sing, T., Rahnenführer, J., Lengauer, T., Selbig, J., Hoffmann, D., and Kaiser, R. (2005). Estimating HIV evolutionary pathways and the genetic barrier to drug resistance. *Journal of Infectious Diseases 191*, 1953-1960.

92. Beerenwinkel, N., Gunthard, H., Roth, V., and Metzner, K.J. (2012). Challenges and opportunities in estimating viral genetic diversity from next-generation sequencing data. *Frontiers in Microbiology 3*, 329.

93. Matthews, P.C., Leslie, A.J., Katzourakis, A., Crawford, H., Payne, R., Prendergast, A., Power, K., Kelleher, A.D., Klenerman, P., Carlson, J., Heckerman, D., Ndung'u, T., Walker, B.D., Allen, T.M., Pybus, O.G., and Goulder, P.J.R. (2009). HLA footprints on human immunodeficiency virus type 1 are associated with interclade polymorphisms and intraclade phylogenetic clustering. *Journal of Virology 83*, 4605-4615.

94. Falugi, P., and Giarré, L. (2009). Identification and validation of quasispecies models for biological systems. *Systems and Control Letters 58*, 529-539.

95. Mora, T., and Bialek, W. (2011). Are biological systems poised at criticality? *Journal of Statistical Physics 144*, 268-302.

96. Tkacik, G., Schneidman, E., Berry II, M.J., and Bialek, W. (2006). Ising models for networks of real neurons. *arXiv*, q-bio/0611072.

97. Tkacik, G., Schneidman, E., Berry II, M.J., and Bialek, W. (2009). Spin glass models for a network of real neurons. *arXiv*, 0912.5409.

98. Bialek, W., Cavagna, A., Giardina, I., Mora, T., Silvestri, E., Viale, M., and Walczak, A.M. (2012). Statistical mechanics for natural flocks of birds. *Proceedings of the National Academy of Sciences of the United States of America 109*, 4786-4791.

99. Weigt, M., White, R.A., Szurmant, H., Hoch, J.A., and Hwa, T. (2009). Identification of direct residue contacts in protein-protein interaction by message passing. *Proceedings of the National Academy of Sciences of the United States of America 106*, 67.

100. Morcos, F., Pagnani, A., Lunt, B., Bertolino, A., Marks, D.S., Sander, C., Zecchina, R., Onuchic, J.N., Hwa, T., and Weigt, M. (2011). Direct-coupling analysis of residue coevolution captures native contacts across many protein families. *Proceedings of the National Academy of Sciences of the United States of America 108*, E1293-E1301.

101. Sułkowska, J.I., Morcos, F., Weigt, M., Hwa, T., and Onuchic, J.N. (2012). Genomics-aided structure prediction. *Proceedings of the National Academy of Sciences of the United States of America 109*, 10340-10345.

102. Cocco, S., Monasson, R., and Weigt, M. (2013). From principal component to direct coupling analysis of coevolution in proteins: Low-eigenvalue modes are needed for structure prediction. *PLOS Computational Biology 9*, e1003176.

103. Lunt, B., Szurmant, H., Procaccini, A., Hoch, J.A., Hwa, T., and Weigt, M. (2010). Chapter Two – Inference of direct residue contacts in two-Component signaling. *Methods in Enzymology 471*, 17-41.

104. Jaynes, E.T. (1957). Information theory and statistical mechanics. *Physical Review 106*, 620-630.

105. Jaynes, E.T. (1957). Information theory and statistical mechanics. II. *Physical Review 108*, 171-190.

106. Binder, K. and Young, A.P. (1986). Spin glasses: Experimental facts, theoretical concepts, and open questions. *Review of Modern Physics 58*, 801-976.

107. Kappen, H.J. and Rodríguez, F.B. (1998). Efficient learning in Boltzmann machines using linear response theory. *Neural Computation 10*, 1137-1156.

108. Thouless, D.J., Anderson, P.W., and Palmer, R.G. (1977). Solution of "Solvable model of a spin glass". *Philosophical Magazine 35*, 593-601.

109. Roudi, Y., Aurell, E., and Hertz, J.A. (2009). Statistical physics of pairwise probability models. *Frontiers in Computational Neuroscience 3*, 22.

110. Roudi, Y., Tyrcha, J., and Hertz, J. (2009). Ising model for neural data: Model quality and approximate methods for extracting functional connectivity. *Physical Review E 79*, 051915.

111. Lezon, T.R., Banavar, J.R., Cieplak, M., Maritan, A., and Fedoroff, N.V. (2006). Using the principle of entropy maximization to infer genetic interaction networks from gene expression patterns. *Proceedings of the National Academy of Sciences of the United States of America 103*, 19033-19038.

112. Cocco, S., and Monasson, R. (2011). Adaptive cluster expansion for inferring Boltzmann machines with noisy data. *Physical Review Letters 106*, 090601.

113. Aurell, E., and Ekeberg, M. (2012). Inverse Ising inference using all the data. *Physical Review Letters 108*, 090201.

114. Dickstein, J.S., Battaglino, P.B., and DeWeese, M.R. (2011). New method for parameter estimation in probabilistic models: Minimum probability flow. *Physical Review Letters 107*, 220601.

115. Habeck, M. (2014). Bayesian approach to inverse statistical mechanics. *Physical Review E 89*, 052113.

116. Machta, B.B., Chachra, R., Transtrum, M.K., and Sethna, J.P. (2013). Parameter space compression underlies emergent theories and predictive models. *Science 342*, 604-607.

117. Halliday, J., Klenerman, P., and Barnes, E. (2011). Vaccination for hepatitis C virus: Closing in on an evasive target. *Expert Review of Vaccines 10*, 659-672.

118. Hajarizadeh, B., Grebely, J., and Dore, G.J. (2013). Epidemiology and natural history of HCV infection. *Nature Reviews Gastroenterology and Hepatology 10*, 553-562.

119. World Health Organization Hepatitis C Fact Sheet (Updated July 2016). World Health Organization. http://www.who.int/mediacentre/factsheets/fs164/en/ (Accessed: January 21, 2017).

120. Alter, M.J. (2007). Epidemiology of hepatitis C virus infection. *World Journal of Gastroenterology 13*, 2436-2441.

121. Liang, T.J. (2013). Current progress in development of hepatitis C virus vaccines. *Nature Medicine 19*, 869-878.

122. Kowdley, K.V., Gordon, S.C., Reddy, K.R., Rossaro, L., Bernstein, D.E., Lawitz, E., Shiffman, M.L., Schiff, E., Ghalib, R., Ryan, M., Rustgi, V., Chojkier, M., Herring, R., Di Bisceglie, A.M., Pockros, P.J., Subramanian, G.M., An, D., Svarovskaia, E., Hyland, R.H., Pang, P.S., Symonds, W.T., McHutchison, J.G., Muir, A.J., Pound, D., and Fried, M.W. (2014). Ledipasvir and Sofosbuvir for 8 or 12 weeks for chronic HCV without cirrhosis. *New England Journal of Medicine 370*, 1879-1888.

123. Swadling, L., Klenerman, P., and Barnes, E. (2013). Ever closer to a prophylactic vaccine for HCV. *Expert Opinion on Biological Therapy 13*, 1109-1124.

124. Lauer, G.M. (2013). Immune responses to hepatitis C virus (HCV) infection and the prospects for an effective HCV vaccine or immunotherapies. *Journal of Infectious Diseases 207*, S7-S12.

125. Page, K., Hahn, J.A., Evans, J., Shiboski, S., Lum, P., Delwart, E., Tobler, L., Andrews, W., Avanesyan, L., Cooper, S., and Busch, M.P. (2009). Acute hepatitis C virus infection in young adult injection drug users: A prospective study of incident infection, resolution, and reinfection. *Journal of Infectious Diseases 200*, 1216-1226.

126. Cox, A.L., Netski, D.M., Mosbruger, T., Sherman, S.G., Strathdee, S., Ompad, D., Vlahov, D., Chien, D., Shyamala, V., Ray, S.C., and Thomas, D.L. (2005). Prospective evaluation of community-acquired acute-phase hepatitis C virus infection. *Clinical Infectious Diseases 40*, 951-958.

127. Murphy, K. and Weaver, C. (2016). *Janeway's Immunobiology* (9th ed.). Garland Science.

128. Akram, A. and Inman, R.D. (2012). Immunodominance: A pivotal principle in host response to viral infections. *Clinical Immunology 143*, 99-115.

129. Streeck, H., Jolin, J.S., Qi, Y., Yassine-Diab, B., Johnson, R.C., Kwon, D.S., Addo, M.M., Brumme, C., Routy, J.-P., Little, S., Jessen, H., Kelleher, A.D., Hecht, F.M., Sekaly, R.-P., Rosenberg, E.S., Walker, D.B., Carrington, M., and Altfeld, M. (2009). Human immunodeficiency virus type 1-specific CD8+ T-cell responses during primary infection are major determinants of the viral set point and loss of CD4+ T cells. *Journal of Virology 83*, 7641-7648.

130. Fischer, W., Liao, H.X., Haynes, B.F., Letvin, N.L., and Korber, B. (2008). Coping with viral diversity in HIV vaccine design: A response to Nickle et al. *PLOS Computational Biology 4*, e15; author reply e25.

131. Arora, J. (2004). *Introduction to Optimum Design*. Academic Press.

18

A wish-list for modeling immunological synapses

MICHAEL L. DUSTIN

18.1 IMMUNOLOGICAL SYNAPSE ORIGINS

18.1.1 LINEAR MODELS FOR CELL ADHESION

When the term immune synapse first appeared in print (Norcross, 1984), I was an undergraduate biologist tasked to measure glucose transport in human red blood cells (RBC). This was no simple task due to the high number of what would become known at Glut1 transporters in the RBC membrane (Lodish, 2013). I was rescued in this effort by a powerful inhibitor that allowed me to establish a time course and a set of published rate equations that allowed me to define Km and Vmax for the transporter under different conditions (Dustin et al., 1984). The lab I was working in was also studying proteins involved in contact inhibition of growth and struggling with isolation of these proteins (Vale et al., 1984). The problem of cell-cell communication through surface receptors captured my interest, and I sought out labs working in this area as a graduate student. I was fortunate to be introduced to Tim Springer just as his lab had identified three lymphocyte function associated (LFA) molecules using function blocking monoclonal antibodies (Springer et al., 1987). The molecules were among the first well-defined cell adhesion molecules as they mediated conjugate formation between cytotoxic T cell and target cells, and their broader roles in the immune response were rapidly becoming apparent. Relationships between the three molecules were established through application of a linear model (Shaw et al., 1986). The model assumed that each antigen was part of a receptor-ligand pair that was completely blocked by its antibody. It was found that effects of anti-LFA-2 (CD2) and anti-LFA-3 (CD58) were non-additive, whereas anti-LFA-1 was additive in its effects with either anti-CD2 or anti-CD58. The hypothesis generated by this model and data was that CD2 and CD58 are a receptor ligand pair and that LFA-1 was part of a distinct pathway. I had the opportunity to be involved in testing this hypothesis with purified CD2 and CD58 and extended it to analysis of LFA-1 ligands in Springer's lab. Intercellular adhesion molecule-1 (ICAM-1) was defined by a monoclonal antibody that inhibited the LFA-1 dependent aggregation of B cell lines (Rothlein et al., 1986). Using culture endothelial cells I showed that the cytokine induced and LFA-1 dependent adhesion of B cells to endothelial cells was dependent on ICAM-1, but also identified at least one LFA-1 dependent, constitutively expressed ligand activity, and a distinct LFA-1 ligand independent activity using quantitative cell adhesion assays (Dustin and Springer, 1988). Based on these predictions we then sought and cloned intercellular adhesion molecule-2 based on binding of cells transfected with an endothelial cell cDNA library to purified LFA-1. ICAM-2 exactly fit the prediction of a constitutively expressed and non-cytokine regulated ligand for LFA-1 on human endothelial cells (Staunton et al., 1989). The LFA-1 independent component turned out to be Very Late Activation Antigen- 4 (VLA-4) interaction with Vascular Cell Adhesion Molecule-1 (Elices et al., 1990), which gave patients suffering with relapsing multiple sclerosis a powerful therapeutic some time later (Polman et al., 2006). The ability to succeed with these linear models was based on an experimental optimization of a very complex non-linear process. While we succeeded in identifying molecular mechanisms based on predictions from linear models, the biophysical process leading to adhesion in these cases was still largely a mystery. We knew that receptors like VLA-5 accumulated at "focal adhesion" in stromal cells and LFA-1 was shown to accumulate at the immunological synapse between helper T cells and B cells (Kupfer and Singer, 1989). We could also use purified LFA-1 and ICAM-1 to carefully analyze the regulation of adhesion systems and define different modes of regulation (Dustin and Springer, 1989). Despite improved quantification, there was no way to directly quantify these interactions the way they normally functioned, as was commonplace for hormones or cytokines. Methods were needed to gain information about interstitial migration and immune recognition by molecules like CD2 and CD58. But the basic parts list was in place for defining an immunological synapse.

18.1.2 SUPPORTED LIPIDS BILAYERS AS A MODEL FOR QUANTIFYING BOND FORMATION

The effort to measure the interactions that mediated migration and immune recognition was also underway, but calibrating these measurements was a challenge. The 1970s saw the description of antibody mediated patching and capping as early events in cellular responses to antibodies (Braun et al., 1978; Braun et al., 1979), but these studies were not translated to interfaces until the early 1980s. Studies of IgE Fc receptor (FcR) were leading the field in many respects with experiments demonstrated a correlation between accumulation of laterally mobile dinitrophenol (DNP) specific IgE- FcR complexes on the surface of a mast cell line and adhesion strength to beads coated with immobile DNP (McCloskey and Poo, 1986). These experiments took advantage of the lateral mobility of the cell surface receptors, but active mechanisms in the cell that could also control movement of the FcR could not be ruled out, complicating the interpretation of receptor distribution changes. While the relationship of fluorescence intensity to adhesion strength was clear, the relatively high affinity interactions led to the contact areas working as perfect traps, further confounding the equilibrium treatments of the data. McConnell's lab examined the interaction of live cells with supported lipid bilayers (SLB) with laterally mobile anti-DNP IgE attached to haptenated phospholipids and found that despite the planar nature of the surface, the FcR that bound to the mobile IgE in an interface underwent discrete clustering similar to what was observed with antibody crosslinking (Balakrishnan et al., 1982). These first observations of microclusters opened a possibility to measure affinities with careful measurement as the laterally mobile IgE was only constrained by Brownian motion in the SLB and its clustering would then only be controlled by the affinity for the FcR and the physical confines of the cell-SLB interface. Transmembrane adhesion molecules were immobile in SLB, probably because the cytoplasmic domains interacted with the underlying glass (McConnell et al., 1986). We utilized SLB to reconstitute purified CD58, which was naturally glycolipid anchored through a co-translational modification, and was laterally mobile in the SLB system similar to the lipid haptens used by McConnell's group (Dustin et al., 1987a; Dustin et al., 1987b; Chan et al., 1991). I was able to label CD58 with a fluorescent dye while protecting the CD2 binding site with the blocking monoclonal antibody and reconstituted the labeled protein in SLB. The fluorescent signals in the SLB could then be calibrated to molecules/μm^2 and images were acquired of cells adhering to the bilayers at three densities of CD58. These images were used to measure the total (inside contact) and free (outside contact) specific fluorescence intensities to calculate the bound CD58 in the contact area (total minus free) for many cells at each CD58 density. The system reached a steady state based on the time-course of contact area development and fluorescence accumulation, making an equilibrium assumption possible. Unlike LFA-1-ICAM-1 interaction, which had a linear temperature dependence (Marlin and Springer, 1987), the CD2-CD58 interaction worked best at low temperature, consistent with a reliance on self-assembly processes that needed to suppress thermal fluctuations of the membrane (Dustin et al., 1987a). The contact areas were roughly circular, suggesting that each contact area existed as a separate, energy minimized physical phase defined by the alignment of the two bilayers. Rearrangement of this data as a Scatchard Plot, which is simply a linearization of the mass action equations for N receptors, reversibly binding to ligands over a range of ligand concentrations with measurements of the receptor-ligand complexes at equilibrium (Scatchard, 1949), led to the estimation of a 2D Kd (Dustin et al., 1996). The use of the Scatchard plot assumes that the CD2 molecules on the cells are all accessible to CD58 and that the system is at equilibrium. An alternative analysis that assumed mass action driven, diffusion-mediated concentration of the mobile fraction (f) of CD2 through interactions with CD58 in the contact area, diffusion of free CD2 over the entire cell surface, and empirically corrected for partial exclusion of free CD58 from the contact area yielded lower Kd values (higher 2D affinity) but similar conclusions as many of the refinements had offsetting effects on the final value of the 2D Kd (Zhu et al., 2006; Dustin et al., 2007; Zhu et al., 2007). The conclusion was that the CD2-CD58 interaction led to self-assembly of ordered interfaces that were strikingly similar to theoretical predictions by Bell and colleagues for the simplest type of adhesion system (Bell, 1978; Bell et al., 1984). For me, it was a beginning to think about highly polyvalent adhesive interfaces in quantitative terms. There were also some fascinating issues regarding how contacts formed on the fluid bilayers, what determined the contact area in the absence of traction, and how forces exerted on the individual interactions were distributed. The individual interactions appeared to be highly dynamic and to undergo rapid exchange of CD2 bound CD58 ligands between the contact area and surrounding bilayer (Dustin, 1997), and modeling these interactions suggested hundreds of rebinding events with multiple CD2 before a CD58 dark CD58 would diffuse out of the typical adhesion zone (Tolentino et al., 2008). We also worked with Byron Goldstein to model the ability of the CD58-Fc chimera to bridge CD2 on effector T cells to CD16 on NK cells to mediate deletion of effector T cell (Dustin et al., 2007). The deletion of effector T cells by a drug based on the CD58-Fc chimera (alefacept) was the basis for the first biologic drug approved to treat psoriasis. A limitation of the mathematical modeling was that we could not accurately predict the number of CD58-Fc bridges that were formed from the total number of laterally mobile CD2 on the effector T cells. The model overestimated the number of bridges formed by >5 fold. Given that this Fc receptor mediated killing remains an important mechanism for many antibody based biologic drugs (Zhang et al., 2003), it would be useful to understand what assumptions lead to this error and to determine if this suggests new regulatory mechanisms that control the number of FcR that are engaged in such settings.

This line of research also led to reconstitution of the helper T cell immunological synapse within a few years (Grakoui et al., 1999), but an important common thread in this work is developing models in which quantification is feasible and biological function (e.g., T cell activation in the case of the immunological synapse) can be achieved.

18.1.3 WHAT IS THE IMMUNOLOGICAL SYNAPSE

The first connection of "immune" and "synapse" in the literature is the above referenced monogram in 1984 in which some commonalities between immune recognition and synaptic communication of neurons are highlighted (Norcross, 1984). The concept proposed was that the TCR might act as a Ca^{2+} channel to activate directed secretion across the adhesion-bridged gap—not unlike a neural synapse. This model was initially conceived for cytotoxic T cells, for which the concept of Ca^{2+} dependent secretion of pore-forming proteins with a requirement for adhesion molecules like LFA-1 was just emerging in 1984. In the absence of specific further data for an organized interface, the concept then lay fallow. Subsequent work on the antigen receptor and adhesion molecules revealed some puzzling structural details regarding the size of the molecules as they were cloned, evolutionary relationships revealed, and structures elucidated. LFA-1 was found to be a member of the integrin family (Hynes, 1987) and ICAM-1 was composed of five tandem immunoglobulin-like domains (Staunton et al., 1990). These were each ~20 nm long—thus potentially spanning up to 40 nm between cells. The cloning of the TCR and structure of the MHC-peptide complex that provided a basis for immunological specificity of T cells were about 7 nm each—spanning a gap of ~13 nm (Davis et al., 1984; Bjorkman et al., 1987). CD2 and CD58 were each composed of two tandem Ig-like domains and appeared to bridge a gap similar in size to the interaction of TCR and MHC-peptide (Seed and Aruffo, 1987). The CD45 tyrosine phosphatase appeared much larger than the TCR-pMHC interaction (Cyster et al., 1991) but was inextricably linked to signaling in both positive and negative ways (Koretzky et al., 1990). Springer sketched out a possible two-tiered contact interface in which TCR-MHC-peptide and CD2-CD58 interactions would share one region and the LFA-1-ICAM-1 interaction and CD45 would occupy an adjacent region separated by a region of membrane bending (Springer, 1990). I was in Springer's lab when this model was formulated, and I recall being very skeptical about it at the time, in part because integrin mediated contacts had been shown by electron microscopy to create very close contacts—even occlusive seals that allow extracellular acidification and the protection of by-stander cells from leakage of cytotoxic agents (Wright and Silverstein, 1984; Schmidt et al., 1988). This issue of integrin mediated close contacts has resurfaced recently and has still not been fully solved (Freeman et al., 2016). However, there are many aspects of this model that have held up admirably. In support, Davis and van der Merwe have provided extensive theoretical and experimental support for the importance of CD45 exclusion from close contacts (Davis and van der Merwe, 1996; Wild et al., 1999; Choudhuri et al., 2005; Chang et al., 2016). Furthermore, I contributed key data in support of this vision. We showed that CD2-CD58 interactions segregate from LFA-1-ICAM-1 interactions in the well controlled SLB system (Dustin et al., 1998). Analysis of this segregation process has later been utilized to derive estimates of relative affinities for the two adhesion systems (Burroughs et al., 2011). We went on to reconstitute the segregation of LFA-1-ICAM-1 interactions from the TCR-MHC-peptide interactions (Grakoui et al., 1999). Our movies of T cell interactions with SLB containing ICAM-1 and agonist MHC-peptide complexes strikingly reconstituted the supramolecular activation clusters (SMACs) visualized for the first time by Kupfer and colleagues in antigen specific T cell-B cell interfaces (Monks et al., 1998). The micron scale bull's eye pattern created a structural definition for the immunological synapse (Bromley et al., 2001b). In both of these studies, the TCR-MHC-peptide interactions in the central (c)SMAC were segregated from the LFA-1-ICAM-1 interactions in the surrounding peripheral (p)SMAC (Figure 18.1). Griffiths and colleagues redefined the cSMAC as including a secretory domain targeted by the granules released by cytotoxic T cells (Stinchcombe et al., 2001). Many other cell types including natural killer cells (Davis et al., 1999), B cells (Batista et al., 2001), mast cells (Carroll-Portillo et al., 2010), and phagocytes (Goodridge et al., 2011) shared this basic organization. Many of these systems shared the bull's eye architecture, but seemed to adapt this to specific functions. However, the bull's eye of antigen receptor and adhesion molecules was too narrow a definition to accommodate all of the relevant biology.

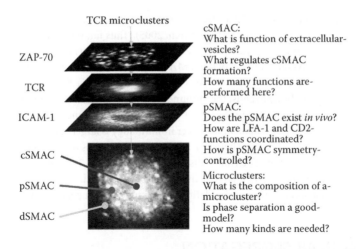

cSMAC:
What is function of extracellular-vesicles?
What regulates cSMAC formation?
How many functions are-performed here?

pSMAC:
Does the pSMAC exist *in vivo*?
How are LFA-1 and CD2-functions coordinated?
How is pSMAC symmetry-controlled?

Microclusters:
What is the composition of a-microcluster?
Is phase separation a good-model?
How many kinds are needed?

Figure 18.1 Wishlist for immunological synapse. Imaging the immunological synapse on SLB involves combining three to four fluorescence channels to identify the three SMACs. The composite image at the bottom combines ICAM-1 on the SLB, anti-TCR Fab on the T cell surface and ZAP-70 imaged in TIRF mode on the cytoplasmic surface of T cell plasma membrane recruited to TCR microclusters. The brightest TCR signal defines the cSMAC, the brightest ICAM-1 signal marks the pSMAC, and the outermost TCR-ZAP-70 microclusters mark the dSMAC. Quantitative models will help address the outstanding questions.

18.1.4 Definition of immunological synapse

While the bull's eye structure was a common motif, particularly with SLB reconstitution models, it was clear that there was a great heterogeneity of structures and T cell behaviors associated with antigen recognition and other types of immune recognition (Brossard et al., 2005; Tseng et al., 2008). There is not a wide consensus on how to define an immunological synapse. We have tried to be consistent in the following criteria (Dustin and Colman, 2002):

1. *The neuron doctrine—cells remain individuals.*
2. *Adhesion.*
3. *Stability.*
4. *Directed secretion.*

Stability is a difficult criterion as its definition is relative and needs a time frame. For example, T cells that form stable interactions with motile B cells *in vivo* such that they move relative to the tissue but can remain connected to each other for hours (Okada et al., 2005), are forming a synapse. Thus, we would say the spatial frame of reference should be the APC when considering stability. T cells move rapidly in the steady state, as I will discuss later: thus, suspending motility for minutes to hours is a significant change that constitutes stability. Functionally, a few minutes may be sufficient for a cytotoxic T cells to deliver a "lethal hit" (Isaaz et al., 1995), whereas hours is the time frame for signal integration needed to prime a naïve T cell and program it for multiple rounds of division (Mayya and Dustin, 2016). If closely aligned interfaces with immunological specificity occur between clearly moving cells, we refer to this as a kinapse, for moving junction (Dustin, 2007; Sims et al., 2007; Azar et al., 2010; Moreau et al., 2015). Recently, we have demonstrated that the kinapse mode of interactions does not preclude a durable interaction with a spatially restricted source of pMHC (Mayya et al., 2018).

18.1.5 The context of the T cell immunological synapse

The immunological synapse concept has been useful in the study of a number of disease states and therapeutic modalities. Two of these are autoimmunity and cancer immunotherapy. Antigen specific therapy of autoimmune disease is an important goal that offers the hope of a cure, rather than current chronic, generally immunosuppressive therapies (Feldmann and Steinman, 2005). Thus far, the pathogenic T cells in autoimmunity disease settings including type 1 diabetes and multiple sclerosis form defective immunological synapses (Schubert et al., 2012). As one function of the cSMAC is to turn off TCR signals (Lee et al., 2003a; Campi et al., 2005; Vardhana et al., 2010), the failure to form a cSMAC may make a T cell more difficult to regulate. The flip side of this coin is the ability to enlist the immune response to fight cancer and chronic infection, situations where tolerance mechanisms that protect most of us from autoimmune disease may increase our susceptibility to some infections. The excitement in cancer immunology is largely driven by biologics that target and modulate the immunological synapse between T cells and cancer cells or lead to formation of synthetic synapses based on T cell engineering (Egen and Allison, 2002; Porter et al., 2011; McCormack et al., 2013; Wu et al., 2015). There is thus enormous potential in being able to predict immunological synapses and to be able to incorporate these predictions into larger simulations of immune system performance.

18.2 MOLECULAR SEGREGATION

18.2.1 BACK OF THE ENVELOPE TO STICKY DETAILS

The speculation by Springer (Springer, 1990) regarding transmembrane tyrosine phosphatase CD45 exclusion from sites of TCR engagement and refinement of this model by Davis and van der Merwe with respect to CD2 (Davis and van der Merwe, 1996) and Shaw and myself with respect to co-stimulation more generally (Shaw and Dustin, 1997) assumed that large proteins would naturally be excluded from close contacts. Engineering of adhesion molecules, MHC molecules, and CD45 itself supported this notion (Wild et al., 1999; Choudhuri et al., 2005; Varma et al., 2006; James and Vale, 2012). Work from Grinstein's lab has reinforced the earlier mentioned observations that integrin can create contacts that exclude CD45 in a manner requiring the actin cytoskeleton (Freeman et al., 2016). In addition, the forces controlling CD45 lateral distribution are complex and may include not only exclusion, but also attractive interactions with Lck kinase, a substrate of CD45, enriched membrane domains that might work against the size based exclusion (Irles et al., 2003). Two studies reported transient exclusion of CD45 from close contact regions followed by enrichment without an obvious change in intermembrane separation, which raises questions about whether observed exclusion was really only based on size or also depended on other factors (Freiberg et al., 2002; Choudhuri et al., 2005). Thus, a method for isolating effects of intermembrane spacing on exclusion of surface protein of various sizes was needed.

Giant unilamellar vesicles offer an approach to isolate the relation of intermembrane spacing to exclusion of proteins of different relative sizes without an active cellular component and on a relevant length scale of micrometers (Reister-Gottfried et al., 2008; Schmid et al., 2016). Schmid et al. utilized synthetic adhesion systems based on green fluorescent protein (GFP) and mCherry oligomers to look at exclusion of proteins from area of close intermembrane apposition (Schmid et al., 2016). Using experimental and simulation approaches they were able to define a parameter, the intermembrane-protein gap, which was positive when the protein was smaller than the gap and negative when the protein is larger than the gap. The gap estimate in this case came from simple models with full extension of proteins. Proteins with positive gaps of greater then 10 nm were not visibly excluded, whereas proteins with negative gaps of 5 nm or greater were optimally excluded (Schmid et al., 2016). Interestingly, the proteins with 0 nm intermembrane protein gap sat at the inflection point—showing half-maximal exclusion (Schmid et al., 2016). A paired-lattice based simulation could capture the key features, including partial exclusion at a 0 nm gap. Thus, molecules that just appear to "fit" can still be partly excluded by steric conflicts and entropic penalties related to interactions with the closely apposed, thermally fluctuating membrane. More recently, studies with GUV-SLB interfaces using extracellular domains of the TCR and pMHC have directly demonstrated partial CD45 exclusion (Carbone et al., 2017). These studies provide a physical basis for CD45 exclusion by size and a notion of binding energy that would be needed to counteract this effect in the context of regulated T cell activation, as mentioned above.

18.2.2 TWO-DIMENSIONAL AFFINITY AND KINETIC RATES—OUT OF EQUILIBRIUM

The thermodynamic underpinning for cells adhesion was well outlined by Bell in 1978, as mentioned above (Bell, 1978). He envisioned the formation of adhesive junctions by low affinity receptor ligand pairs (3D Kd ~1–10 μM) that would interact in hundreds or thousands/μm² with a "confinement length" ~1 nm deep. Bell and colleagues defined the confinement length, σ = 2D Kd ÷ 3D Kd. σ is a phenomenological parameter that will be discussed further below. We performed measurements on the interaction of live T cells expressing CD2 with supported planar bilayers containing different densities of laterally mobile, fluorescent CD58 and obtained equilibrium binding data that perfectly fulfilled Bell's expectations for a simple adhesion system (Dustin et al., 1996; Dustin et al., 1997b; Dustin et al., 2007). Molecular dynamic simulations that incorporate adhesion molecules and phospholipids of apposed membranes suggest that σ can be broken down into terms of translational and rotational entropy and membrane roughness, which is measured in nm (Hu et al., 2013).

Immune cell antigen recognition and costimulation is dominated by interactions that span an intermembrane gap of ~12–13 nm (the length of three Ig-like domains). Why is this? Some clues have come from experiments that increase the length of CD2 ligands. Initial efforts in this direction were focused on understanding the role of CD45 exclusion and did not address any change in adhesion efficiency, because ligands were overexpressed and no titration was performed to evaluate if adhesion efficiency was increased or decreased by making one of the molecules longer (Wild et al., 1999). Also, there was an earlier notion from studies of erythrocyte adhesion to T cells that the small size of the CD2-CD58 adhesion molecules made them sensitive to inhibition by charge based repulsion between cells, and the general thought was that extending adhesion molecules might make them better. Early studies, however, suggested that there was actually an offsetting disadvantage to making CD2 ligands longer at physiological temperature (Selvaraj et al., 1987; Chan and Springer, 1992). Using purified versions of extended CD2 ligands in SLB, we later learned that adding two or three Ig-like domains resulted in a 10-fold deterioration in the 2D affinity (Milstein et al., 2008). Adding each Ig domain added ~4 nm in size to the protein, but only increased the intermembrane spacing by 1 nm per Ig-domain, as found previously for pMHC based synthetic adhesion systems (Choudhuri et al., 2005). This suggests that adding Ig-domains beyond the three-domain span of the wild type pair (the N-terminal domains of CD2 and CD58 overlap when interacting) increases tilting of the receptor-ligand pair to allow a shorter intermembrane distance. The increase in length of CD2 ligands apparently increased σ by ~10-fold. As discussed above, this parameter incorporates translational and rotational entropy differences and thermal membrane roughness. If this is the case, then how do larger adhesion molecules like E-cadherin, which is five domains long and interacts primarily through the N-terminal domains spanning ~40 nm if fully extended, work in cell-cell junctions? It seems that E-cadherin overcomes this in two ways. First, the binding of Ca^{2+} between the domains rigidifies the molecule and this may contribute to reducing σ (Pokutta et al., 1994) Second, simulations indicate that the large entropy loss associated with trans binding of the E-cadherin is offset by cis interactions, which minimize σ by nucleating a 2D lattice (Wu et al., 2011). While cadherin junctions sometimes appear highly ordered in electron micrographs (Harrison et al., 2011; Le Bihan et al., 2015), experimental verification of this lattice structure is still pending. It is not clear how other large adhesion receptors like integrins manage σ, although one solution may be to have a high on-rate and somewhat higher binding affinity or force-dependent allostery (catch bonds) to offset larger σ values (Zhu et al., 2008; Chen et al., 2012).

Many receptors bind to multiple ligands that may generate different intermembrane separations, for example, CD6-ALCAM and ALCAM-ALCAM (Chappell et al., 2015). While potential competition in this system has not been explored, the interaction of CD2 with engineered ligands of different sizes leading to differences in intermembrane separation of only 2 nm (or 15%) resulted in lateral phase separation in contact areas (Milstein et al., 2008). Finding single contact areas with coexisting small and large separation phases was technically difficult because the vast majority of contacts were either all small or all large separation phases in experiments that were near the tipping point for the competition between the small and large ligands (Milstein et al., 2008). A model for this process predicted that coexisting phases were impossible at equilibrium and that interaction of the single receptor with one of the small or large ligands would always dominate a single contact area given sufficient time (Krobath et al., 2011). Thus, the rare situations where we observed phase separation within a contact probably arose from discrete nucleation events with the long and short ligands and once merged into one contact would move toward dominance by one pair or the other if given sufficient time. Thus, the model predictions explained our difficulty of finding examples of single contacts with co-existing long and short ligand interactions with one receptor (Krobath et al., 2011). In a biological situation the relative expression level of long and short ligands of a single receptor is predicted to act in a switch-like manner to favor one ligand.

In an article in 1991, Alan Williams commented on immunologist's fascination with affinity, an equilibrium concept, in immunological settings that are kept out of equilibrium by forces of blood flow and endocytosis (Williams, 1991). While 2D affinity is discussed in the context of the immunological synapse (Grakoui et al., 1999; Huppa et al., 2010), these systems are clearly kept out of equilibrium by many energy dependent processes such that even if the 2D affinity is allowed to vary locally, any calculation that depends on equilibrium assumptions may be misleading. This is not to say that measurements are not valuable. The adhesion frequency assays pioneered by Zhu and colleagues utilize very dilute ligands on the surface of an ultrasoft red blood cell to probe for bond formation on the surface of a cell of interest (Chesla et al., 1998). The conditions are titrated to avoid progression to multivalent interactions and ideally reach an "equilibrium" between formation and breakage of single bonds with a sufficiently long test period in a defined contact area. The ideal scenario for analysis of this type of data would be for recombinant proteins attached to two RBC that are used to test each other, as the contact area between the smooth, soft surfaces would be straightforward to determine. The Zhu lab has shown that recombinant FcR bound to RBC surface shows a 50-fold higher on-rate than the same protein attached to the surface of CHO cells (stromal cells with an irregular surface) (Williams et al., 2001). This suggests that there is a 50-fold reduction in real contact area compared to the apparent contact due to surface roughness. It should be noted that the surface roughness associated with the surface of a lymphocyte can be measured in 10s or 100s of nm, rather than ~1-10 nm as in the ordered contacts mediated by CD2-CD58 interactions. The adhesion frequency and related biomembrane force probe experiments have been used to assess the interaction of RBC bound MHC-peptide complexes to TCR on live T cells (Huang et al., 2010; Liu et al., 2014). In contrast to the example above, the on-rate for MHC-peptide encounter with TCR is five-fold greater on a T cell than when recombinant TCR is attached to an RBC (Liu et al., 2015). One way to interpret these results is that the distribution of the TCR on T cells improves the effective on-rate by 250-fold (if we assume similar 50-fold reduction in actual surface contact as for CHO cell). Accordingly, when the native membrane organization of the T cell was disrupted with latrunculin A or cholesterol oxidation, the k_{on} was reduced 20- to 100-fold. A recent 3D super-resolution microscopy study suggests that the TCR is concentrated on the ends of small projections on the T cell surface (Jung et al., 2016). Such concentration of TCR on projections that are most likely to make contact with an antigen-presenting surface is expected to increase the k_{on}. 3D measurements tend to emphasize correlation of activation with off-rates. There is currently controversy as to whether *in situ* off-rates will be the same, greater than, or equal to the 3D off-rates (Huppa et al., 2010; O'Donoghue et al., 2013; Liu et al., 2014). The dwell-time, a parameter that incorporates both k_{on} and k_{off}, may take on greater significance in membrane interfaces as increasing k_{on} makes re-binding more likely. Such serial molecular interactions may be functionally similar to a single longer interaction (Klammt et al., 2015). Its likely that different, complementary approaches to single bond measurements will be needed to address outstanding issues that account for the sensitive and rapid nature of TCR recognition and triggering.

18.2.3 EMERGENT PATTERNS

Initial models for the immunological synapse bull's eye focused on the role of the actinomyosin system in moving TCR complexes inward in a process related to the earlier described "capping" and adhesion systems being displaced outward (Grakoui et al., 1999; Dustin and Cooper, 2000). However, it was also suggested that the self-assembly processes related to the drive for receptor segregation could also contribute to this process (Qi et al., 2001). The self-assembly models could account for some differences in T cell response by TCR-pMHC interactions of different kinetics (Lee et al., 2002; Weikl and Lipowsky, 2004) and were further coupled to underlying signaling networks to further predict T cell responses (Lee et al., 2003b; Cemerski et al., 2007).

The role of the actinomyosin system was further reinforced by higher resolution studies that broke the SMACs down into smaller microclusters and thus decreased the length scales for relevant membrane bending events (Mossman et al., 2005; Varma et al., 2006; Kaizuka et al., 2007) (Figure 18.1). Mathematical models for synapse patterning through introduction of diffusion barriers in the bilayer made further specific predictions about how patterned bilayers would impact synaptic patterns formed by different mechanisms (Figge and Meyer-Hermann, 2006). More recently, it has become clear that the actinomyosin cytoskeleton is not the only contributor to T cell activation and synaptic patterning (Ilani et al., 2009; Kumari et al., 2012), but that the microtubule based transport (Hashimoto-Tane et al., 2011) and the endosomal sorting complexes required for transport (ESCRT) (Vardhana et al., 2010) are also important for establishing patterns. While microtubule based transport was well known to deliver intracellular vesicular cargo to the center of the synapse, the ESCRT machinery was shown to extrude TCR enriched extracellular vesicles into the cSMAC (Choudhuri et al., 2014). The extracellular vesicles fundamentally change the topology of the synapse to one in which the cSMAC develops a large separation between the T cell and antigen presenting substrates to accommodate the 60-200 nm extracellular vesicles, or synaptic ectosomes (Dustin, 2014b, a). This large central cleft may also be contributed to by exocytic events related to directed secretion. This new element has yet to be incorporated into self-assembly models with regards to how it impacts cSMAC formation and interpretation. However, it is too early to conclude that all cSMACs are filled with extracellular vesicles as the initial studies mostly focused on full agonist pMHC, and weak agonists at high densities can also form cSMACs. The function of the extracellular vesicles is currently a mystery, but similar vesicles released by regulatory T cells have been implicated in the ability of these cells to control the activity of other T cell types through transfer of microRNAs (Okoye et al., 2014). A recent study has demonstrated that the helper T cells transfer CD40L to B cells in a TCR signaling and CD40 dependent manner. This study has suggested that helper T cells release CD40L in extracellular vesicles (Dustin, 2017; Gardell and Parker, 2017).

The behavior of the CD2-CD58 and CD28-CD80 system in the synapse has also remained somewhat enigmatic. As described above, CD2-CD58 was expected to co-localize with the TCR-pMHC recognition in the immunological synapse, but initial studies suggested that CD2-CD58 interactions strongly segregate from both the LFA-1-ICAM-1 and the TCR-pMHC interactions in the periphery of the synapse (Grakoui et al., 1999). The CD2-CD48 (the ligand for CD2 in rodents is CD48) interactions were further concentrated in the pSMAC, although still segregated from LFA-1-ICAM-1 interactions (http://www.sciencemag.org/site /feature/data/Grakoui/1040037s1_large.jpeg). It was also shown that CD2-CD58 interactions on their own induced a partial TCR signal when engaged by CD58 in bilayers or proteins micelles (Bockenstedt et al., 1988; Dustin et al., 1989; Kaizuka et al., 2009). The CD28-CD80 interaction appeared to partially overlap with TCR in early wide-field imaging studies (Bromley et al., 2001a), but with improved axial resolution it became clear that there was typically a highly TCR-pMHC enriched core surrounded by a CD28-CD80 enriched, TCR-pMHC intermediate collar in the cSMAC (Tseng et al., 2008; Yokosuka et al., 2008). Protein kinase C-θ was strongly recruited to this CD28 rich collar (Yokosuka et al., 2008). TCR movement from this collar domain into the core, which corresponds to extracellular vesicle formation, is mediated by the ESCRT machinery and appears to promote sustained co-stimulation (Vardhana et al., 2010; Choudhuri et al., 2014). Thus, while we have some understanding of the mechanism by which the CD28-CD80 costimulatory collar of the cSMAC is formed, it is not clear why CD2-ligand interactions segregate from the TCR and compete with LFA-1-ICAM-1 interactions for space in the synapse periphery.

18.2.4 SYNAPSES AND KINAPSES

Different model systems have been utilized to study the formation of immunological synapses and kinapses. The classical studies of Kupfer mostly focused on the D10 T cell line interacting with transformed B cell lines presenting conalbumin peptides to generate the famous bull's eye pattern with a ring of LFA-1 surrounding a central cluster of TCR (Monks et al., 1998). Live cell imaging from the Davis lab similarly employed B cell tumors as APCs, although they typically utilized primary T cells (Wulfing et al., 1998). We observed that functional reconstitution of T cell activation with SLB containing ICAM-1 and agonist MHC-peptide reconstituted the bull's eye pattern defined by Kupfer (Grakoui et al., 1999). A challenge to the view of a radially symmetric and stable synapse was mounted by Gunzer and colleagues using a collagen gel model, in which T cells migrated continuously on antigen presenting dendritic cell networks without stopping (Gunzer et al., 2000). *In vitro* studies with dendritic cells emphasized a multifocal pattern of receptor clustering and greater dynamics, perhaps reflecting the dramatic dynamics of the dendritic cell surface (Donnadieu et al., 1994; Brossard et al., 2005; Tseng et al., 2008). These studies suggested a limit of sort for *in vitro* studies and required a "reality check" with *in vivo* analysis of the range of physiological interactions to better set the goals for *in vitro* reconstitutions.

18.3 IN VIVO VERITAS AND BLUEPRINT FOR IN VITRO STUDY DESIGN

18.3.1 INTRAVITAL MICROSCOPY STUDIES

In vitro model systems that allow quantitative data to be obtained are invaluable, but eventually we want to take these elements back into an *in vivo* setting, which has been a major goal of intravital microscopy studies over many decades (Arfors et al., 1969; Miller et al., 2002). Another important axiom is that quantitative analysis of *in vivo* immune system dynamics provides a blueprint for design of *in vitro* platforms (Lawrence and Springer, 1991; Woolf et al., 2007). Two-photon laser scanning microscopy enables tracking of cell dynamics in intact tissues *ex vivo* (organ cultures) or *in vivo*. Striking work from Cahalan and colleagues, initially in explants but then *in vivo*, revealed rapid T cell and B cells movement through lymphoid tissues at ~12 μm/min and 5 μm/min, respectively, in the steady state (Miller et al., 2002). Against this highly dynamic steady state, priming by dendritic cells was shown to involve dramatic deceleration over a period of hours, suggesting a dramatic change in the mode of interaction triggered by antigen recognition (Stoll et al., 2002; Bousso and Robey, 2003; Mempel et al., 2004; Shakhar et al., 2005). The scenario described by Gunzer and colleagues in collagen gels appeared to correspond most closely to some modes of antigen specific tolerance induction in vivo, which proceed without any T cell deceleration as long as the weak agonist antigens are distributed throughout the lymphoid tissue (Hugues et al., 2004; Skokos et al., 2007). Priming T-DC interaction *in vivo* involved dramatic deceleration and local confinement of the T cell, but detailed observations suggested continued local exploration by antigen specific T cells (Azar et al., 2010). Priming of naïve T cells on SLBs revealed a T cell autonomous program of symmetry breaking and relocation that paralleled dynamics in vivo and was promoted by activity of PKCθ (Sims et al., 2007). We referred this slow exploration of the DC that was distinct from the rapid steady state migration as a kinapse, for "moving junction" (Dustin, 2007). There is a debate as to whether the kinapse is a discrete mode of interaction or part of a continuum, but recent data suggest that steady state migration is largely integrin independent, whereas the kinapse mode is distinguished by its integrin dependence and large contact area (Woolf et al., 2007; Moreau et al., 2012; Moreau et al., 2015). It will be important to understand the implications of this T cell behavior during priming and how these relate to similar data on T-APC interactions in later stages. The best evidence at this point is for stable synapses to play an important role in effector function in defense against pathogens (Waite et al., 2011) and cancer (Ruocco et al., 2012), but also in immunopathology (Shaw et al., 2015). Even in effector phases, it has been suggested that serial hits from rapidly moving cytotoxic T cells may be as good a strategy for target killing as a single stable synapse (Halle et al., 2016). Dynamic interactions of CTL in tissues have also been associated with immunopathology (Kim et al., 2009), and arrest of these cells in a PD-1 dependent paralytic synapse is an evolved solution to this challenge of pathogens that attach vulnerable niches (Zinselmeyer et al., 2013). Development of appropriate models should help to shed light on optimizing interaction strategies for different functions.

18.3.2 SEARCH STRATEGIES

In vivo microscopy studies dramatically changed the models for how immune cells searched for their targets. Cahalan and colleagues proposed a random search that was well modeled by Brownian motion, such that a

T cell could be described to diffuse in the T cell zone in its search for APCs with individual DC contacting up to 5000 T cells per hour (Miller et al., 2003; Miller et al., 2004). Optimizing such a search process is a fantastic modeling problem. The biological scaffold for T cells and DC organization is a remarkable stromal cell network that is induced within mucosal tissues and the lymphatic and the vascular systems by innate lymphocytes (Mebius, 2003). These cells create a unique 3D tissue space supported by a enclosed collagen bundle network and the stromal cells also produce chemokines that stimulate T and B cell motility in different compartments (Ebnet et al., 1996; Bajenoff et al., 2006). While T and B cell movement can give a linear fit in a mean-square displacement plot, this is a relatively weak test for correlated behavior that might suggest more sophisticated search strategies. Within T cell zone its been shown that activated dendritic cells that have been helped by CD4 T cell produce chemokines that induce local swarming of CD8 T cells to increase the chance for encountering cells within that subset (Castellino et al., 2006). Inflammatory chemokines may also help to concentrate memory T cells in locations where they will have a first look at entering DC (Kastenmuller et al., 2013). It has also been proposed that T cells use Levy walks to find pathogens in a tissue setting, a strategy in which directional changes are random, but the distance moved prior to the next changes in direction is taken from a power law distribution (Harris et al., 2012). These longer runs interspersed with more extensive searches allow more unique area to be investigated. However, the movement of T cells in lymphoid tissues is better approximated by a composite-correlated random walk (Beltman et al., 2007). Furthermore, it has become clear from genetic experiments that the turning angle distribution is not determined entirely by lymph node architecture, but is also regulated by specific gene products in the T cell (Gerard et al., 2014). Because correlated random walks can approximate Levy walks, its possible that T cells will always use a combination of environmental cues and cell autonomous strategies to regulate their searching behavior in the absence of explicit chemotactic information—an area ripe for modeling.

18.4 SYSTEMATIC ANALYSIS

18.4.1 SYSTEMATIC ANALYSIS OF CELL-CELL SYNAPSES

An important future direction for analysis of the immunological synapse is to take advantage of powerful genetic tools like shRNA and CRISPR libraries and high content screens to get a more comprehensive view of the immunological synapse. Wuelfing and colleagues have performed some impressive screens with cellular systems to investigate signaling proteins (Singleton et al., 2011). Automating the image processing and classification of the synapses will facilitate these studies. Its possible that guiding such analysis with models for the 3D structures would facilitate orientation and classification of images. Most cell-cell conjugates are viewed from the side, and this information about the depth of various signals in the cytoplasm of the apposed cells can be useful. However, rapid analysis of synapse patterns also benefits from end-on views with significant throughput. A low throughput approach to this is to use a laser trap to orient the conjugates, which was successful in generating an en face view of the IS in cell-cell conjugates that could be scanned with a confocal microscope (Oddos et al., 2008). Somewhat higher throughput, but lower loading efficiency, was obtained using micropit arrays, but this is only feasible if cells are plentiful and of similar size (Biggs et al., 2011). A microfluidic-based system that combines the micropit approach with a mechanism to specifically capture the second cell looks promising (Jang et al., 2015). Combining a robust positioning methodology with a high resolution and high-speed methods like lattice light sheet microscope could put cell-cell imaging on a more even playing field with imaging cells at interfaces with glass substrates (Ritter et al., 2015). Since the cell-cell setting is undoubtedly closer to nature, closing this gap substantially would be a major advance.

18.4.2 SOLID PHASE LIGAND PRESENTATION

The most accessible and effective T cell activating substrates for most researchers are beads or planar surfaces coated with anti-CD3 and anti-CD28 antibodies. The formation of TCR microclusters and translocation of SLP-76 based signaling complexes are well documented on these substrates, although these phenotypes are strongly modulated by addition of adhesion molecules like ICAM-1, VCAM-1, or fibronectin (Bunnell et al., 2006; Nguyen et al., 2008). While sub-optimal for pattern formation that requires ligand mobility, these substrates have the potential advantage in that several large gene expression studies have utilized these substrates to provide standardized T cell stimulation and costimulation (Ciofani et al., 2012; Yosef et al., 2013). Magnetic beads coated with anti-CD3 and anti-CD28 are also a standard for expansion of human T cells in clinical protocols for immunotherapy, such that understanding T cell responses to these substrates is of significant practical interest (Levine et al., 1997). Better models for how synapses are patterned on immobile substrates and how information can be mapped between easy to establish solid phase substrates and more fragile SLB systems would help speed analysis. Some concerns have been raised about the non-specific activation potential of highly interactive surfaces like poly-L-lysine coated glass (Chang et al., 2016). I have spent many years working on developing planar substrates that optimize imaging parameters while retaining biological specificity (Dustin and Springer, 1989; Dustin et al., 1997a; Grakoui et al., 1999). Therefore, while great care is needed, I remain convinced that such substrate based system will generate useful quantitative data so help gain a deeper understanding of in vivo and in vitro cell-cell interaction data.

18.4.3 HIGH THROUGHPUT ANALYSIS ON SLB

SLBs are a complex substrate system and are somewhat cumbersome for high throughput analysis, but there is no doubt that robotics will be able to increase the throughput of these systems beyond the current practice (Nair et al., 2015). Currently, a big day for my lab might be to examine 10–20 conditions in detail. The analysis of this data would then take weeks. The use of 96 well plates, robotic SLB assembly, and automated analysis can increase this throughput to 100–200 samples per day while greatly reducing the potential for human error and total time to results to two days. The use of screening microscopes with dry objectives (max NA of ~0.7) limits resolution, but this is adequate for scoring of supramolecular activation clusters at moderate densities of anti-CD3 or MHC-peptide complexes. The identification and analysis of cellular phenotypes may be aided by custom software development to get accurate cell counts and analysis of associated fluorescent signals (Mayya et al., 2015). Performing imaging-based analysis of small numbers of cells from patient samples is a current challenge, and methods that make efficient use of cells and offer reasonable throughput are needed but not currently available. One potential direction is nanowell technologies, which can also be used to identify synaptic phenotypes of single cells that can then be subjected to further analysis through micromanipulation (Torres et al., 2013). Recently, Ibidi has marketed microwell inserts that would allow imaging of ~1000 lymphocytes distributed over a single 20× imaging field (http://ibidi.com/xtproducts/en/ibidi-Labware/Open-Slides-Dishes:-Removable-Chambers /micro-Insert-4-Well-FulTrac).

The bottom-up approach to reconstitution of the immunological synapse has thus far investigated only a small fraction of the molecules expressed on the surface of antigen presenting cells that guide responses, mostly restricted to MHC-peptide complexes, ICAM-1 and B7 family co-stimulatory molecules, and NKG2D ligands (Bromley et al., 2001a; Somersalo et al., 2004; Yokosuka et al., 2012). In order to guide these investigations further, it will be of great interest to document molecules on the surface of different types of antigen presenting cells using quantitative methods in order to express and present these molecules on surface to test for function and synaptic patterning (Weekes et al., 2010). Hybrid systems in which supported bilayers with mobile (lipid anchored) and immobile (transmembrane) components can be easily generated would provide opportunities for more physiological presentation of many transmembrane proteins with both mobile and immobile fractions on the cell surface.

An important aspect of screening studies that focus on the immunological synapse is a data format that would work for investigators interested in modeling. In our work on SLB, we have a standard approach to calibration and report ligands densities in molecules/μm^2. Methods to classify patterns and provide quantitative summaries of large imaging data sets will also aid modeling efforts by making data more publically accessible through databases, perhaps built on platforms like Omero (http://www.openmicroscopy.org/site /products/omero).

18.4.4 SIGNALING COMPLEXES AND INTEGRATION

Quantitative proteomics that can generate real estimates of protein abundance are an exciting direction and are potentially of great value in design of bottom-up experimental programs and for parametizing modeling efforts. The Cantrell group has performed phosphoproteomics and total proteome analysis of cytotoxic T cells (Navarro et al., 2014). Putting general phosphoproteomics data into the context of supramolecular organization will be greatly aided by immunoisolation of molecular assemblies and their analysis by quantitative proteomics. A challenge here is having reliable antibodies to signaling molecules that allow consistent isolation and comparison. The Malissen group has generated a series of knock-in mice in which different candidate signaling adapters were epitope tagged such that they could also be isolated with the same, well characterized and highly specific monoclonal antibodies (Roncagalli et al., 2014). The results of such analyses can be extended by reconstitution on liposomes or SLBs to better mimic the *in situ* signaling at triggered receptors (Hui and Vale, 2014). These methods can be combined with patterning of SLBs and imaging to study issues of compartmentalization and phase separation associated with reconstituted signaling networks (Iversen et al., 2014; Su et al., 2016). Initial efforts to couple TCR signaling to down-stream signaling did not explicitly take into account lateral phase separation, which we now know is also driven by extracellular interactions, the lipid core of the plasma membrane, and the signaling complexes in the cytoplasmic space (Dustin and Muller, 2016). Incorporating these principles into signaling models (Das et al., 2009; Mukherjee et al., 2013) should generate new opportunities to understand immune system regulation. Coupling cell surface signaling with signals conveyed through extracellular vesicles and cytokines will lead to integration of these inputs in transcriptional networks. Time courses for T cell activation in response to infection *in vivo* have generated a number of new ideas for the role of immunological synapse (Best et al., 2013). Collection of gene expression data in mouse and human models may generally benefit from either joining or adopting the SOPs of consortia such as IMMGEN, as the use of a common SOPs to collect data across the entire immune system clearly creates fantastic opportunities for modeling efforts with a high confidence (Heng and Painter, 2008; Ciofani et al., 2012). It is likely that issues of immunological synapse duration and kinapse based integration of information from antigen rich clusters within lymphoid tissues will be encoded in expressed transcription factors and chromatin modifications (Tkach et al., 2014; Mayya and Dustin, 2016). To more explicitly connect what we know about events in the synapse to events in the nucleus should be an exciting area for modeling in the future.

18.4.5 INTEGRATION WITH SINGLE CELL REVOLUTION

Faster progress in human immunology has been fueled by methods that allow analysis of rare or single cells (Hataye et al., 2006; Brusic et al., 2014; Yu et al., 2015; Ryan et al., 2016). Single cell phenotyping incorporating both imaging and nucleic acid analysis also offers further power in relating single cell phenotypes to synaptic architecture (Buettner et al., 2015; Proserpio et al., 2016: Torres, 2013 #9696). For example, it should be possible to relate synaptic phenotypes of CD2 patterning to a response to pathogens or a susceptibility to autoimmune disease (McKinney et al., 2015). Such approaches will benefit from robust models for quantitative hypothesis testing and should provide considerable raw material for data driven modeling.

18.5 CONCLUSIONS

Data driven quantitative immunology will play an important role in refining the questions that we ask in basic immunology and our ability to take what we have learned and apply this to therapy. The acquisition of the data needed for this will require further efforts to standardize methods and formatting beyond initial successes in analysis of gene expression. Efforts to "harden" the relatively soft data reporting for flow cytometry and imaging and making these types of data available to the community more efficiently should be a future goal. How successful examples of strong standard operating procedures and standards can be applied beyond small consortia to entire fields is a future challenge for collaborative science. I would wish for a holistic model that takes into account all of the relevant interactions needed to generate an immunological synapse.

This model could then be incorporated as an element in a larger model of the immune response that depends upon these elements. The benefit of such efforts will be a deeper understanding of the immune response and the ways in which immunological synapses and kinapses operate in decisions that impact patient health.

ACKNOWLEDGMENTS

I thank my mentors S. Peterson, T. Springer, S. Kornfeld, E. Unanue, D. Littman, and M. Feldmann and members of my lab for their inspiration. I thank S. Vardhana for the original image for Figure 18.1. A Wellcome Trust Principal Research Fellowship supports MLD.

REFERENCES

Arfors KE, Dhall DP, Engeset J, Hint H, Matheson NA, Tangen O (1969) In vivo quantitation of platelet activity using biolaser-induced endothelial injury. Bibl Anat 10:502-506.

Azar GA, Lemaitre F, Robey EA, Bousso P (2010) Subcellular dynamics of T cell immunological synapses and kinapses in lymph nodes. Proc Natl Acad Sci U S A 107:3675-3680.

Bajenoff M, Egen JG, Koo LY, Laugier JP, Brau F, Glaichenhaus N, Germain RN (2006) Stromal cell networks regulate lymphocyte entry, migration, and territoriality in lymph nodes. Immunity 25:989-1001.

Balakrishnan K, Hsu FJ, Cooper AD, McConnell HM (1982) Lipid hapten containing membrane targets can trigger specific immunoglobulin E-dependent degranulation of rat basophil leukemia cells. J Biol Chem 257:6427-6433.

Batista FD, Iber D, Neuberger MS (2001) B cells acquire antigen from target cells after synapse formation. Nature 411:489-494.

Bell GI (1978) Models for the specific adhesion of cells to cells. Science 200:618-627.

Bell GI, Dembo M, Bongrand P (1984) Cell adhesion. Competition between nonspecific repulsion and specific bonding. Biophys J 45:1051-1064.

Beltman JB, Maree AF, de Boer RJ (2007) Spatial modelling of brief and long interactions between T cells and dendritic cells. Immunol Cell Biol 85:306-314.

Best JA, Blair DA, Knell J, Yang E, Mayya V, Doedens A, Dustin ML, Goldrath AW (2013) Transcriptional insights into the CD8(+) T cell response to infection and memory T cell formation. Nat Immunol 14:404-412.

Biggs MJ, Milone MC, Santos LC, Gondarenko A, Wind SJ (2011) High-resolution imaging of the immunological synapse and T-cell receptor microclustering through microfabricated substrates. J R Soc Interface 8:1462-1471.

Bjorkman PJ, Saper MA, Samraoui B, Bennett WS, Strominger JL, Wiley DC (1987) Structure of the human class I histocompatibility antigen, HLA-A2. Nature 329:506-512.

Bockenstedt LK, Goldsmith MA, Dustin M, Olive D, Springer TA, Weiss A (1988) The CD2 ligand LFA-3 activates T cells but depends on the expression and function of the antigen receptor. J Immunol 141:1904-1911.

Bousso P, Robey E (2003) Dynamics of CD8+ T cell priming by dendritic cells in intact lymph nodes. Nat Immunol 4:579-585.

Braun J, Sha'afi RI, Unanue ER (1979) Crosslinking by ligands to surface immunoglobulin triggers mobilization of intracellular 45Ca2+ in B lymphocytes. J Cell Biol 82:755-766.

Braun J, Fujiwara K, Pollard TD, Unanue ER (1978) Two distinct mechanisms for redistribution of lymphocyte surface macromolecules. I. Relationship to cytoplasmic myosin. J Cell Biol 79:409-418.

Bromley SK, Iaboni A, Davis SJ, Whitty A, Green JM, Shaw AS, Weiss A, Dustin ML (2001a) The immunological synapse and CD28-CD80 interactions. Nat Immunol 2:1159-1166.

Bromley SK, Burack WR, Johnson KG, Somersalo K, Sims TN, Sumen C, Davis MM, Shaw AS, Allen PM, Dustin ML (2001b) The immunological synapse. Annu Rev Immunol 19:375-396.

Brossard C, Feuillet V, Schmitt A, Randriamampita C, Romao M, Raposo G, Trautmann A (2005) Multifocal structure of the T cell - dendritic cell synapse. Eur J Immunol 35:1741-1753.

Brusic V, Gottardo R, Kleinstein SH, Davis MM, committee Hs (2014) Computational resources for high-dimensional immune analysis from the Human Immunology Project Consortium. Nat Biotechnol 32:146-148.

Buettner F, Natarajan KN, Casale FP, Proserpio V, Scialdone A, Theis FJ, Teichmann SA, Marioni JC, Stegle O (2015) Computational analysis of cell-to-cell heterogeneity in single-cell RNA-sequencing data reveals hidden subpopulations of cells. Nat Biotechnol 33:155-160.

Bunnell SC, Singer AL, Hong DI, Jacque BH, Jordan MS, Seminario MC, Barr VA, Koretzky GA, Samelson LE (2006) Persistence of cooperatively stabilized signaling clusters drives T-cell activation. Mol Cell Biol 26:7155-7166.

Burroughs NJ, Kohler K, Miloserdov V, Dustin ML, van der Merwe PA, Davis DM (2011) Boltzmann energy-based image analysis demonstrates that extracellular domain size differences explain protein segregation at immune synapses. PLoS Comput Biol 7:e1002076.

Campi G, Varma R, Dustin ML (2005) Actin and agonist MHC-peptide complex-dependent T cell receptor microclusters as scaffolds for signaling. J Exp Med 202:1031-1036.

Carbone CB, Kern N, Fernandes RA, Hui E, Su X, Garcia KC, Vale RD (2017) In vitro reconstitution of T cell receptor-mediated segregation of the CD45 phosphatase. Proc Natl Acad Sci U S A. 114:E9338-E45.

Carroll-Portillo A, Spendier K, Pfeiffer J, Griffiths G, Li H, Lidke KA, Oliver JM, Lidke DS, Thomas JL, Wilson BS, Timlin JA (2010) Formation of a mast cell synapse: Fc epsilon RI membrane dynamics upon binding mobile or immobilized ligands on surfaces. J Immunol 184:1328-1338.

Castellino F, Huang AY, Altan-Bonnet G, Stoll S, Scheinecker C, Germain RN (2006) Chemokines enhance immunity by guiding naive CD8+ T cells to sites of CD4+ T cell-dendritic cell interaction. Nature 440:890-895.

Cemerski S, Das J, Locasale J, Arnold P, Giurisato E, Markiewicz MA, Fremont D, Allen PM, Chakraborty AK, Shaw AS (2007) The stimulatory potency of T cell antigens is influenced by the formation of the immunological synapse. Immunity 26:345-355.

Chan PY, Springer TA (1992) Effect of lengthening lymphocyte function-associated antigen 3 on adhesion to CD2. Mol Biol Cell 3:157-166.

Chan PY, Lawrence MB, Dustin ML, Ferguson LM, Golan DE, Springer TA (1991) Influence of receptor lateral mobility on adhesion strengthening between membranes containing LFA-3 and CD2. J Cell Biol 115:245-255.

Chang VT, Fernandes RA, Ganzinger KA, Lee SF, Siebold C, McColl J, Jonsson P, Palayret M, Harlos K, Coles CH, Jones EY, Lui Y, Huang E, Gilbert RJ, Klenerman D, Aricescu AR, Davis SJ (2016) Initiation of T cell signaling by CD45 segregation at 'close contacts'. Nat Immunol 17:574-582.

Chappell PE, Garner LI, Yan J, Metcalfe C, Hatherley D, Johnson S, Robinson CV, Lea SM, Brown MH (2015) Structures of CD6 and Its Ligand CD166 Give Insight into Their Interaction. Structure 23:1426-1436.

Chen W, Lou J, Evans EA, Zhu C (2012) Observing force-regulated conformational changes and ligand dissociation from a single integrin on cells. J Cell Biol 199:497-512.

Chesla SE, Selvaraj P, Zhu C (1998) Measuring two-dimensional receptor-ligand binding kinetics by micropipette. Biophys J 75:1553-1572.

Choudhuri K, Wiseman D, Brown MH, Gould K, van der Merwe PA (2005) T-cell receptor triggering is critically dependent on the dimensions of its peptide-MHC ligand. Nature 436:578-582.

Choudhuri K, Llodra J, Roth EW, Tsai J, Gordo S, Wucherpfennig KW, Kam LC, Stokes DL, Dustin ML (2014) Polarized release of T-cell-receptor-enriched microvesicles at the immunological synapse. Nature 507:118-123.

Ciofani M et al. (2012) A validated regulatory network for Th17 cell specification. Cell 151:289-303.

Cyster JG, Shotton DM, Williams AF (1991) The dimensions of the T lymphocyte glycoprotein leukosialin and identification of linear protein epitopes that can be modified by glycosylation. EMBO J 10:893-902.

Das J, Ho M, Zikherman J, Govern C, Yang M, Weiss A, Chakraborty AK, Roose JP (2009) Digital signaling and hysteresis characterize ras activation in lymphoid cells. Cell 136:337-351.

Davis DM, Chiu I, Fassett M, Cohen GB, Mandelboim O, Strominger JL (1999) The human natural killer cell immune synapse. Proc Natl Acad Sci U S A 96:15062-15067.

Davis MM, Chien YH, Gascoigne NR, Hedrick SM (1984) A murine T cell receptor gene complex: Isolation, structure and rearrangement. Immunol Rev 81:235-258.

Davis SJ, van der Merwe PA (1996) The structure and ligand interactions of CD2: Implications for T-cell function. Immunol Today 17:177-187.

Donnadieu E, Bismuth G, Trautmann A (1994) Antigen recognition by helper T cells elicits a sequence of distinct changes of their shape and intracellular calcium. Curr Biol 4:584-595.

Dustin ML (1997) Adhesive bond dynamics in contacts between T lymphocytes and glass supported planar bilayers reconstituted with the immunoglobulin related adhesion molecule CD58. J Biol Chem 272:15782-15788.

Dustin ML (2007) Cell adhesion molecules and actin cytoskeleton at immune synapses and kinapses. Curr Opin Cell Biol 19:529-533.

Dustin ML (2014a) The immunological synapse. Cancer Immunology Research 2:1023-1033.

Dustin ML (2014b) What Counts in the Immunological Synapse? Mol Cell 54:255-262.

Dustin ML (2017) Help to go: T cells transfer CD40L to antigen-presenting B cells. Eur J Immunol 47:31-34.

Dustin ML, Springer TA (1988) Lymphocyte function-associated antigen-1 (LFA-1) interaction with intercellular adhesion molecule-1 (ICAM-1) is one of at least three mechanisms for lymphocyte adhesion to cultured endothelial cells. J Cell Biol 107:321-331.

Dustin ML, Springer TA (1989) T cell receptor cross-linking transiently stimulates adhesiveness through LFA-1. Nature 341:619-624.

Dustin ML, Cooper JA (2000) The immunological synapse and the actin cytoskeleton: Molecular hardware for T cell signaling. Nat Immunol 1:23-29.

Dustin ML, Colman DR (2002) Neural and immunological synaptic relations. Science 298:785-789.

Dustin ML, Muller J (2016) CELL SIGNALING. Liquidity in immune cell signaling. Science 352:516-517.

Dustin ML, Jacobson GR, Peterson SW (1984) Effects of insulin receptor down-regulation on hexose transport in human erythrocytes. J Biol Chem 259:13660-13663.

Dustin ML, Olive D, Springer TA (1989) Correlation of CD2 binding and functional properties of multimeric and monomeric lymphocyte function-associated antigen 3. J Exp Med 169:503-517.

Dustin ML, Sanders ME, Shaw S, Springer TA (1987a) Purified lymphocyte function-associated antigen 3 binds to CD2 and mediates T lymphocyte adhesion. J Exp Med 165:677-692.

Dustin ML, Selvaraj P, Mattaliano RJ, Springer TA (1987b) Anchoring mechanisms for LFA-3 cell adhesion glycoprotein at membrane surface. Nature 329:846-848.

Dustin ML, Ferguson LM, Chan PY, Springer TA, Golan DE (1996) Visualization of CD2 interaction with LFA-3 and determination of the two-dimensional dissociation constant for adhesion receptors in a contact area. J Cell Biol 132:465-474.

Dustin ML, Bromley SK, Kan Z, Peterson DA, Unanue ER (1997a) Antigen receptor engagement delivers a stop signal to migrating T lymphocytes. Proc Natl Acad Sci U S A 94:3909-3913.

Dustin ML, Golan DE, Zhu DM, Miller JM, Meier W, Davies EA, van der Merwe PA (1997b) Low affinity interaction of human or rat T cell adhesion molecule CD2 with its ligand aligns adhering membranes to achieve high physiological affinity. J Biol Chem 272:30889-30898.

Dustin ML, Starr T, Coombs D, Majeau GR, Meier W, Hochman PS, Douglass A, Vale R, Goldstein B, Whitty A (2007) Quantification and Modeling of Tripartite CD2-, CD58FC Chimera (Alefacept)-, and CD16-mediated Cell Adhesion. J Biol Chem 282:34748-34757.

Dustin ML, Olszowy MW, Holdorf AD, Li J, Bromley S, Desai N, Widder P, Rosenberger F, van der Merwe PA, Allen PM, Shaw AS (1998) A novel adapter protein orchestrates receptor patterning and cytoskeletal polarity in T cell contacts. Cell 94:667-677.

Ebnet K, Kaldjian EP, Anderson AO, Shaw S (1996) Orchestrated information transfer underlying leukocyte endothelial interactions. Annu Rev Immunol 14:155-177.

Egen JG, Allison JP (2002) Cytotoxic T lymphocyte antigen-4 accumulation in the immunological synapse is regulated by TCR signal strength. Immunity 16:23-35.

Elices MJ, Osborn L, Takada Y, Crouse C, Luhowskyj S, Hemler ME, Lobb RR (1990) VCAM-1 on activated endothelium interacts with the leukocyte integrin VLA-4 at a site distinct from the VLA-4/fibronectin binding site. Cell 60:577-584.

Feldmann M, Steinman L (2005) Design of effective immunotherapy for human autoimmunity. Nature 435:612-619.

Figge MT, Meyer-Hermann M (2006) Geometrically repatterned immunological synapses uncover formation mechanisms. PLoS Comput Biol 2:e171.

Freeman SA, Goyette J, Furuya W, Woods EC, Bertozzi CR, Bergmeier W, Hinz B, van der Merwe PA, Das R, Grinstein S (2016) Integrins Form an Expanding Diffusional Barrier that Coordinates Phagocytosis. Cell 164:128-140.

Freiberg BA, Kupfer H, Maslanik W, Delli J, Kappler J, Zaller DM, Kupfer A (2002) Staging and resetting T cell activation in SMACs. Nat Immunol 3:911-917.

Gardell JL, Parker DC (2017) CD40L is transferred to antigen-presenting B cells during delivery of T-cell help. Eur J Immunol 47:41-50.

Gerard A, Patino-Lopez G, Beemiller P, Nambiar R, Ben-Aissa K, Liu Y, Totah FJ, Tyska MJ, Shaw S, Krummel MF (2014) Detection of rare antigen-presenting cells through T cell-intrinsic meandering motility, mediated by Myo1g. Cell 158:492-505.

Goodridge HS, Reyes CN, Becker CA, Katsumoto TR, Ma J, Wolf AJ, Bose N, Chan AS, Magee AS, Danielson ME, Weiss A, Vasilakos JP, Underhill DM (2011) Activation of the innate immune receptor Dectin-1 upon formation of a 'phagocytic synapse'. Nature 472:471-475.

Grakoui A, Bromley SK, Sumen C, Davis MM, Shaw AS, Allen PM, Dustin ML (1999) The immunological synapse: A molecular machine controlling T cell activation. Science 285:221-227.

Gunzer M, Schafer A, Borgmann S, Grabbe S, Zanker KS, Brocker EB, Kampgen E, Friedl P (2000) Antigen presentation in extracellular matrix: Interactions of T cells with dendritic cells are dynamic, short lived, and sequential. Immunity 13:323-332.

Halle S et al. (2016) In Vivo Killing Capacity of Cytotoxic T Cells Is Limited and Involves Dynamic Interactions and T Cell Cooperativity. Immunity 44:233-245.

Harris TH, Banigan EJ, Christian DA, Konradt C, Tait Wojno ED, Norose K, Wilson EH, John B, Weninger W, Luster AD, Liu AJ, Hunter CA (2012) Generalized Levy walks and the role of chemokines in migration of effector CD8+ T cells. Nature 486:545-548.

Harrison OJ, Jin X, Hong S, Bahna F, Ahlsen G, Brasch J, Wu Y, Vendome J, Felsovalyi K, Hampton CM, Troyanovsky RB, Ben-Shaul A, Frank J, Troyanovsky SM, Shapiro L, Honig B (2011) The extracellular architecture of adherens junctions revealed by crystal structures of type I cadherins. Structure 19:244-256.

Hashimoto-Tane A, Yokosuka T, Sakata-Sogawa K, Sakuma M, Ishihara C, Tokunaga M, Saito T (2011) Dynein-driven transport of T cell receptor microclusters regulates immune synapse formation and T cell activation. Immunity 34:919-931.

Hataye J, Moon JJ, Khoruts A, Reilly C, Jenkins MK (2006) Naive and memory CD4+ T cell survival controlled by clonal abundance. Science 312:114-116.

Heng TS, Painter MW (2008) The Immunological Genome Project: Networks of gene expression in immune cells. Nat Immunol 9:1091-1094.

Hu J, Lipowsky R, Weikl TR (2013) Binding constants of membrane-anchored receptors and ligands depend strongly on the nanoscale roughness of membranes. Proc Natl Acad Sci U S A 110:15283-15288.

Huang J, Zarnitsyna VI, Liu B, Edwards LJ, Jiang N, Evavold BD, Zhu C (2010) The kinetics of two-dimensional TCR and pMHC interactions determine T-cell responsiveness. Nature 464:932-936.

Hugues S, Fetler L, Bonifaz L, Helft J, Amblard F, Amigorena S (2004) Distinct T cell dynamics in lymph nodes during the induction of tolerance and immunity. Nat Immunol 5:1235-1242.

Hui E, Vale RD (2014) In vitro membrane reconstitution of the T-cell receptor proximal signaling network. Nat Struct Mol Biol 21:133-142.

Huppa JB, Axmann M, Mortelmaier MA, Lillemeier BF, Newell EW, Brameshuber M, Klein LO, Schutz GJ, Davis MM (2010) TCR-peptide-MHC interactions in situ show accelerated kinetics and increased affinity. Nature 463:963-967.

Hynes RO (1987) Integrins: A family of cell surface receptors. Cell 48:549-554.

Ilani T, Vasiliver-Shamis G, Vardhana S, Bretscher A, Dustin ML (2009) T cell antigen receptor signaling and immunological synapse stability require myosin IIA. Nat Immunol 10:531-539.

Irles C, Symons A, Michel F, Bakker TR, van der Merwe PA, Acuto O (2003) CD45 ectodomain controls interaction with GEMs and Lck activity for optimal TCR signaling. Nat Immunol 4:189-197.

Isaaz S, Baetz K, Olsen K, Podack E, Griffiths GM (1995) Serial killing by cytotoxic T lymphocytes: T cell receptor triggers degranulation, re-filling of the lytic granules and secretion of lytic proteins via a non-granule pathway. Eur J Immunol 25:1071-1079.

Iversen L, Tu HL, Lin WC, Christensen SM, Abel SM, Iwig J, Wu HJ, Gureasko J, Rhodes C, Petit RS, Hansen SD, Thill P, Yu CH, Stamou D, Chakraborty AK, Kuriyan J, Groves JT (2014) Molecular kinetics. Ras activation by SOS: Allosteric regulation by altered fluctuation dynamics. Science 345:50-54.

James JR, Vale RD (2012) Biophysical mechanism of T-cell receptor triggering in a reconstituted system. Nature 487:64-69.

Jang JH, Huang Y, Zheng P, Jo MC, Bertolet G, Zhu MX, Qin L, Liu D (2015) Imaging of Cell-Cell Communication in a Vertical Orientation Reveals High-Resolution Structure of Immunological Synapse and Novel PD-1 Dynamics. J Immunol 195:1320-1330.

Jung Y, Riven I, Feigelson SW, Kartvelishvily E, Tohya K, Miyasaka M, Alon R, Haran G (2016) Three-dimensional localization of T-cell receptors in relation to microvilli using a combination of superresolution microscopies. Proc Natl Acad Sci U S A 113:E5916-E5924.

Kaizuka Y, Douglass AD, Varma R, Dustin ML, Vale RD (2007) Mechanisms for segregating T cell receptor and adhesion molecules during immunological synapse formation in Jurkat T cells. Proc Natl Acad Sci U S A 104:20296-20301.

Kaizuka Y, Douglass AD, Vardhana S, Dustin ML, Vale RD (2009) The coreceptor CD2 uses plasma membrane microdomains to transduce signals in T cells. J Cell Biol 185:521-534.

Kastenmuller W, Brandes M, Wang Z, Herz J, Egen JG, Germain RN (2013) Peripheral prepositioning and local CXCL9 chemokine-mediated guidance orchestrate rapid memory CD8+ T cell responses in the lymph node. Immunity 38:502-513.

Kim JV, Kang SS, Dustin ML, McGavern DB (2009) Myelomonocytic cell recruitment causes fatal CNS vascular injury during acute viral meningitis. Nature 457:191-195.

Klammt C, Novotna L, Li DT, Wolf M, Blount A, Zhang K, Fitchett JR, Lillemeier BF (2015) T cell receptor dwell times control the kinase activity of Zap70. Nat Immunol 16:961-969.

Koretzky GA, Picus J, Thomas ML, Weiss A (1990) Tyrosine phosphatase CD45 is essential for coupling T-cell antigen receptor to the phosphatidyl inositol pathway. Nature 346:66-68.

Krobath H, Rozycki B, Lipowsky R, Weikl TR (2011) Line tension and stability of domains in cell-adhesion zones mediated by long and short receptor-ligand complexes. PLoS ONE 6:e23284.

Kumari S, Vardhana S, Cammer M, Curado S, Santos L, Sheetz MP, Dustin ML (2012) T Lymphocyte Myosin IIA is Required for Maturation of the Immunological Synapse. Frontiers in immunology 3:230.

Kupfer A, Singer SJ (1989) The specific interaction of helper T cells and antigen-presenting B cells. IV. Membrane and cytoskeletal reorganizations in the bound T cell as a function of antigen dose. J Exp Med 170:1697-1713.

Lawrence MB, Springer TA (1991) Leukocytes roll on a selectin at physiologic flow rates: Distinction from and prerequisite for adhesion through integrins. Cell 65:859-873.

Le Bihan O, Decossas M, Gontier E, Gerbod-Giannone MC, Lambert O (2015) Visualization of adherent cell monolayers by cryo-electron microscopy: A snapshot of endothelial adherens junctions. J Struct Biol 192:470-477.

Lee KH, Dinner AR, Tu C, Campi G, Raychaudhuri S, Varma R, Sims TN, Burack WR, Wu H, Wang J, Kanagawa O, Markiewicz M, Allen PM, Dustin ML, Chakraborty AK, Shaw AS (2003a) The immunological synapse balances T cell receptor signaling and degradation. Science 302:1218-1222.

Lee SJ, Hori Y, Groves JT, Dustin ML, Chakraborty AK (2002) Correlation of a dynamic model for immunological synapse formation with effector functions: Two pathways to synapse formation. Trends Immunol 23:492-499.

Lee SJE, Hori Y, Chakraborty AK (2003b) Low T cell receptor expression and thermal fluctuations contribute to formation of dynamic multifocal synapses in thymocytes. Proc Natl Acad Sci U S A 100:4383-4388.

Levine BL, Bernstein WB, Connors M, Craighead N, Lindsten T, Thompson CB, June CH (1997) Effects of CD28 costimulation on long-term proliferation of CD4+ T cells in the absence of exogenous feeder cells. J Immunol 159:5921-5930.

Liu B, Chen W, Evavold BD, Zhu C (2014) Accumulation of Dynamic Catch Bonds between TCR and Agonist Peptide-MHC Triggers T Cell Signaling. Cell 157:357-368.

Liu B, Chen W, Natarajan K, Li Z, Margulies DH, Zhu C (2015) The cellular environment regulates in situ kinetics of T-cell receptor interaction with peptide major histocompatibility complex. Eur J Immunol 45:2099-2110.

Lodish H (2013) Cloning expeditions: Risky but rewarding. Mol Cell Biol 33:4620-4627.

Marlin SD, Springer TA (1987) Purified intercellular adhesion molecule-1 (ICAM-1) is a ligand for lymphocyte function-associated antigen 1 (LFA-1). Cell 51:813-819.

Mayya V, Dustin ML (2016) What Scales the T Cell Response? Trends Immunol 37:513-522.

Mayya V, Neiswanger W, Medina R, Wiggins CH, Dustin ML (2015) Integrative analysis of T cell motility from multi-channel microscopy data using TIAM. J Immunol Methods 416:84-93.

Mayya V, Judokusumo E, Abu Shah E, Peel CG, Neiswanger W, Depoil D, Blair DA, Wiggins CH, Kam LC, Dustin ML (2018) Durable Interactions of T Cells with T Cell Receptor Stimuli in the Absence of a Stable Immunological Synapse. Cell Reports 22:340-349.

McCloskey MA, Poo MM (1986) Contact-induced redistribution of specific membrane components: Local accumulation and development of adhesion. J Cell Biol 102:2185-2196.

McConnell HM, Watts TH, Weis RM, Brian AA (1986) Supported planar membranes in studies of cell-cell recognition in the immune system. Biochim Biophys Acta 864:95-106.

McCormack E, Adams KJ, Hassan NJ, Kotian A, Lissin NM, Sami M, Mujic M, Osdal T, Gjertsen BT, Baker D, Powlesland AS, Aleksic M, Vuidepot A, Morteau O, Sutton DH, June CH, Kalos M, Ashfield R, Jakobsen BK (2013) Bi-specific TCR-anti CD3 redirected T-cell targeting of NY-ESO-1- and LAGE-1-positive tumors. Cancer Immunol Immunother 62:773-785.

McKinney EF, Lee JC, Jayne DR, Lyons PA, Smith KG (2015) T-cell exhaustion, co-stimulation and clinical outcome in autoimmunity and infection. Nature 523:612-616.

Mebius RE (2003) Organogenesis of lymphoid tissues. Nat Rev Immunol 3:292-303.

Mempel TR, Henrickson SE, Von Andrian UH (2004) T-cell priming by dendritic cells in lymph nodes occurs in three distinct phases. Nature 427:154-159.

Miller MJ, Wei SH, Parker I, Cahalan MD (2002) Two-photon imaging of lymphocyte motility and antigen response in intact lymph node. Science 296:1869-1873.

Miller MJ, Wei SH, Cahalan MD, Parker I (2003) Autonomous T cell trafficking examined in vivo with intravital two-photon microscopy. Proc Natl Acad Sci U S A 100:2604-2609.

Miller MJ, Hejazi AS, Wei SH, Cahalan MD, Parker I (2004) T cell repertoire scanning is promoted by dynamic dendritic cell behavior and random T cell motility in the lymph node. Proc Natl Acad Sci U S A 101:998-1003.

Milstein O, Tseng SY, Starr T, Llodra J, Nans A, Liu M, Wild MK, van der Merwe PA, Stokes DL, Reisner Y, Dustin ML (2008) Nanoscale increases in CD2-CD48-mediated intermembrane spacing decrease adhesion and reorganize the immunological synapse. J Biol Chem 283:34414-34422.

Monks CR, Freiberg BA, Kupfer H, Sciaky N, Kupfer A (1998) Three-dimensional segregation of supramolecular activation clusters in T cells. Nature 395:82-86.

Moreau HD, Lemaitre F, Garrod KR, Garcia Z, Lennon-Dumenil AM, Bousso P (2015) Signal strength regulates antigen-mediated T-cell deceleration by distinct mechanisms to promote local exploration or arrest. Proc Natl Acad Sci U S A 112:12151-12156.

Moreau HD, Lemaitre F, Terriac E, Azar G, Piel M, Lennon-Dumenil AM, Bousso P (2012) Dynamic in situ cytometry uncovers T cell receptor signaling during immunological synapses and kinapses in vivo. Immunity 37:351-363.

Mossman KD, Campi G, Groves JT, Dustin ML (2005) Altered TCR signaling from geometrically repatterned immunological synapses. Science 310:1191-1193.

Mukherjee S, Rigaud S, Seok SC, Fu G, Prochenka A, Dworkin M, Gascoigne NR, Vieland VJ, Sauer K, Das J (2013) In silico modeling of Itk activation kinetics in thymocytes suggests competing positive and negative IP4 mediated feedbacks increase robustness. PLoS One 8:e73937.

Nair PM, Ngu H, Torres E, Marsters S, Lawrence DA, Stephan JP, Komuves L, Ashkenazi A (2015) Membrane display and functional analysis of juxtacrine ligand-receptor signaling. Biotechniques 59:231-238, 240.

Navarro MN, Goebel J, Hukelmann JL, Cantrell DA (2014) Quantitative phosphoproteomics of cytotoxic T cells to reveal protein kinase d 2 regulated networks. Molecular & cellular proteomics: MCP 13:3544-3557.

Nguyen K, Sylvain NR, Bunnell SC (2008) T cell costimulation via the integrin VLA-4 inhibits the actin-dependent centralization of signaling microclusters containing the adaptor SLP-76. Immunity 28:810-821.

Norcross MA (1984) A synaptic basis for T-lymphocyte activation. Ann Immunol (Paris) 135D:113-134.

O'Donoghue GP, Pielak RM, Smoligovets AA, Lin JJ, Groves JT (2013) Direct single molecule measurement of TCR triggering by agonist pMHC in living primary T cells. eLife 2:e00778.

Oddos S, Dunsby C, Purbhoo MA, Chauveau A, Owen DM, Neil MA, Davis DM, French PM (2008) High-speed high-resolution imaging of intercellular immune synapses using optical tweezers. Biophys J.

Okada T, Miller MJ, Parker I, Krummel MF, Neighbors M, Hartley SB, O'Garra A, Cahalan MD, Cyster JG (2005) Antigen-engaged B cells undergo chemotaxis toward the T zone and form motile conjugates with helper T cells. PLoS Biol 3:e150.

Okoye IS, Coomes SM, Pelly VS, Czieso S, Papayannopoulos V, Tolmachova T, Seabra MC, Wilson MS (2014) MicroRNA-containing T-regulatory-cell-derived exosomes suppress pathogenic T helper 1 cells. Immunity 41:89-103.

Pokutta S, Herrenknecht K, Kemler R, Engel J (1994) Conformational changes of the recombinant extracellular domain of E-cadherin upon calcium binding. Eur J Biochem 223:1019-1026.

Polman CH, O'Connor PW, Havrdova E, Hutchinson M, Kappos L, Miller DH, Phillips JT, Lublin FD, Giovannoni G, Wajgt A, Toal M, Lynn F, Panzara MA, Sandrock AW, Investigators A (2006) A randomized, placebo-controlled trial of natalizumab for relapsing multiple sclerosis. N Engl J Med 354:899-910.

Porter DL, Levine BL, Kalos M, Bagg A, June CH (2011) Chimeric antigen receptor-modified T cells in chronic lymphoid leukemia. N Engl J Med 365:725-733.

Proserpio V, Piccolo A, Haim-Vilmovsky L, Kar G, Lonnberg T, Svensson V, Pramanik J, Natarajan KN, Zhai W, Zhang X, Donati G, Kayikci M, Kotar J, McKenzie AN, Montandon R, Billker O, Woodhouse S, Cicuta P, Nicodemi M, Teichmann SA (2016) Single-cell analysis of CD4+ T-cell differentiation reveals three major cell states and progressive acceleration of proliferation. Genome Biol 17:103.

Qi SY, Groves JT, Chakraborty AK (2001) Synaptic pattern formation during cellular recognition. Proc Natl Acad Sci U S A 98:6548-6553.

Reister-Gottfried E, Sengupta K, Lorz B, Sackmann E, Seifert U, Smith AS (2008) Dynamics of specific vesicle-substrate adhesion: From local events to global dynamics. Phys Rev Lett 101:208103.

Ritter AT, Asano Y, Stinchcombe JC, Dieckmann NM, Chen BC, Gawden-Bone C, van Engelenburg S, Legant W, Gao L, Davidson MW, Betzig E, Lippincott-Schwartz J, Griffiths GM (2015) Actin depletion initiates events leading to granule secretion at the immunological synapse. Immunity 42:864-876.

Roncagalli R, Hauri S, Fiore F, Liang Y, Chen Z, Sansoni A, Kanduri K, Joly R, Malzac A, Lahdesmaki H, Lahesmaa R, Yamasaki S, Saito T, Malissen M, Aebersold R, Gstaiger M, Malissen B (2014) Quantitative proteomics analysis of signalosome dynamics in primary T cells identifies the surface receptor CD6 as a Lat adaptor-independent TCR signaling hub. Nat Immunol 15:384-392.

Rothlein R, Dustin ML, Marlin SD, Springer TA (1986) A human intercellular adhesion molecule (ICAM-1) distinct from LFA-1. J Immunol 137:1270-1274.

Ruocco MG, Pilones KA, Kawashima N, Cammer M, Huang J, Babb JS, Liu M, Formenti SC, Dustin ML, Demaria S (2012) Suppressing T cell motility induced by anti-CTLA-4 monotherapy improves antitumor effects. J Clin Invest 122:3718-3730.

Ryan JF, Hovde R, Glanville J, Lyu SC, Ji X, Gupta S, Tibshirani RJ, Jay DC, Boyd SD, Chinthrajah RS, Davis MM, Galli SJ, Maecker HT, Nadeau KC (2016) Successful immunotherapy induces previously unidentified allergen-specific CD4+ T-cell subsets. Proc Natl Acad Sci U S A 113:E1286-1295.

Scatchard G (1949) The attractions of proteins for small molecules and ions. Ann NY Acad Sci 51:660-672.

Schmid EM, Bakalar MH, Choudhuri K, Weichsel J, Ann H, Geissler PL, Dustin ML, Fletcher DA (2016) Size-dependent protein segregation at membrane interfaces. Nat Phys 12:704-711.

Schmidt RE, Caulfield JP, Michon J, Hein A, Kamada MM, MacDermott RP, Stevens RL, Ritz J (1988) T11/CD2 activation of cloned human natural killer cells results in increased conjugate formation and exocytosis of cytolytic granules. J Immunol 140:991-1002.

Schubert DA, Gordo S, Sabatino JJ, Jr., Vardhana S, Gagnon E, Sethi DK, Seth NP, Choudhuri K, Reijonen H, Nepom GT, Evavold BD, Dustin ML, Wucherpfennig KW (2012) Self-reactive human CD4 T cell clones form unusual immunological synapses. J Exp Med 209:335-352.

Seed B, Aruffo A (1987) Molecular cloning of the CD2 antigen, the T-cell erythrocyte receptor, by a rapid immunoselection procedure. Proc Natl Acad Sci U S A 84:3365-3369.

Selvaraj P, Plunkett ML, Dustin M, Sanders ME, Shaw S, Springer TA (1987) The T lymphocyte glycoprotein CD2 (LFA-2/T11/E-Rosette receptor) binds the cell surface ligand LFA-3. Nature 326:400-403.

Shakhar G, Lindquist RL, Skokos D, Dudziak D, Huang JH, Nussenzweig MC, Dustin ML (2005) Stable T cell-dendritic cell interactions precede the development of both tolerance and immunity in vivo. Nat Immunol 6:707-714.

Shaw AS, Dustin ML (1997) Making the T cell receptor go the distance: A topological view of T cell activation. Immunity 6:361-369.

Shaw S, Luce GE, Quinones R, Gress RE, Springer TA, Sanders ME (1986) Two antigen-independent adhesion pathways used by human cytotoxic T-cell clones. Nature 323:262-264.

Shaw TN, Stewart-Hutchinson PJ, Strangward P, Dandamudi DB, Coles JA, Villegas-Mendez A, Gallego-Delgado J, van Rooijen N, Zindy E, Rodriguez A, Brewer JM, Couper KN, Dustin ML (2015) Perivascular Arrest of CD8+ T Cells Is a Signature of Experimental Cerebral Malaria. PLoS Pathog 11:e1005210.

Sims TN, Soos TJ, Xenias HS, Dubin-Thaler B, Hofman JM, Waite JC, Cameron TO, Thomas VK, Varma R, Wiggins CH, Sheetz MP, Littman DR, Dustin ML (2007) Opposing effects of PKCtheta and WASp on symmetry breaking and relocation of the immunological synapse. Cell 129:773-785.

Singleton KL, Gosh M, Dandekar RD, Au-Yeung BB, Ksionda O, Tybulewicz VL, Altman A, Fowell DJ, Wulfing C (2011) Itk controls the spatiotemporal organization of T cell activation. Sci Signal 4:ra66.

Skokos D, Shakhar G, Varma R, Waite JC, Cameron TO, Lindquist RL, Schwickert T, Nussenzweig MC, Dustin ML (2007) Peptide-MHC potency governs dynamic interactions between T cells and dendritic cells in lymph nodes. Nat Immunol 8:835-844.

Somersalo K, Anikeeva N, Sims TN, Thomas VK, Strong RK, Spies T, Lebedeva T, Sykulev Y, Dustin ML (2004) Cytotoxic T lymphocytes form an antigen-independent ring junction. J Clin Invest 113:49-57.

Springer TA (1990) Adhesion receptors of the immune system. Nature 346:425-434.

Springer TA, Dustin ML, Kishimoto TK, Marlin SD (1987) The lymphocyte function-associated LFA-1, CD2, and LFA-3 molecules: Cell adhesion receptors of the immune system. Annu Rev Immunol 5:223-252.

Staunton DE, Dustin ML, Springer TA (1989) Functional cloning of ICAM-2, a cell adhesion ligand for LFA-1 homologous to ICAM-1. Nature 339:61-64.

Staunton DE, Dustin ML, Erickson HP, Springer TA (1990) The arrangement of the immunoglobulin-like domains of ICAM-1 and the binding sites for LFA-1 and rhinovirus. Cell 61:243-254.

Stinchcombe JC, Bossi G, Booth S, Griffiths GM (2001) The immunological synapse of CTL contains a secretory domain and membrane bridges. Immunity 15:751-761.

Stoll S, Delon J, Brotz TM, Germain RN (2002) Dynamic imaging of T cell-dendritic cell interactions in lymph nodes. Science 296:1873-1876.

Su X, Ditlev JA, Hui E, Xing W, Banjade S, Okrut J, King DS, Taunton J, Rosen MK, Vale RD (2016) Phase separation of signaling molecules promotes T cell receptor signal transduction. Science 352:595-599.

Tkach KE, Barik D, Voisinne G, Malandro N, Hathorn MM, Cotari JW, Vogel R, Merghoub T, Wolchok J, Krichevsky O, Altan-Bonnet G (2014) T cells translate individual, quantal activation into collective, analog cytokine responses via time-integrated feedbacks. eLife 3:e01944.

Tolentino TP, Wu J, Zarnitsyna VI, Fang Y, Dustin ML, Zhu C (2008) Measuring diffusion and binding kinetics by contact area FRAP. Biophys J 95:920-930.

Torres AJ, Contento RL, Gordo S, Wucherpfennig KW, Love JC (2013) Functional single-cell analysis of T-cell activation by supported lipid bilayer-tethered ligands on arrays of nanowells. Lab Chip 13:90-99.

Tseng SY, Waite JC, Liu M, Vardhana S, Dustin ML (2008) T cell-dendritic cell immunological synapses contain TCR-dependent CD28-CD80 clusters that recruit protein kinase Ctheta. J Immunol 181:4852-4863.

Vale RD, Peterson SW, Matiuck NV, Fox CF (1984) Purified plasma membranes inhibit polypeptide growth factor-induced DNA synthesis in subconfluent 3T3 cells. J Cell Biol 98:1129-1132.

Vardhana S, Choudhuri K, Varma R, Dustin ML (2010) Essential role of ubiquitin and TSG101 protein in formation and function of the central supramolecular activation cluster. Immunity 32:531-540.

Varma R, Campi G, Yokosuka T, Saito T, Dustin ML (2006) T cell receptor-proximal signals are sustained in peripheral microclusters and terminated in the central supramolecular activation cluster. Immunity 25:117-127.

Waite JC, Leiner I, Lauer P, Rae CS, Barbet G, Zheng H, Portnoy DA, Pamer EG, Dustin ML (2011) Dynamic imaging of the effector immune response to listeria infection in vivo. PLoS Pathog 7:e1001326.

Weekes MP, Antrobus R, Lill JR, Duncan LM, Hor S, Lehner PJ (2010) Comparative analysis of techniques to purify plasma membrane proteins. J Biomol Tech 21:108-115.

Weikl TR, Lipowsky R (2004) Pattern formation during T-cell adhesion. Biophys J 87:3665-3678.

Wild MK, Cambiaggi A, Brown MH, Davies EA, Ohno H, Saito T, van der Merwe PA (1999) Dependence of T cell antigen recognition on the dimensions of an accessory receptor-ligand complex. J Exp Med 190:31-41.

Williams AF (1991) Cellular interactions. Out of equilibrium. Nature 352:473-474.

Williams TE, Nagarajan S, Selvaraj P, Zhu C (2001) Quantifying the impact of membrane microtopology on effective two-dimensional affinity. J Biol Chem 276:13283-13288.

Woolf E, Grigorova I, Sagiv A, Grabovsky V, Feigelson SW, Shulman Z, Hartmann T, Sixt M, Cyster JG, Alon R (2007) Lymph node chemokines promote sustained T lymphocyte motility without triggering stable integrin adhesiveness in the absence of shear forces. Nat Immunol 8:1076-1085.

Wright SD, Silverstein SC (1984) Phagocytosing macrophages exclude proteins from the zones of contact with opsonized targets. Nature 309:359-361.

Wu CY, Roybal KT, Puchner EM, Onuffer J, Lim WA (2015) Remote control of therapeutic T cells through a small molecule-gated chimeric receptor. Science 350:aab4077.

Wu Y, Vendome J, Shapiro L, Ben-Shaul A, Honig B (2011) Transforming binding affinities from three dimensions to two with application to cadherin clustering. Nature 475:510-513.

Wulfing C, Sjaastad MD, Davis MM (1998) Visualizing the dynamics of T cell activation: Intracellular adhesion molecule 1 migrates rapidly to the T cell/B cell interface and acts to sustain calcium levels. Proc Natl Acad Sci U S A 95:6302-6307.

Yokosuka T, Takamatsu M, Kobayashi-Imanishi W, Hashimoto-Tane A, Azuma M, Saito T (2012) Programmed cell death 1 forms negative costimulatory microclusters that directly inhibit T cell receptor signaling by recruiting phosphatase SHP2. J Exp Med 209:1201-1217.

Yokosuka T, Kobayashi W, Sakata-Sogawa K, Takamatsu M, Hashimoto-Tane A, Dustin ML, Tokunaga M, Saito T (2008) Spatiotemporal regulation of T cell costimulation by TCR-CD28 microclusters and protein kinase C theta translocation. Immunity 29:589-601.

Yosef N et al. (2013) Dynamic regulatory network controlling TH17 cell differentiation. Nature 496:461-468.

Yu W, Jiang N, Ebert PJ, Kidd BA, Muller S, Lund PJ, Juang J, Adachi K, Tse T, Birnbaum ME, Newell EW, Wilson DM, Grotenbreg GM, Valitutti S, Quake SR, Davis MM (2015) Clonal Deletion Prunes but Does Not Eliminate Self-Specific alphabeta CD8(+) T Lymphocytes. Immunity 42:929-941.

Zhang Z, Zhang M, Goldman CK, Ravetch JV, Waldmann TA (2003) Effective therapy for a murine model of adult T-cell leukemia with the humanized anti-CD52 monoclonal antibody, Campath-1H. Cancer Res 63:6453-6457.

Zhu DM, Dustin ML, Cairo CW, Golan DE (2007) Analysis of two-dimensional dissociation constant of laterally mobile cell adhesion molecules. Biophys J 92:1022-1034.

Zhu DM, Dustin ML, Cairo CW, Thatte HS, Golan DE (2006) Mechanisms of Cellular Avidity Regulation in CD2-CD58-Mediated T Cell Adhesion. ACS Chem Biol 1:649-658.

Zhu J, Luo BH, Xiao T, Zhang C, Nishida N, Springer TA (2008) Structure of a complete integrin ectodomain in a physiologic resting state and activation and deactivation by applied forces. Mol Cell 32:849-861.

Zinselmeyer BH, Heydari S, Sacristan C, Nayak D, Cammer M, Herz J, Cheng X, Davis SJ, Dustin ML, McGavern DB (2013) PD-1 promotes immune exhaustion by inducing antiviral T cell motility paralysis. J Exp Med 210:757-774.

Index

Page numbers followed by f and t indicate figures and tables, respectively.

T - #0212 - 071024 - C0 - 254/178/19 - PB - 9780367780920 - Gloss Lamination